ANABOLIC STEROIDS

and

MAKING THEM

Professor Frank

Order this book online at www.trafford.com
or email orders@trafford.com

Most Trafford titles are also available at major online book retailers.

Print information available on the last page.

ISBN: 978-1-4120-7859-7 (sc)
ISBN: 978-1-4122-4027-7 (e)

Trafford rev. 01/15/2019

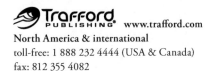

www.trafford.com

North America & international
toll-free: 1 888 232 4444 (USA & Canada)
fax: 812 355 4082

INDEX

CHAPTER ONE

1

2,875,196

6β,19-SELENO-1-DEHYDROTESTOSTERONE AND ESTERS THEREOF

Klaus G. Florey, Westfield, N. J., assignor to Olin Mathieson Chemical Corporation, New York, N. Y., a corporation of Virginia

No Drawing. Application September 18, 1956
Serial No. 610,641

7 Claims. (Cl. 260—239.5)

This application is a continuation-in-part of my parent application, Serial No. 547,315, filed November 16, 1955, now abandoned.

This invention relates to the synthesis of steroids and, more particularly, to new selenium-containing steroid derivatives of testosterone and to process for preparing and using them.

The new steroids of this invention comprise 6β,19-seleno-1-dehydrotestosterone and esters thereof.

These new steroids are prepared by heating to a temperature below 200° C. testosterone or an ester thereof [particularly a hydrocarbon carboxylic acid ester, wherein the acyl radical has less than ten carbon atoms, as exemplified by lower alkanoyl (e. g., formyl, acetyl, propionyl, butyryl and enanthoyl), hydrocarbon aroyl (e. g., benzoyl and toluyl) and hydrocarbon aralkanoyl (e. g., phenylacetyl and β-phenylpropionyl)], with selenium dioxide, preferably in a suitable organic solvent for the steroid reactant, which is unattacked by selenium dioxide under the reaction conditions employed. Suitable organic solvents include ethers (e. g., dioxane), acid anhydrides (e. g., acetic anhydride), tertiary alcohols (e. g., tertiary butanol) and preferably organic acids (especially liquid lower fatty acids, such as acetic acid). The reaction is carried out at an elevated temperature below 200° C., such as one in the range of about 80° C. to about 140° C. (optimally at reflux of the organic solvent, if one is used). At least one mole of selenium dioxide is required for the reaction, but preferably an excess (about 3 to 4 moles) is used. If an ester of testosterone is employed as a reactant, the corresponding ester derivative is initially formed. This ester can then be converted to the free 17-hydroxyl compound by treatment with a base, such as methanolic potassium carbonate.

The product formed is 6β,19-seleno-1-dehydrotestosterone (or an ester thereof) and can be represented by the structural formula

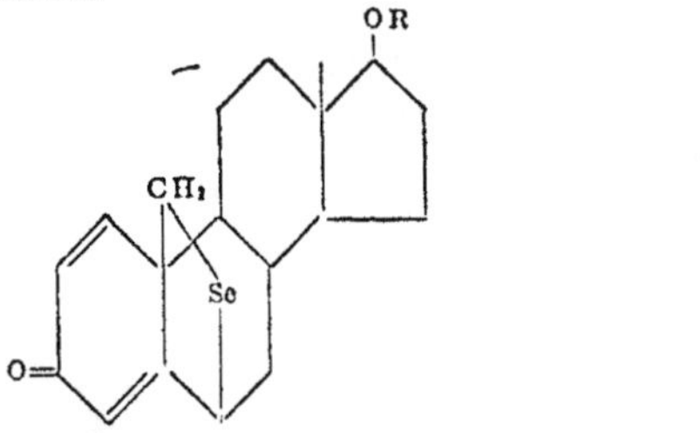

wherein R is hydrogen or an acyl radical (particularly an acyl radical of a hydrocarbon carboxylic acid containing less than ten carbon atoms).

The new seleno steroids of this invention can be employed as intermediates in the preparation of 1-dehydrotestosterone. This conversion can be effected by either of two methods. Employing one of the alternative procedures, 6β,19-seleno-1-dehydrotestosterone (or an ester thereof) is heated with a pyrophoric form of nickel (e. g., Raney nickel). According to the other alternative pro-

2

cedure, 6β,19-seleno-1-dehydrotestosterone (or an ester thereof) is pyrolized by heating to a temperature of about 300° C. to about 500° C. (optimally about 350° C. to about 370° C. in vacuo) to yield 1-dehydrotestosterone.

The following examples illustrate the invention:

EXAMPLE 1

6β,19-seleno-1-dehydrotestosterone acetate

A mixture of 2.0 g. of testosterone acetate (Δ⁴-androstene-17β-ol-3-one 17-acetate) and 2.0 g. of selenium dioxide in 8 ml. of acetic acid is refluxed for one hour, cooled to room temperature and filtered from selenium. The filtrate is diluted with 50 ml. of chloroform and washed with water and sodium bicarbonate solution. The solvent is evaporated, and the resulting residue, upon crystallization from acetone-hexane, yields about 700 mg. of a crystalline substance, 6β,19-seleno-1-dehydrotestosterone acetate, having the following properties: M. P. about 152–157° C.; $[\alpha]_D^{25} + 125$ (c., 0.62 in chloroform):

$\lambda_{max.}^{ale.}$ 244 mμ ($\epsilon = 7,930$); 257 mμ ($\epsilon = 7,800$); 306 mμ ($\epsilon = 889$); $\lambda_{max.}^{Nujol}$ 5.76μ (acetyl), 6.10μ, 6.17μ, 6.27μ (Δ¹·⁴-3-keto).

Analysis.—Calculated for $C_{21}H_{26}O_3Se$ (405.38): C, 62.22; H, 6.47; Se, 19.49. Found: C, 63.06; H, 7.07; Se, 17.85.

In a similar manner, upon the substitution of other esters of testosterone (e. g., testosterone propionate and testosterone enanthate) for testosterone acetate in the procedure of Example 1, the corresponding ester derivatives (e. g., the propionate and enanthate analogues) are formed. Furthermore, when the process is repeated with dioxane substituted for the acetic acid, the same product is obtained.

EXAMPLE 2

6β,19-seleno-1-dehydrotestosterone

To 400 mg. of 6β,19-seleno-1-dehydrotestosterone acetate in 40 ml. of ethanol was added 2 ml. of a 10% aqueous potassium carbonate solution. The mixture is refluxed for 3 hours, diluted with chloroform and washed with water. Evaporation of the solvent and subsequent crystallization from methanol yields about 180 mg. of the crystalline substance, 6β,19-seleno-1-dehydrotestosterone, having the following properties: M. P. about 273–275° C.; $[\alpha]_D^{23}$ —4.6° (c., 0.54 in chloroform);

$\lambda_{max.}^{ale.}$ 245 mμ ($\epsilon = 10,800$); 257 mμ ($\epsilon = 10,700$); 307 mμ ($\epsilon = 1,170$); $\lambda_{max.}^{Nujol}$ 2.87μ (17–OH), 6.10μ, 6.20μ, 6.28μ (Δ¹·⁴-3-keto).

Analysis.—Calculated for $C_{19}H_{24}O_2Se$ (363.34): C, 62.80; H, 6.66; Se, 21.73. Found: C, 62.58; H, 6.76; Se, 22.12.

EXAMPLE 3

1-dehydrotestosterone

To 200 mg. of 6β,19-seleno-1-dehydrotestosterone in 18 ml. of benzene is added 4 ml. of Raney nickel in 4 ml. of ethanol. The mixture is refluxed for 5 hours. The mixture is filtered from nickel, washed with water and concentrated to dryness in vacuo. The residue, upon crystallization from etherhexane, yields 1-dehydrotestosterone, identical with an authentic sample.

EXAMPLE 4

1-dehydrotestosterone acetate and 6-dehydrotestosterone acetate

300 mg. of 6β,19-seleno-1-dehydrotestosterone acetate is heated to 350–370° C. at 1 mm. pressure for 30 minutes. The reaction mixture is diluted with chloroform, filtered from selenium, washed with water and concen-

3

trated to dryness in vacuo. The residue is chromatographed on alumina, and the following portions in order of elution are obtained with hexane-benzene and benzene-ether solvent mixtures: (a) 1-dehydrotestosterone acetate, M. P. 151–153° C., identical with authentic material, and (b) mixtures of 1-dehydrotestosterone acetate and 6-dehydrotestosterone acetate, identified by ultra-violet maxima in the 240 mμ and 280 mμ regions.

The invention may be otherwise variously embodied within the scope of the appended claims.

I claim:

1. A compound selected from the group consisting of 6β,19-seleno-1-dehydrotestosterone and esters thereof with hydrocarbon carboxylic acids of less than ten carbon atoms.

2. 6β,19-seleno-1-dehydrotestosterone.

3. An ester of 6β,19-seleno-1-dehydrotestosterone with a hydrocarbon carboxylic acid of less than ten carbon atoms.

4. 6β,19-seleno-1-dehydrotestosterone acetate.

5. A process for preparing a compound selected from the group consisting of 6β,19-seleno-1-dehydrotestosteron and esters thereof with hydrocarbon carboxylic acids of less than ten carbon atoms, which comprises heat-

4

ing to a temperature below 200° C. selenium dioxide and a steroid selected from the group consisting of testosterone and esters of testosterone with hydrocarbon carboxylic acids of less than ten carbon atoms, at least one mole of selenium dioxide being present per mole of steroid, and recovering the product thus formed.

6. The process of claim 5, wherein the steroid is an ester of testosterone with a hydrocarbon carboxylic acid of less than ten carbon atoms.

7. The process of claim 5, wherein the steroid is testosterone acetate.

References Cited in the file of this patent

UNITED STATES PATENTS

2,422,904	Inhoffen	June 24, 1947
2,695,286	Dearborn	Nov. 23, 1954
2,705,237	Djerassi	Mar. 29, 1955
2,729,634	Dearborn	Jan. 3, 1956

OTHER REFERENCES

Chem. Reviews by Watkins, vol. 36 (1945), page 249.
Schwenk: Arch. Biochem. 14, 125 (1947).
McKenzie: J. Biol. Chem. 173, 271 (1947).

1

2,837,464

PROCESS FOR PRODUCTION OF DIENES BY CORYNEBACTERIA

Arthur Nobile, Belleville, N. J., assignor to Schering Corporation, Bloomfield, N. J., a corporation of New Jersey

No Drawing. Application January 11, 1955
Serial No. 481,279

19 Claims. (Cl. 195—51)

The present invention relates to the microbiological treatment of 10,13-dimethyl steroids whereby selective chemical modification of such steroid compounds is effected in a simple and inexpensive manner, and in good yield.

More particularly, the invention relates to the microbiological treatment of 10,13-dimethyl steroids whereby desirable chemical changes are effected without undesired degradation of the steroid molecule, such as splitting of the D-ring, or degradation of a side chain when present.

It is the general object of the invention to effect chemical modification of steroid compounds by a microbiological treatment thereof or by treatment with an enzymatic extract of the microbial culture.

More specifically, it is an object of the invention to accomplish one or more of the operations of oxidation, dehydrogenation, and hydrolysis, and including the introduction of a second double bond into the A-ring of steroids already having a double bond in such ring, by subjecting them to the action of a culture of a member of the family of Corynebactriaceae, preferably of the genus Corynebacterium, and particularly of the species *Corynebacterium simplex* (American Type Culture Collection No. 6946), or of *Corynebacterium hoagii* (A. T. C. C. 7005) or of an enzymatic extract of such cultures.

A number of chemical transformations of steroids by by microorganisms have recently been developed which have involved the introduction of one or more hydroxyl groups into the steroid nucleus, or oxidation of hydroxyl groups to keto groups but without affecting the degree of saturation of the steroid nucleus. More recently there has been published the chemical transformation of progesterone by the use of microorganisms, such conversions involving the introduction of a double bond in ring A, but with scission of carbon-linkages in the side chain as well as in ring D (Fried, Thoma and Klingsberg, "Oxidation of Steroids by Microorganisms. III. Side Chain Degradation, Ring D Cleavage and Dehydrogenation in Ring A," J. A. C. S. 75, 5764 (1953). As described in this publication, fermentation of progesterone with *Streptomyces lavendulae* afforded 1,4-androstadien-3,17-dione, and also 1,4-androstadien-17β-ol-3-one, known to be useful as intermediates in the synthesis of estradiol and estrone. This process thus involves the introduction of a Δ¹-double bond into progestrone, but with complete degradation of the side chain. With other microorganisms there was obtained not only elimination of the side chain, but also cleavage between carbon atoms 13 and 17. Thus, fermentation of progestrone with *Penicillium chrysogenum* gave the known testololactone, without introduction of a new double bond into ring A.

The above-named authors state further that "Biooxidation involving both lactone formation in ring D and dehydrogenation in ring A is less widespread and has been observed with but a small number of organisms." They refer to the fermentation of progesterone, Reichstein's Compound S or testosterone with *Cylindrocarbon radicola*, and report that in each case they obtained Δ¹-dehydrotestololactone, i. e., the dehydrogenation was ac-

2

complished both by elimination of the side chain of the starting compound and by opening up of the D-ring.

It is accordingly a still further object of the present invention to provide a process for the introduction of a second double bond into the A-ring of steroid compounds already possessing a double bond in such ring between the 4,5-carbons without simultaneous degradation of the side chain and without splitting of the D-ring, by fermenting them in a culture of a microorganism of the family Corynebactriaceae, or by treating them with an enzymatic extract of such culture, whereby compounds of improved physiological activity, and also compounds capable of conversion by known means into physiologically active compounds, are obtained.

It is also an object of the invention to provide a simple and inexpensive process for effecting other chemical transformations in steroid compounds with the aid of the above-named microorganisms, both with and without the introduction of a double bond into ring A, all without splitting of the carbon skeleton of the original starting compound.

A further object of the invention is to provide more effective Δ¹-dehydroderivatives of the anti-arthritic adrenocortical hormones cortisone (Kendall's Compound E, 4-pregnene-17α,21-diol-3,11,20-trione) and hydrocortisone (Kendall's Compound F, 4-pregnene-11β,17α,21-triol-3,20-dione) and of their esters, and likewise the Δ¹-dehydro derivative of the epimer of hydrocortisone (4-pregnene-11α,17α,21 - triol-3,20 - dione) which can serve as an intermediate for the preparation of the corresponding 11-keto compound (Δ¹-dihydrocortisone).

Other objects and advantages of the invention will become apparent to those skilled in the art from the following more detailed description and the features of novelty will be set forth in the appended claims.

I have found that the chemical modification of 10,13-dimethyl steroids, and especially and most importantly the A-ring dehydrogenation of steroid compounds already singly unsaturated in the A-ring, with or without one or more of the operations of oxidation, reduction, and ester-hydrolysis, can be accomplished in an efficient and inexpensive manner by incubating or fermenting the starting steroid with a culture medium containing an organism of the family Corynebactriaceae (or the enzymatic extract thereof), the nature of the chemical transformation or transformations depending upon the character of the starting compound.

In the preferred manner of carrying out the present invention there is accordingly employed a culture (or its enzymatic extract) of a dehydrogenating member of the family Corynebactriaceae, which includes the genera Corynebacterium, Listeria, and Erysipelothrix, which will introduce a 1,2-double bond without degrading the molecule of the substrate. The last two of these genera include the species *monocytogenes, rhusiopathiae, muriseptica* and *erysipeloids*, which are highly pathogenic bacteria, and their commercial use consequently introduces the problem of protecting the personnel against infection. While, therefore, the members of these two genera which act to dehydrogenate the A-ring of 10,13-dimethyl steroids can be employed in the process of this invention if proper precautions are taken, it is preferred to employ members of the genus Corynebacterium, as the latter includes many species which are non-pathogenic in character. Good results have been obtained with the species *Corynebacterium simplex* and *Corynebacterium hoagii*, the first of which is a soil bacterium, while the second is found in the human throat (where it apparently produces no pathologic condition) and sometimes as a contaminant of cultures exposed to the atmosphere, although its real or original habitat is not known. As highly satisfactory results have been obtained with *Coryne-*

bacterium simplex, the invention will be further described mainly with particular reference to this organism, but it will be understood that other steroid-modifying, and particularly dehydrogenating members of the family Corynebacteriaceae can be employed in place of *Corynebacterium simplex*.

The starting steroid compounds can be of great variety, and I have been unable to discover any group of suitably substituted 10,13-dimethyl steroids which is not transformed chemically by the named microorganism. Thus, as disclosed more in detail hereinbelow, the culture is effective on various pregnenes androstenes, including 17-methyl and 17-ethyl androstenes, and on sapogenins. The presence of a free hydroxyl group appears to promote the chemical transformations, but such transformations occur even though the hydroxy group is itself oxidized to a keto group.

The starting compounds can have hydroxyl, keto, halogen, and ester groups in various positions of the nucleus or side chain; thus, hydroxyl groups may be present in the 3, 11, 17, 20 or 21-positions; keto groups may occupy the 3, 11, 17, 20 or 21-(aldehydo) positions, while halogen, such as fluorine or chlorine may be attached to the 9-carbon, or at other points of the nucleus or side chain. Ester groups of great variety, and preferably the esters of acids usually employed in steroid synthesis and in preparing steroid hormones for therapeutic use, and particularly of the lower alkanoic acids, may be located at the 3, 11, 17, 20 or 21-positions. The hydroxyl groups at the 3, 11, and 17-positions can be either the α- or β-epimers.

By the process of the present invention it has been possible to convert, for example, 4-pregnene-17α,21-diol-3,11,20-trione (cortisone) into 1,4-pregnadiene-17α,21-diol - 3,11,20 - trione; 4-pregnene-11β,17α,21-triol-3,20-dione (hydrocortisone) into 1,4-pregnadiene-11β,17α,21-triol - 3,20 - dione; 4 - pregnene-17α-21-diol-3,20-dione (Reichstein's Compound S) into 1,4-pregnadiene-17α,21-diol - 3,20 - dione; 5 - pregnene-3β,20-diol into 1,4-pregnadiene-3,20-dione; 17-ethinyltestosterone into 17-ethinyl-1,4 - androstadiene - 17β-ol-3-one; 17-methyltestosterone into 17 - methyl-1,4-androstadiene-17β-ol-3-one; 4-pregnene-11β,21-diol-3,20-dione into 1,4-pregnadiene-11β,21-diol - 3,20-dione; 4-pregnene-21-ol-3,20-dione into 1,4-pregnadiene-21-ol-3,20-dione; and 4-pregnene-21-ol-3,11,20-trione into 1,4-pregnadiene-21-ol-3,11,20-trione.

In place of the 3-keto starting compounds, the corresponding 3-hydroxy compounds and their 3-esters can be employed, like 5-pregnene-3,11β,17α,21-tetrol-20-one and 5-pregnene-3,17α,21-triol-11,20-dione and their 3-acetates or 3,21-diacetates, to produce the same 3-keto diene and products.

An ester group may be present not only in the 3-position but also in one or more of the 11, 17 and 21-positions. Where an ester group is present in the 3-position, it is hydrolyzed and the resulting hydroxyl group oxidized to a keto group in the course of the reaction. The ester groups in the 11- and 17-positions are generally not hydrolyzed, at least not to any significant extent; while an ester group in the 21-position may or may not be hydrolyzed, depending on the reaction conditions. Thus, where the starting compound is a 3,21-diester, the reaction product may be a 3-keto-21-ester compound, or a 3-keto-21-hydroxy compound. Along with 3-hydroxyl, also 20-hydroxyl will be oxidized to a keto group. It will thus be seen that the organism employed in the present invention is selective with respect to the oxidation step, this being limited practically completely to the 3- and 20-positions, while the hydrolysis may be restricted to 3-ester groups.

I have found that deacetylation at the 21-position occurs most readily at a pH of 6.8–7.1, and at a temperature of about 26° to 29° C. Hydrolysis is greatly diminished below a pH of 6.5 and at a temperature above

32° C. On the other hand, the introduction of the Δ¹-double bond proceeds satisfactorily outside of the pH and temperature ranges at which deacetylation proceeds most actively; that is, the dehydrogenation occurs at a satisfactory rate at a pH of 7.6-8.0 and at a temperature of 32° to 37° C. These conditions are therefore to be employed if hydrolysis of a 21-ester is to be minimized.

My process is applicable also to the treatment of the 11α-hydroxy epimers of the above-mentioned 11β-hydroxy starting compounds, such as 4-pregnen-11α,17α,21-triol-3,20 - dione, 4-pregnen-11α,17α,20,21-tetrol-3-one, 5-pregnen-3,11α17α-21-tetrol-20-one, 5-pregnen-3,11α,17α,20,21-pentol and their mono- and poly-esters like the 3-acetates, 3,21 - diacetates, and 3,17α,21 - triacetates, these starting compounds yielding 1,4-pregnadien-11α,17α,21-triol-3,20-dione or an ester thereof. The 11-epimers of the 1,4-diene of Compound F and its esters can be converted into the 1,4-diene of cortisone and its esters by oxidation of the 11α-hydroxyl group in known manner, as with the theoretical amount of chromic acid, with or without pyridine or acetic acid, at room temperature or below (5 to 15° C.) preferably after esterifying the 21-hydroxyl if it is free. These 11α-hydroxy starting compounds are relatively easily prepared in high yield as is known in the art, and therefore represent desirable starting compounds for the preparation of the Δ¹-dehydro derivatives of cortisone and hydrocortisone.

Additional transformations that may be accomplished with the microorganism employed in the process of the present invention include the conversion of testosterone, 5 - androstene - 3,17 - diol, 4-androstene-3α,17-diol, and 4-androstene-3β,17-diol into a mixture of 1,4-androstadiene - 17 - ol-3-one and 1,4-androstadiene-3,17-dione; of 5 - androstene - 3 - ol - 17-one into 1,4-androstadiene-3,17-dione; of 5-pregnene-3,17α,21-triol-20-one 3-21-diacetate into a mixture of 1,4-pregnadiene-17α,21-diol-3,20-dione and 5-pregnen-17α,21-diol-3,20-dione 21-acetate; and of diosgenin into 1,4-diosgedienone. By alteration of the fermenting medium, Compound S can be made to yield not only 1,4-pregnadiene-17α,21-diol-3,20-dione but also 1,4-pregnadiene-17α,20β,21-triol-3-one, i. e., reduction is effected on the 20-keto group. However, the microorganism can also effect oxidation of a 20-secondary hydroxyl group, as in the conversion of 5-pregnene-3,20-diol into 1,4-pregadiene-3,20-dione.

The process of the invention is applicable also to 9α-fluoro and 9α-chloro steroids and will yield the corresponding substituted reaction products. The various transformations may be represented by the following equations:

(1)

wherein X is H_2, =O or $\begin{cases} H \\ OH \end{cases}$ (α or β); $\begin{cases} Y \text{ is } -OH \\ Z \text{ is } ... C \equiv CH \text{ or } ... CH_3 ... H. \end{cases}$

$\begin{cases} Y \text{ is } -CO \cdot CH_2OH \\ Z \text{ is } ... OH \text{ or } ... H; \end{cases}$

(2)

wherein W is F, Cl, or H; X is $\begin{cases} H \\ OH \end{cases}$, =O or H_2; Y is $-CO \cdot CH_2OH$, $CO \cdot CH_2OOCR'$, or $-CHOH \cdot CH_2OH$; Z is OH or H; and R' is lower alkyl radical;

(3)

wherein R is lower alkanoyl group; Y is $CO \cdot CH_2OH$, $-CHOH \cdot CH_3$, $-CO \cdot CH_2OOCR'$, or $CHOH \cdot CH_2OH$; Z is $=O$ or OH; and R' is lower alkyl radical.

Typical products obtained in accordance with the invention, and their corresponding starting materials are designated in the following table.

TABLE I

OBSERVED TRANSFORMATIONS

Starting material		Products
Technical name	Common name	
5-androstene-3β-ol-17-one	Dehydroepiandrosterone	4-androstene-3,17-dione.
4-androstene-17β-ol-3-one	Testosterone	1,4-androstadiene-3,17-dione; 1,4-androstadiene-17β-ol-3-one.
5-pregnene-3β, 20-diol		1,4-pregnadiene-3,20-dione.
4-pregnene-17α,21-diol-3,20-dione	Reichstein's Compound S	1,4-pregnadiene-17α,21-diol-3,20-dione, and 1,4-pregnadiene-17α,20β,21-triol-3-one.
5-androstene-3β,17β-diol		1,4-androstadiene-3,17-dione; 1,4-androstadiene-17β-ol-3-one.
17-methyl-4-androstene-17β-ol-3-one	Methyltestosterone	17-methyl-1,4-androstadiene-17β-ol-3-one.
17-ethinyl-4-androstene-17β-ol-3-one	Ethinyltestosterone	17-ethinyl-1,4-androstadiene-17β-ol-3-one.
4-pregnene-21-ol-3,20-dione	Desoxycorticosterone	1,4-pregnadiene-21-ol-3,20-dione.
9α-fluoro-4-pregnene-11β,17α,21-triol-3,20-dione	Fluoro Compound F	9α-fluoro-1,4-pregnadiene-11β,17α,21-triol-3,20-dione.
4-pregnene-11β,21-diol-3,20-dione	Corticosterone	1,4-pregnadiene-11β,21-diol-3,20-dione.
4-pregnene-21-ol-3,11,20-trione	Kendall's Compound A	1,4-pregnadiene-21-ol-3,11,20-trione.
5-pregnene-3β,17α,21-triol-20-one 3-21-diacetate		1,4-pregnadiene-17α,21-diol-3,20-dione; 4-pregnene-17α,21-diol-3,20-dione 21-acetate.
4-pregnene-20-ol-3-one		1,4-pregnadiene-3,20-dione.
4-pregnene-11β,17α,21-triol-3,20-dione	Kendall's Compound F	1,4-pregnadiene-11β,17α,21-triol-3,20-dione.
4-pregnene-17α,21-diol-3,11,20-trione	do	1,4-pregnadiene-17α,21-diol-3,11,20-trione.

The importance of my invention is many-fold. It is now possible to prepare easily and directly previously unknown, as well as known, steroid hormone substances containing an additional Δ^1-unsaturation. The heretofore unknown compounds include the Δ^1-derivative of Kendall's Compound E, Kendall's Compound F, corticosterone, Kendall's Compound A, testosterone and methyl and ethinyl testosterone, and progesterone. The products of the above-described reactions posses the same pharmacodynamic properties as do the corresponding hormones Compound E, Compound F and their esters, progesterone, ethinyl-testosterone, methyltestosterone, corticosterone, desoxycorticosterone and 4-pregnene-21-ol-3,11,20-trione (in all of which the Δ^1-unsaturation is absent), but to a considerably enhanced degree, which makes them valuable agents in the treatment of the various diseases and conditions for which the parent substances are employed. For example, in the widely accepted eosinophile test (Rosenberg, E. et al., Endocrinology 54, 363 (1954)), for cortical hormone activity, the dienes corresponding to Compounds E and F are several times as potent as Compounds E and F, and this has been confirmed by the treatment of human arthritic patients.

In clinical testing, the diene derivative of Compound F has been found to be considerably more effective in a daily dose of 50 mg. than 75 to 100 mg. of cortisone acetate or of Compound F. Whereas a patient standardized on a 75 to 100 mg. dosage of cortisone acetate, or Compound F, would require 90 to 100 mg. of codeine per day to be relieved of pain when the dosage of the cortisone acetate or Compound F was reduced to 50 mg. per day, this dosage (50 mg.) of the diene derivative of Compound F required no supplemental treatment with codeine and gave complete relief from pain. In a fact, a daily oral dose of 50 mg. of the diene derivative of Compound F had even more favorable results than a daily oral dose of 75 to 100 mg. of cortisone acetate, or Compound F, as it gave greater relief from pain, as evidenced by the ability of the patient to clench the fist,

walk briskly, and engage in other muscular activity without pain. Similar improved clinical results are obtainable with the diene derivative of cortisone acetate and of hydrocortisone acetate.

This pronounced enhancement of activity is of tremendous importance since it permits a reduced dose of the new Δ^1-dehydro derivatives of cortisone and hydrocortisone to accomplish the same beneficial actions for which cortisone and hydrocortisone have been employed at higher dosage levels in arthritis and other human afflictions. At the same time, the incidence of side effects commonly associated with the known compounds is very markedly diminished.

Furthermore, it is now possible to convert 5-androstene-3β,20-diol directly and in one step to $\Delta^{1,4}$-androstadiene-17β-ol-3-one and $\Delta^{1,4}$-androstadiene-3,17-dione, which are valuable intermediates in the preparation of estradiol and estrone. The process of the present invention provides a much more efficient way of preparing these intermediates than has been described heretofore.

In order to obtain a desirable growth of *Corynebacterium simplex* (American Type Culture Collection 6946) for the process of this invention, a suitable nutrient medium is prepared containing carbohydrate, organic nitrogen, cofactors, and inorganic salts. It is possible to omit the use of carbohydrate without completely impairing the growth of the organism. The steroid compound as a solid or dissolved or suspended in ethanol, acetone or any other water-miscible solvent which is non-toxic toward the organism, is added to the cultivated microorganism in a broth medium under sterile conditions. This culture is then shaken, aerated, or simultaneously aerated and agitated, in order to enhance the growth of the *Corynebacterium simplex* and the biochemical conversion of the steroid substrate. The steroid may be added to the broth medium and then inoculated with the bacterium, or the cultivated microorganism in broth medium may be added to the steroid. In certain cases, depending on the conditions of the reaction medium, it may be more desirable to obtain optimum growth of the microorganism before the addition of the steroid. Alternatively, enzyme preparations obtained in known manner from cultures of *Corynebacterium simplex* may be used for carrying out the process.

A useful method for carrying out the process is the cultivation of *Corynebacterium simplex* on a suitable nutrient medium under aerobic conditions. After cultivation of the microorganism, the cell mass may be harvested by centrifuging the nutrient broth, decanting the supernatant liquid and suspending the cell mass in saline. A suitable volume of the cell suspension is then seeded into a desirable nutrient medium for supporting growth of the microorganism. The nutrient medium

7

employed may be a yeast extract (Difco), casein hydrolysate (N–Z–Amine) (Type B Sheffield), corn steep liquor, water extract of soybean oil meal, lactalbumin hydrolysate (Edamine-Sheffield Enzymatic), fish solubles, and the like.

Inorganic salts are desirable to maintain a pH level in the reaction medium of between 6.8 and 7.2. However, the use of inorganic salts for buffering the reaction mixture may be omitted. The omission of inorganic salts causes the pH to rise from an initial value of 6.8 to about 7.7-8. This, however, will still permit the formation of the desired steroidal end products. The optimum temperature for growth of the selected microorganism is 37° C., but the temperatures may vary between 25° and 37°, and even between 20° and 40° C. The time of reaction may vary from as little as 3 hours to as much as 48 hours. The length of time which is employed will depend on the steroid which is being transformed. Any water miscible, non-toxic (to the organism) solvent may be employed to dissolve or suspend the steroid. I prefer to use ethanol or acetone in such amounts that the final concentration of these solvents in the reaction mixture is no higher than about 7% and may amount to only traces; owing to evaporation, the final concentration of the organic solvent may even be practically zero.

Following the completion of the oxidation or dehydrogenation process, which may be accompanied by partial or complete hydrolysis when mono- or poly-esters are used, the products of reaction may be recovered from the mixture by extraction with a suitable water-immiscible solvent, by filtration, by adsorption on a suitable adsorbent, or by any of the other procedures commonly used in the art. For extraction, chlorinated lower hydrocarbons, ketones, and alcohols are useful. These include chloroform, methylene chloride, trichloroethane, ethylene dichloride, butanol, diethylketone, and others. I prefer to use extraction as the method for isolating the steroidal products. Following extraction, the products may be isolated by concentration of the extracts to a small volume or to dryness. Purification of the residues may be then accomplished in several ways. In many instances, as with the dienes of Compound E, Compound F and Compound S, simple recrystallizations from a suitable solvent or solvent mixture, such as acetone, methylene chloride, ethanol, acetone-hexane, methylene chloride-hexane, etc., affords the desired dienone in excellent yield and high state of purity. Where there are several products formed in the same reaction, such as the conversion of testosterone to $\Delta^{1,4}$-androstadiene-17β-ol-3-one and $\Delta^{1,4}$-androstadiene-3,17-dione, a separation is conveniently achieved by chromatography on silica gel, magnesium silicate (Florisil), alumina or other commonly employed adsorbents. For example, to achieve the separation of the products derived from testosterone, a column of Florisil is prepared by adding Florisil portion-wise to a tube half-filled with hexane until the visible free liquid has almost vanished. Then a solution of the steroid in ether, methylene chloride, or some other non-polar solvent is added to the column and the effluent liquid is collected in suitable fractions. The column is then washed successively with hexane, hexane-10% ether, hexane-20% ether, hexane-30% ether, etc. $\Delta^{1,4}$-androstadiene-3,17-dione appears in the fractions of lower ether concentration (10-20%) and $\Delta^{1,4}$-androstadiene-17β-ol-3-one in the fractions of higher ether content (30–100% ether). It should be understood that where a mixture of more polar steroids is to be separated, more polar eluents will be required in chromatographic separation. Furthermore, the activity of the adsorbent varies from batch to batch and consequently the same steroids may be more strongly or more weakly held in parallel experiments which will result in variation of the value of the concentration of the eluents which will elute a given steroid. In any case, the order of elution will remain the same for a given adsorbent and a given solvent system.

8

The 1,4-diene structure of the products has been established in various ways. Many of the steroids described herein are new substances and careful attention has been paid to the proof of their structures. Infrared analyses, ultra-violet analyses, rotational analyses, degradative studies, and carbon-hydrogen analyses have been employed where necessary to establish the nature of the products. For example, the product derived from Compound S, namely $\Delta^{1,4}$-pregnadiene-17α,21-diol-3,20-dione, was degraded to the known $\Delta^{1,4}$-androstadiene-3,17-dione by an unequivocal method establishing beyond question the presence of the dienone structure in ring A. Furthermore, introduction of the Δ^1-unsaturation in a 3-keto-Δ^4-unsaturated steroid is known to have a characteristic negative effect on the molecular rotation of the product. I have observed this shift in rotation in the dienones which I have prepared from Compounds E and F among others. In similar fashion, all of the other products have been carefully identified.

The chemical transformations which can be accomplished by subjecting the various 10,13-dimethyl steroids to the action of a culture of *Corynebacterium simplex* (the term "culture of *Corynebacterium simplex*" is to be understood in this specification and in the claims as including the enzymatic extract of such culture) are thus of widely different kinds, and can take place singly, or two or more of such transformations can occur simultaneously or in sequence. The various reactions appear to be unaffected by other substituents in the steroid nucleus or in the side chain, when present.

As applied specifically to the manufacture of the Δ^1-dehydro derivative of Compounds E, F and epi-F, the reactions may be summarized by the following equation:

wherein R is H or acyl,

X is $=O$ or $<^{OR}_H$ or $<^{OR}_H$; while Y is $=O$ or $<^{OR}_H$; and

Z is $=O$ or $<^{OH}_H$; the dotted line indicating the alternative position of the double bond.

These reactions include the conversion of 5-pregnene-3,17α,20,21-tetrol-11-one and its 3- and/or 21-esters into 1,4-pregnadiene-17α,21-diol-3,11,20-trione, and its 21-ester; and of 5-pregnene-3,11,17α,20,21-pentol and its 3- and/or 21-esters into 1,4-pregnadiene-11α,17α,21-triol-3,20-dione and its 21-ester. The 11α-hydroxy compounds can be readily oxidized to the 11-keto compound (Δ^1-cortisone and its esters).

While the lower alkanoic esters are generally preferred, and particularly the acetates, as above indicated, it will be understood that the specific character of the ester is not controlling in my process and that other esters, both of organic and inorganic acids may be employed, such as cyclopentyl and cyclohexyl acetates, propionates and butyrates, and also the phosphates, polyphosphates and sulfates, it being necessary only that the esters be nontoxic toward the microorganism. The hydroxylated products of my process can, if desired, be converted into their corresponding esters by known procedures, for example, into their lower alkanoic and particularly their acetic acid esters.

As will be evident from the foregoing, the unsaturated starting compound can have a Δ^5-3-hydroxy or Δ^5-3-ester structure in place of the 3-keto-Δ^4-structure; upon conversion of the 3-hydroxyl or ester group to ketonic oxygen, the double bond will shift to the Δ^4-position.

The therapeutically active dienes of the present invention are preferably administered by mouth in the form of tablets containing a full daily dosage, say 50 mg. or a sub-multiple of such dosage, say 25 or 20 mg., or even 10 mg. mixed with a solid carrier containing one or more of the usual ingredients, such as starch, sugar, gums, clays and the like. They may, however, be also administered by intravenous and intramuscular injection, dissolved or suspended in a suitable non-toxic liquid vehicle; or they can be administered in the solid form by subcutaneous implantation, or in the form of suppositories dissolved or suspended in a fatty or waxy vehicle which melts at approximately body temperature. They can also be administered topically in the form of an ointment or cream dissolved in an unguent or cream base of known composition.

The fish solubles referred to hereinabove are presently available commercially as an extract of herring, menhaden, and various mixtures thereof, which has been subjected to an enzymatic hydrolysis. This material can be added directly to the culture broth for supplying the nutrient material. Where fish solubles (50% solid content) are available which have not been subjected to enzymatic hydrolysis, such extracts should be diluted with water and steamed for about 10 minutes at 90° C., followed by filtration, preferably with the aid of Filter-Cel.

The invention will be described in further detail in the following examples which are presented by way of illustration only and not as indicating the scope of the invention.

EXAMPLE 1

Conversion of Compound E to $\Delta^{1,4}$-pregnadiene-17α,21-diol-3,11,20-trione

From a solution of 30 g. of yeast extract (Difco) in 3.0 l. of tap water containing 13.2 g. of potassium dihydrogen phosphate and 26.4 g. of disodium hydrogen phosphate (pH of the solution 6.9) 27 portions of 100 ml. each are withdrawn, placed in 300 ml. Erlenmeyer flasks and sterilized by autoclaving for 15 minutes at 15 lb. steam pressure (120° C.). After autoclaving and cooling of the broth one ml. of a suspension of *Corynebacterium simplex* (A. T. C. C. 6946) is placed in each flask. The flasks are then shaken on a shake table at 220 R. P. M. and 28° C. for 24 hours.

Into each of 27 Erlenmeyer flasks are placed 150 mg. of Kendall's Compound E. The flasks and contents are then sterilized for 15 minutes at 15 lb. steam pressure (120° C.). To each flask are then added 5.0 ml. of ethanol. The 24-hour bacterial culture is then transferred aseptically and the resulting suspensions are shaken on a shake table at 220 R. P. M. and 28° C. for 48 hours. The final pH is 7.2.

The contents of all the flasks are combined and extracted with a total of 9.0 l. of chloroform in three equal portions. The combined extracts are then concentrated to a residue which is crystallized from acetone-hexane. There results 1.1 g. of $\Delta^{1,4}$-pregnadiene-17α,21-diol-3,11,20-trione, M. P. 210–215° (dec.). Several additional recrystallizations raised the M. P. to 230–232° (dec.); $[\alpha]_D^{25} + 175.3$ (dioxane); ϵ_{238} 15,400 (methanol).

Anal.: Calcd. for $C_{21}H_{26}O_5$; C, 70.37; H, 7.31. Found: C, 70.38; H, 7.67.

The infrared spectrum of the product shows the presence of a $\Delta^{1,4}$-diene-3-one system, hydroxyl and additional carbonyl (6-membered ring or side-chain). The structure of the product is established as $\Delta^{1,4}$-pregnadiene-17α,21-diol-3,11,20-trione by degradation to $\Delta^{1,4}$-androstadiene-3,11,17-trione (identical with an authentic sample) and by formation of a monoacetate by the action of acetic anhydride-pyridine which shows a characteristic interaction of the C-20 carbonyl with the C-21 acetate in the infrared spectrum.

21-acetylation of $\Delta^{1,4}$-pregnadiene-17α,21-diol-3,11,20-trione

To a solution of 0.5 g. of $\Delta^{1,4}$-pregnadiene-17α,21-diol-3,11,20-trione in 5 ml. of anhydrous pyridine are added 3 ml. of acetic anhydride. The reaction mixture is permitted to stand overnight at room temperature, and is then diluted with ice and water. The resulting precipitate is filtered and recrystallized from acetone-hexane. There is obtained 0.35 g. of $\Delta^{1,4}$-pregnadiene-17α,21-diol 3,11,20-trione 21-acetate, M. P. 227–228° d. After several recrystallizations from acetone-hexane it melted at 233–236° (dec.).

EXAMPLE 2

Conversion of Compound F to $\Delta^{1,4}$-pregnadiene-11β,17α,21-triol-3,20-dione

From a solution of 3 g. of yeast extract (Difco) in 3.0 l. of tap water containing 13.2 g. of potassium dihydrogen phosphate and 26.4 g. of disodium hydrogen phosphate (pH of the solution, 6.9) 27 portions of 100 ml. each are withdrawn, placed in 300 ml. Erlenmeyer flasks and sterilized by autoclaving for 15 minutes at 15 lb. steam pressure (120° C.). After autoclaving and cooling of the broth, one ml. of suspension of *Corynebacterium simplex* (A. T. C. C. 6946) is placed in each flask. The flasks are then shaken on a shake table at 220 R. P. M. and 28° C. for 24 hours.

Into each of 27 Erlenmeyer flasks are placed 150 mg. of Kendall's Compound F. The flasks and contents are then sterilized for 15 minutes at 15 lb. steam pressure (120° C.). To each flask are then added 5.0 ml. of ethanol. The 24-hour bacterial culture is then transferred aseptically and the resulting suspensions are shaken on a shake table at 220 R. P. M. and 28° C. for 48 hours. The pH at the end of the shake period is 7.0.

The contents of all the flasks are combined and extracted with a total of 9.0 l. of chloroform in three equal portions. The combined extracts are then concentrated to a residue which weighs 3.75 g. The M. P. of the residue is 227–232°. From 2.75 g. of this crude material on sludging with 50 ml. of acetone and cooling, there is recovered on filtration 1.35 g. of $\Delta^{1,4}$-pregnadiene-11β,17α,21-triol-3,20-dione, M. P. 237–239° (dec.). Additional product can be recovered from the mother liquor. Recrystallization from acetone raised the M. P. to 239–241° (dec.); $[\alpha]_D^{25} + 107°$ (dioxane); ϵ_{243} 14,600 (methanol).

Anal.: Calcd. for $C_{21}H_{28}O_5$; C, 69.97; H, 7.83. Found: C, 70.24; H, 8.13.

The infrared spectrum indicates the presence of a $\Delta^{1,4}$-diene-3-one system, hydroxyl and a 6-membered ring or side-chain ketone (in addition to the dienone carbonyl). From this evidence and the fact that a monoacetate is formed with acetic anhydride-pyridine whose infrared spectrum shows the expected interaction between the C–21 acetate and the C–20 carbonyl group, the product of fermentation is proven to possess the assigned structure.

21-acetylation of $\Delta^{1,4}$-pregnadiene-11β,17α,21-triol-3,20-dione

To a solution of 0.85 g. of $\Delta^{1,4}$-pregnadiene-11β,17α,21-triol-3,20-dione in 5 ml. of pyridine are added 3 ml. of acetic anhydride. The reaction mixture is allowed to stand at room temperature overnight and is then diluted with ice water. The resulting precipitate is filtered from the mixture and recrystallized from acetone-hexane. There is recovered 0.45 g. of $\Delta^{1,4}$-pregnadiene-11β,17α,21-triol-3,20-dione 21-acetate. M. P. 235–239°. On recrystallization, the M. P. rose to 237–239°; $[\alpha]_D^{25} + 116°$ (dioxane); ϵ_{243} 15,000 (methanol).

Anal.—Calcd. for $C_{23}H_{30}O_6$; C, 68.63; H, 7.51. Found: C, 68.62; H, 7.78.

11

EXAMPLE 3

Conversion of Compound S to Δ^{1,4}-pregnadiene-17α,21-diol-3,20-dione, and Δ^{1,4}-pregnadiene-17α,20,21-triol-3-one

One hundred ml. of a 1.0% yeast extract concentrate including 9.0 ml. of 0.2 M KH$_2$PO$_4$ and 9.0 ml. of 0.2 M Na$_2$HPO$_4$ is sterilized as before and inoculated with a 1.0% suspension of *Corynebacterium simplex* (A. T. C. C. 6946) from a 24-hour broth culture. The newly seeded culture is incubated and shaken (shake table) for 20 hours at 28° C. After incubation, the broth culture is transferred aseptically to a second sterile 300 ml. Erlenmeyer flask containing 150.0 mg. of sterile Cpd. S (4 - pregnen - 17α,21 - diol - 3,20-dione) in 5.0 ml. methanol or acetone. The pH of the reaction mixture is 7.0. The bacterial culture containing steroid and solvent is incubated and shaken for a period of 48 hours at 28° C. The final pH of the reaction mixture is 7.2–7.4. The culture is then extracted thoroughly with chloroform. The extracts are pooled and concentrated on a steam bath to dryness. The crude extract weighs 196.0 mg.

The total crude extract is sludged with methanol and there is obtained 80 mg. of crystalline solid, M. P. 246–250°. After two crystallizations from acetone, the M. P. is 246–249° dec., (α)$_D^{25}$+76° (CHCl$_3$), ε$_{245}$ 15,500 (C$_2$H$_5$OH).

Calcd. for C$_{21}$H$_{28}$O$_4$: C, 73.22; H, 8.19. Found: C, 73.56; H, 8.40.

The infrared spectrum indicates the presence of the Δ^{1,4}-diene-3-one system, hydroxyl and another carbonyl (6-membered ring or side-chain). The product is therefore Δ^{1,4}-pregnadiene-17α,21-diol-3,20-dione.

The structure is proved by degradation with sodium bismuthate in aqueous acetic acid to Δ^{1,4}-androstadiene-3,17-dione and by acetylation to a 21-monoacetate (interaction between 21-acetate and 20-carbonyl apparent in the infrared spectrum).

21-acetylation of Δ^{1,4}-pregnadiene - 17α,21 - diol - 3,20-dione.—To a solution of 0.25 g. of Δ^{1,4}-pregnadiene-17α,21-diol-3,20-dione in 2 ml. of pyridine was added 1 ml. of acetic anhydride. The reaction mixture was allowed to stand at room temperature overnight and was then diluted with ice and water. The resulting precipitate was filtered and recrystallized from methylene chloride-hexane, affording 0.20 g. of Δ^{1,4}-pregnadiene-17α, 21-diol-3,20-dione 21-acetate, M. P. 226.5–228°.

EXAMPLE 3a

Conversion of Compound S to Δ^{1,4}-pregnadiene-17α,21-diol-3,20-dione, and Δ^{1,4}-pregnadiene-17α,20,21-triol-3-one

One hundred ml. of a medium consisting of 1% fish solubles (prepared as described above), 0.1% yeast extract, 9.0 ml. of 0.2 M KH$_2$PO$_4$ and 9.0 ml. of 0.2 M Na$_2$HPO$_4$ are sterilized as described hereinabove and inoculated with a suspension of *Corynebacterium simplex* from a 24-hour broth culture. The newly seeded culture is incubated and shaken (shake table) for 20 hours at 28° C. After incubation, the broth culture is transferred aseptically to a second sterile 300 ml. Erlenmeyer flask containing 150 mg. of sterile Compound S in 5.0 ml. of ethanol. The pH of the reaction mixture is 6.9. The bacterial culture containing steroid and solvent is incubated and shaken for 48 hours at 28° C. The final pH is 7.3. The culture is extracted with 2 l. of chloroform in 5 equal portions, the extracts are pooled, and the pool is concentrated on the steam bath.

The crude residue is taken up in methylene chloride and chromatographed over Florisil. There is isolated from the chromatogram, starting material (15 mg.), Δ^{1,4}-pregnadiene-17α,21-diol-3,20-dione (30 mg.) and Δ^{1,4}-pregnadiene-17α,20,21-triol - 3 - one (90 mg.). The previously unidentified triol is recrystallized from acetone-

12

hexane and melts at 195–196°, [α]$_D^{25}$+33° (methanol).

Anal. — Calcd. for C$_{21}$H$_{30}$O$_4$: C, 72.80; H, 8.73. Found: C, 72.79; H, 9.08.

The structure of the triol is proved by acetylation with acetic anhydride-pyridine to a 20,21-diacetate and degradation to Δ^{1,4}-androstadiene-3,17-dione. The infrared spectrum of the triol shows a Δ^{1,4}-diene-3-one band, strong hydroxyl band and the absence of anything corresponding to a 20-carbonyl band.

In place of ethanol there can be employed other water-soluble organic solvents which are non-toxic to the microorganism, such as acetone, mixtures of ethanol and acetone, and the like.

EXAMPLE 4

Reaction of Δ^5-pregnen-3β,20-diol

One hundred ml. of 0.1% yeast extract concentrate including 9.0 ml. of 0.2 M KH$_2$PO$_4$ and 9.0 ml. of 0.2 M Na$_2$HPO$_4$ is autoclaved in a 300 ml. Erlenmeyer flask. After autoclaving for 15 minutes at 15 lbs. (120° C.), the flask is allowed to cool to room temperature. The flask is then seeded with a suspension of *Corynebacterium simplex* (A. T. C. C. 6946). The seeded flask is incubated and shaken (shake table) for 24 hours at 28° C.

A second 300 ml. Erlenmeyer flask containing 150 mg. of Δ^5-pregnene-3α,20-diol is sterilized in an autoclave for 15 minutes at 15 lbs. (120° C.). To this flask is then added 5.0 ml. of acetone or ethanol to dissolve the steroid. The 24-hour growth culture of *Corynebacterium simplex* is transferred aseptically to the flask containing the steroid and the reaction mixture is shaken (shake table) for 36 hours at 28° C. At the end of the transformation period, the pH is 7.1–7.2.

The reaction mixture is then extracted thoroughly with chloroform, the chloroform extracts are pooled and the resulting solution is concentrated to a residue (0.20 g.). The crude extract is crystallized from ether as long prisms, M. P. 135–138°. Two crystallizations from methylene chloride-hexane afford 0.06 g. of Δ^{1,4}-pregnadiene-3,20-dione, M. P. 152–153°, [α]$_D^{25}$+122° (CHCl$_3$), ε$_{245}$ 15,000 (C$_2$H$_5$OH). The infrared spectrum indicated the presence of a Δ^{1,4}-diene-3-one system, another carbonyl (6-membered ring or side-chain), and the complete absence of hydroxyl.

EXAMPLE 5

Reaction of dehydroisoandrosterone

One hundred ml. of a 24-hour broth culture of *Corynebacterium simplex* (A. T. C. C. 6946) grown in a 0.1% yeast extract (Difco) and 9.0 ml. of a 0.2 M KH$_2$PO$_4$ and 9.0 ml. of a 0.2 M Na$_2$HPO$_4$ are transferred to a 300 ml. Erlenmeyer flask containing 150.0 mg. of dehydroisoandrosterone in 5.0 ml. ethanol. The flask containing the steroid and bacterial culture is placed on a shaking machine and allowed to shake for a period of 24 hours at a temperature of 28° C. to 30° C.

From an initial pH of 6.8, in 48 hours, the reaction medium has a final pH of 7.1 to 7.2.

After the transformation period, the 100 ml. broth culture is extracted with 3 equal volumes of CHCl$_3$. The CHCl$_3$ volumes are combined and concentrated to dryness on a steam bath. The solid crude residue weighs 193.0 mg.

The total crude residue from the extraction of the broth is sludged with methanol, whereupon there result 30 mg. of elongated prisms, M. P. 155–165°. The infrared spectrum of this compound is identical with that of 4-androstene-3,17-dione.

From the mother liquors of the sludge on further concentration and crystallization from ether-hexane there is obtained 70 mg. of solid M. P. 110–143°. Recrystallization from ether gives 53 mg., M. P. 147–152°. The infrared spectrum of this material is identical with that of 4-androstene-3,17-dione.

The products from the two crystallizations are combined and crystallized from ether. There result 70 mg. of 4-androstene-3,17-dione, M. P. 167–169°; there is no depression of melting point on admixture with an authentic sample.

EXAMPLE 6

Reaction of 5-androsten-3β,17β-diol

One hundred ml. of a 20-hour broth culture of *Corynebacterium simplex* (A. T. C. C. 6946) containing a 0.1% yeast extract, 9.0 ml. of 0.2 M KH₂PO₄ and 9.0 ml. of 0.2 M Na₂HPO₄ are transferred to a 300 ml. Erlenmeyer flask containing 150 mg. of androstenediol in 5.0 ml. ethanol. The flask is placed on a shaking machine and incubated at 28° C. and is allowed to run for a period of 48 hours, the final pH of this reaction mixture being 7.1.

The broth culture is extracted with three equal volumes of CHCl₃. The solvent volumes are combined and concentrated to dryness on a steam bath. The solid crude extract weighs 158.0 mg.

The total crude extract is crystallized from ether and there result 40 mg. of solid M. P. 128–135°, [a]_D^25 + 69° (CHCl₃), whose infrared spectrum contains bands characteristic of a Δ^1,4-diene-3-one system (strong), hydroxyl (strong) and five-membered ring carbonyl (moderate). Repeated crystallization from ether-hexane and methylene chloride-hexane afford ultimately 11 mg. of Δ^1,4-androstadiene-17β-ol-3-one, M. P. 164–166°, [a]_D^25 + 25° (CHCl₃). The infrared spectrum of this sample is identical with that of an authentic sample.

The mother liquor from the original ether crystallization is chromatographed over Florisil which had been prepared with hexane. Material eluted from the column with 10–20% ether in hexane contains only traces of hydroxyl in the infrared spectrum and shows a strong five-membered ring carbonyl together with the Δ^1,4-diene-3-one bands. Crystallization of the pooled eluates of this group from ether-hexane affords 25 mg. of Δ^1,4-androstadiene-3,17-dione, M. P. 139–140°, [a]_D^25 + 110° (CHCl₃). The infrared spectrum of this material is identical with that of an authentic sample.

EXAMPLE 7

Reaction of testosterone

A one hundred ml. broth culture containing a 0.1% yeast extract concentration. 9.0 ml. of 0.2 M KH₂PO₄ and 9.0 ml. of 0.2 M Na₂HPO₄, contained in a 300 ml. Erlenmeyer flask, is seeded with 1 ml. of a 24-hour broth culture of *Corynebacterium simplex* (A. T. C. C. 6946). The flask is incubated at 28° C. for 24 hours. A second 300 ml. Erlenmeyer flask containing 150 mg. of sterile testosterone in 5.0 ml. acetone is inoculated with the 24-hour culture of *Corynebacterium simplex* (A. T. C. C. 6946). The culture-containing steroid solution is incubated for 48 hours at 28° to 30° C.

After termination of the transformation period, the pH is 7.2–7.3. The culture is now directly extracted with 3 equal volumes of CHCl₃, the solvent volumes combined and concentrated to dryness on a steam bath. The crude extract weighs 153.0 mg.

The total crude is chromatographed on Florisil prepared with hexane. The fractions collected with 10–20% ether-hexane eluate are pooled and crystallized from ether-hexane, affording 12 mg. of a solid, M. P. 134–138°, which is shown to be identical with Δ^1,4-androstadiene-3,17-dione by comparison of the infrared spectra and absence of depression of melting point on admixture with an authentic sample. The fractions collected with 30–50% ether-hexane eluate are pooled and crystallized from ether-hexane, affording 32 mg. of a solid, M. P. 159–165°, which is shown to be identical with Δ^1,4-androstadiene-17β-ol-3-one by comparison of the infrared

spectra and absence of depression of melting point on admixture with an authentic sample.

EXAMPLE 8

Reaction of diosgenin

To a 300 ml. Erlenmeyer flask, containing 9.0 ml. each of 0.2 M KH₂PO₄ and 0.2 M Na₂HPO₄ in 1.0% yeast extract (Difco) is added an inoculum in the form of 1 ml. of a bacterial suspension of *Corynebacterium simplex* (A. T. C. C. 6946). The bacterial culture is placed on a shaking machine and incubated at 28° C. for 24 hours.

After 24 hours of incubation, the culture is transferred aseptically to a second flask containing 150 mg. of diosgenin in 5.0 ml. of ethanol. The flask is then shaken for a period of from 24–36 hours.

At the end of the transformation period, the flask is extracted with 3 equal volumes of CHCl₃. The CHCl₃ volumes are combined and concentrated to dryness on a steam bath. The crude extract weighs 175.0 mg.

The total crude extract is crystallized from methanol and there is isolated a product whose infrared spectrum shows the presence of a Δ^1,4-diene-3-one system, a 3-keto-Δ^4 system and the spiroketal side-chain. The products are chromatographed over Florisil and there are isolated diosgenone and Δ-1,4-diosgedienone.

EXAMPLE 9

Reaction of 5-pregnene-3β,17α,21-triol-20-one 3,21-diacetate

The reaction medium and organism are prepared as described in Example 7. 150 mg. of 5-pregnene-3β,17α,-21-triol-20-one 3,21-diacetate are added, and the reaction is permitted to proceed as previously described.

The products are extracted with chloroform, the chloroform extracts are concentrated to a small volume and chromatographed on Florisil. The order of elution is unreacted starting material (75 mg.) first, then Compound S 21-acetate (15 mg.) and finally Δ^1,4-pregnadiene-17α,21-diol-3,20-dione (30 mg.). The products were all identified by comparison of their infrared spectra with those of authentic samples.

EXAMPLE 10

Reaction of 4-pregnene-3β-ol-20-one

The reaction medium and organism are prepared as described in Example 7. 150 mg. of 4-pregnene-3β-ol-20-one are added, and the reaction is permitted to proceed as previously described. The product is extracted with chloroform and isolated by evaporation to dryness. Recrystallization of the residue from ether-hexane affords 73 mg. of Δ^1,4-pregnadiene-3,20-dione, M. P. 150–152°.

EXAMPLE 11

Reaction of 17-ethinyltestosterone

To the reaction medium and organism prepared as described in Example 7, there are added 150 mg. of 17-ethinyltestosterone and the reaction is permitted to proceed as previously described.

The product is extracted with chloroform and isolated by evaporation to dryness. Recrystallization of the residue yields 17-ethinyl-Δ^1,4-androstadiene-17β-ol-3-one as a crystalline solid.

EXAMPLE 12

Reaction of 17-methyltestosterone

The reaction medium and organism are prepared as described in Example 7. 150 mg. of 17-methyltestosterone are added and the reaction is permitted to proceed as above described.

The product is extracted with chloroform and isolated by evaporation to dryness. Recrystallization of the residue gives crystalline 17-methyl-Δ^1,4-androstadiene-17β-ol-3-one.

15

EXAMPLE 13

Reaction of corticosterone

The reaction medium and organism are prepared as described in Example 7. 150 mg. of 4-pregnene-11β,21-diol-3,20-dione are added and the reaction is permitted to proceed as above described.

The product is extracted with chloroform and isolated by evaporation to dryness. Recrystallization of the residue affords crystalline Δ¹,⁴-pregnadiene-11β,21-diol-3,20-dione.

EXAMPLE 14

Reaction of desoxycorticosterone

The reaction medium and organism are prepared as described in Example 7. 150 mg. of 4-pregnene-21-ol-3,20-dione are added and the reaction is permitted to proceed as above described.

The product is extracted with chloroform and isolated by evaporation to dryness. Recrystallization of the residue affords Δ¹,⁴-pregnadiene-21-ol-3,20-dione as a crystalline solid.

EXAMPLE 15

Reaction of 11-dehydrocorticosterone

To the reaction medium and organism prepared as described in Example 7, 150 mg. of 4-pregnene-21-ol-3,11,20-trione are added and the reaction is permitted to proceed as above described.

The product is extracted with chloroform and isolated by evaporation to dryness. Recrystallization of the residue yields crystalline Δ¹,⁴-pregnadiene-21-ol-3,11,20-trione.

EXAMPLE 16

Reaction with 9α-fluoro-4-pregnene-11β,17α,21-triol-3,20-dione

The reaction medium and organism are prepared as described in Example 7. 150 mg. of 9α-fluoro-4-pregnene-11β,17α,21-triol-3,20-dione are added and the reaction is permitted to proceed as previously described.

The product is extracted with chloroform and isolated by evaporation to dryness. Recrystallization of the residue affords 9α-fluoro-Δ¹,⁴-pregnadiene-11β,17α,21-triol-3,20-dione as a crystalline solid.

With reference to the acetylation of the dienes described in Examples 1, 2 and 3, it will be evident that other esters of the diene derivatives can be similarly prepared by reaction with the anhydride of the acid or with its chloride in known manner. While the acetates of the adrenal hormones are those most commonly used in therapy, other lower alkanoyl esters of the various hydroxylated dienes may be produced, such as the formates, propionates, butyrates, and valerates, and likewise the esters of other non-toxic acids, like the benzoates, and also the neutral and acid esters of polybasic acids, like succinic, maleic, malic, citric, tartaric, phthalic and hexahydrophthalic. In the case of the acid esters, the metal salts can be formed in the usual manner by reaction with the hydroxide, carbonate or bicarbonate of the metal, as of the alkali and alkaline earth metals.

Instead of forming the 1,4-dienes of Compounds E and F and subsequently esterifying the products, the corresponding esters of Compounds E and F and of their intermediates can be subjected to the process of the present invention and will yield the dienes of the esters of Compounds E and F; however, as above indicated, by suitable control of the reaction conditions, the 21-alcohols can also be obtained from the 21-esters. Thus, in Example 1, Compound E can be replaced by its 21-ester or by its 17α,21-diester (such as the acetate ester), or by 5-pregnene-3,17α,21-triol-11,20-dione 21-acetate or 17α,21-diacetate, or 3,17α,21-triacetate or other esters; while in Example 2, Compound F can be replaced by its 21-acetate, or 17α,21-diacetate, or 11β,17α,21-triacetate;

16

or by 5-pregnene-3,11β,17α,21-tetrol-20-one 3,21-diacetate, 3,17α,21-triacetate or 3,11β,17α,21-tetraacetate. The latter group of compounds can be replaced by the corresponding 11α-hydroxy epimers, to yield the 11-epimers of the diene of Compound F and its 21-esters and 17α,21-diesters. The polyesters can in all cases be mixed esters, like 3-propionate-21-acetate.

Examples of these variations of our process are presented by way of illustration in the following:

EXAMPLE 17

Conversion of Compound F 21-acetate to the 1,4-diene and its 21-acetate

The reaction is run exactly as described for the transformation of Compound F (4-pregnene-11β,17α,21-triol-3,20-dione) to the corresponding diene (Example 2), and the product is isolated by chloroform extraction and crystallization from acetone. From 1.0 g. of Compound F 21-acetate there is obtained 0.22 g. of 1,4-pregnadiene-11β,17α,21-triol-3,20-dione, M. P. 239–241° (dec.).

When it is desired to suppress the deacetylation reaction, the same conditions as above are used with the exception that the temperature of the environment for the growth and reaction phases of the process is raised to 36° C. The product is isolated in the usual way. From 1.0 g. of Compound F 21-acetate there results 0.13 g. of Compound F diene-21-acetate, M. P. 237–239° (dec.).

EXAMPLE 18

Conversion of cortisone 21-acetate to the 1,4-diene and its 21-acetate

The reaction is conducted as described for the transformation of cortisone (4-pregnene-17α,21-diol-3,11,20-trione) to the corresponding diene (Example 1), and the product is isolated by chloroform extraction and crystallized from acetone-hexane. From 1.0 g. of cortisone acetate there is isolated 0.17 g. of Δ¹,⁴-pregnadiene-17α,21-diol-3,11,20-trione, M. P. 230–232°.

When it is desired to suppress the deacetylation, the same conditions as above are used with the exception that the temperature of the environment for the growth and reaction phases of the process is raised to 36° C. The product is isolated in the usual way. From 1.0 g. of cortisone acetate there results 0.11 g. of cortisone diene-21-acetate, M. P. 230–233° (dec.).

EXAMPLE 19

Conversion of 4-pregnene-11α,17α,21-triol-3,20-dione to 1,4-pregnadiene-11α,17α,21-triol-3,20-dione

The reaction is run exactly as described in the transformation of 4-pregnene - 11β,17α,21 - triol - 3,20 - dione (Compound F) to the corresponding diene, the product is isolated by chloroform extraction and crystallized from acetone-hexane. From 1.0 g. of 11-epi Compound F there is isolated 0.25 g. of Δ¹,⁴-pregnadiene-11α,17α,21-triol-3,20-dione as a crystalline solid. M. P. 245–246° (dec.).

Acetylation of 11-epi Compound F diene (1.0 g.) is accomplished by solution in 15 ml. of anhydrous pyridine followed by the addition of 0.3 g. of acetic anhydride. The reaction mixture is allowed to stand at room temperature overnight and is then poured into ice-water. The resulting precipitate is separated by filtration and recrystallized as a crystalline solid (Δ¹,⁴-pregnadiene-11α,17α,21-triol-3,20-dione 21-acetate) from acetone-hexane.

As already stated, where a 3-hydroxy intermediate is employed, the formation of the diene derivative will be accompanied by an oxidation of the hydroxyl group to a keto group with a shifting of the double bond to the 4,5-position; while in the case of a 3-ester, such oxidation step will be preceded by a hydrolysis of the 3-ester group.

In place of Compound E, there can be employed as starting material 5-pregnen-3,17α,21-triol,11,20-dione, 5-pregnen-3,17α,20,21-tetrol-11-one or their 3-acetates or other esters which are non-toxic toward the microorganism or inhibiting toward its enzyme; while similarly, in place of Compound F, there can be used 5-pregnen-3,11β,17α,21-tetrol-20-one, 5 - pregnen - 3,11β,17α,20,21-pentol, or their 3-acetates or other esters. As indicated above, the 20-hydroxy group will in each case be oxidized to a keto group.

EXAMPLE 20

Conversion of Compound F to 1,4-pregnadiene-11β,17α,21-triol-3,20-dione

From a solution of 1 gram yeast extract (Difco) in 1.0 liter of tap water containing 4.4 gm. of potassium dihydrogen phosphate and 8.8 g. of disodium hydrogen phosphate (pH of the solution 6.9), 10 portions of 100 ml. each are withdrawn, placed in 300 ml. Erlenmeyer flasks and sterilized by autoclaving for 15 minutes at 15 lbs. steam pressure (120° C.). After autoclaving and cooling of the broth, one ml. of suspension of *Corynebacterium hoagii* (American Type Culture Collection 7005) is placed in each flask. The flasks are then shaken on a shake table at 220 R. P. M. and 28° C. for 16½ hours.

Into each of the 10 Erlenmeyer flasks, 50 mg. of Kendall's Compound F, dissolved in 1 ml. of 90% methanol is added aseptically. The flasks are replaced on the shaker and incubated for 7 hours. The pH at the end of the shake period is 6.82.

The contents of all flasks are combined and extracted with a total of 3 liters of chloroform in 3 equal portions. The combined extracts are concentrated to a residue of 425 mg. Crystallization of the residue from acetone affords 248 mg. of 1,4-pregnadiene-11β,17α,21-triol-3,20-dione.

EXAMPLE 21

Conversion of Compound F to 1,4-pregnadiene-11β,17α,21-triol-3,20-dione

From a solution of 0.5 gram Basamin Busch (Anheuser-Busch) in 1 liter of tap water, 10 portions of 100 ml. each are withdrawn, placed in 300 ml. Erlenmeyer flasks and sterilized by autoclaving for 15 minutes at 15 lb. steam pressure (120° C.). After autoclaving and cooling of the broth, one ml. of a suspension of *Corynebacterium simplex* is placed in each flask. The flasks are then shaken on a shake table at 220 R. P. M. and at 28° C. for 24 hours.

Into each of the 10 Erlenmeyer flasks 50 mg. of Kendall's Compound F, dissolved in 0.8 ml. of absolute methanol, are added aseptically. The flasks are replaced on the shaker and incubated for an additional 4–7 hours. The pH at the end of the shake period is 7.2–7.6.

The contents of all flasks are combined and extracted with a total of 3 liters of chloroform in 3 equal portions. The combined extracts are concentrated to a residue of 490 mg. Crystallization of the residue from acetone affords 403 mg. of 1,4-pregnadiene-11β,17α,21-triol-3,20-dione, M. P. 238–240° C. (dec); $(\alpha)_D^{25} +105°$ (dioxane): ϵ_{243} 14,500 (methanol).

EXAMPLE 22

Conversion of Compound E to 1,4-pregnadiene-17α,21-diol-3,11,20-trione

The procedure described in Example 21 is followed except that Compound E is used in place of Compound F, while the conversion time is increased to 6–12 hrs. The crude diene is obtained in a yield of 85%.

Examples 21 and 22 show that the yield is increased with reduction in the concentration of the starting compound.

As will be evident from the foregoing, the carbon

side chain remains undisturbed in our process, i.e., it is not split off in whole or in part, whether it contains but a single carbon atom, as in 17-methyl-testosterone, or contains two carbon atoms, saturated or unsaturated, as in pregnane compounds and in ethinyl testosterone, or contains more complex side chains, as in the sapogenins and psuedo-sapogenins, and as experiments have indicated, in other steroids, like cholenic acids generally and their nor- and bisnor-derivatives.

It will be understood that where in the claims reference is made to the action of a culture of the specified organism or group of organisms, there is included also the treatment with an enzymatic extract of a culture of the organism as an equivalent procedure.

The present application is a continuation-in-part of my co-pending applications Serial No. 449,257, filed August 11, 1954, and Serial No. 464,159, filed October 22, 1954.

Having now particularly described and ascertained the nature of my said invention and in what manner the same is to be performed. I declare that what I claim is:

1. Process for the manufacture of Δ^1,4-pregnadienes which comprises subjecting a Δ^4-3-keto pregnene to the action of a culture of a member of the group consisting of *Corynebacterium simplex* and *Corynebacterium hoagii*.

2. The process which comprises subjecting a 3-hydroxy-10,13-dimethyl steroid of the androstane and pregnane series having a double bond attached to the 5-carbon, to the action of a culture of a member of the group consisting of *Corynebacterium simplex* and *Corynebacterium hoagii*, until a 3-keto-10,13-dimethyl-steroid-1,4-diene is obtained.

3. Process for the manufacture of 1,4-pregnadien-17α,21-diol-3,11,20-trione which comprises subjecting cortisone to the action of a culture of a member of the group consisting of *Corynebacterium simplex* and *Corynebacterium hoagii*.

4. Process for the manufacture of 1,4-pregnadien-17α,21-diol-3,11,20-trione and of the esters of such diene, which comprises subjecting a lower alkanoyl ester of 5-pregnen-3,17α,25-triol-11,20-dione to the action of a culture of a member of the group consisting of *Corynebacterium simplex* and *Corynebacterium hoagii*.

5. Process for the manufacture of 1,4-pregnadien-17α,21-diol-3,11,20-trione which comprises subjecting the 21-acetate of cortisone to the action of a culture of *Corynebacterium simplex* at a pH of 6.8 to 7.1 and a temperature of about 26 to 29° C.

6. Process for the manufacture of 1,4-pregnadien-11β,17α,21-triol-3,20-dione, which comprises subjecting hydrocortisone to the action of a culture of a member of the group consisting of *Corynebacterium simplex* and *Corynebacterium hoagii*.

7. Process for the manufacture of 1,4-pregnadien-11β,17α,21-triol-3,20-dione and of the esters of such diene, which comprises subjecting a lower alkanoyl ester of 5-pregnen-3,11β,17α,21-tetrol-20-one to the action of a culture of a member of the group consisting of *Corynebacterium simplex* and *Corynebacterium hoagii*.

8. Process for the manufacture of 1,4-pregnadien-17α,21-diol-3,11,20-trione and its 21-lower alkanoyl esters, which comprises subjecting 4-pregnen-11α,17α,21-triol-3,20-dione and its 21-lower alkanoyl esters to the action of a culture of a member of the group consisting of *Corynebacterium simplex* and *Corynebacterium hoagii*, and thereafter oxidizing the 11α-hydroxyl to a keto group.

9. Process for the manufacture of 3-keto-1,4-pregnadienes, which comprises subjecting a pregnene compound having a nuclear double bond attached to the 5-carbon, said pregnene having methylene groups at the 1- and 2-carbons and a member of the class consisting of ketonic oxygen, hydroxyl and ester groups at the 3-carbon, to the action of a culture of a microorganism of the group

19

consisting of *Corynebacterium simplex* and *Corynebacterium hoagii*.

10. Process according to claim 9, wherein the steroid is substituted by a member of the class consisting of hydroxyl and ester groups, at least at one of the 11-, 17-, 20-, and 21-positions.

11. Process according to claim 9, wherein the pregnene has a 20-hydroxy group which is oxidized to a 20-keto group by the microorganism.

12. Process according to claim 9, wherein the pregnen has a 20-keto group which is reduced to a 20-hydroxy group by the microorganism.

13. Process for the manufacture of pregnadienes of the formula

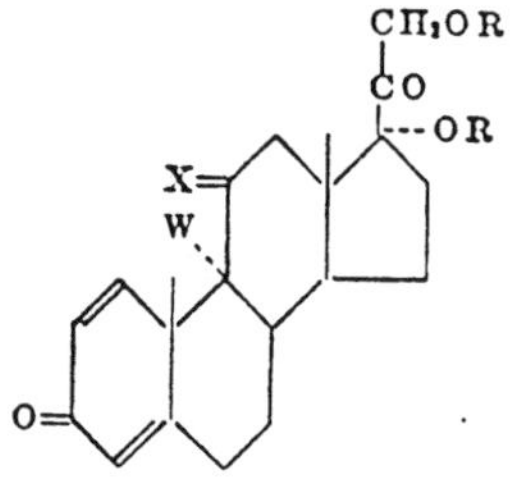

wherein R is a member of the group consisting of H and lower alkanoyl, and X is a member of the group consisting of

while W is a member of the group consisting of H, F and Cl, which comprises subjecting a pregnene compound of the formula

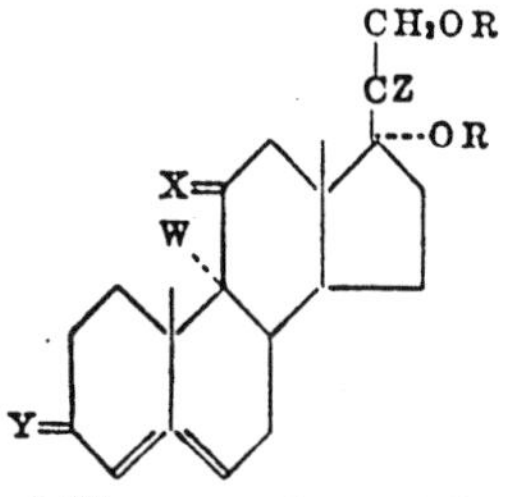

wherein R, X and W are as above defined, while Y is a member of the group consisting of

and Z is a member of the group consisting of

20

the dotted lines indicating the alternative location of the double bond, to the action of a culture of a member of the group consisting of *Corynebacterium simplex* and *Corynebacterium hoagii*.

14. The process which comprises subjecting a lower alkanoyl ester of cortisone to the action of a culture of a member of the group consisting of *Corynebacterium simplex* and *Corynebacterium hoagii*.

15. The process which comprises subjecting a lower alkanoyl ester of hydrocortisone to the action of a culture of a member of the group consisting of *Corynebacterium simplex* and *Corynebacterium hoagii*.

16. Process for the manufacture of 1,4-pregnadiene-17α,21-diol-3,20-dione which comprises subjecting 4-pregnene-17α.21-diol-3,20-dione to the action of a culture of a member of the group consisting of *Corynebacterium simplex* and *Corynebacterium hoagii*.

17. Process for the manufacture of 1,4-androstadienes which comprises subjecting an androstene compound having a double bond attached to the 5-carbon and a hydroxyl group at least at one of the 3- and 17-carbons, to the action of a culture of a member of the group consisting of *Corynebacterium simplex* and *Corynebacterium hoagii*.

18. Process for the manufacture of 9α-fluoro-1,4-pregnadien-17α.21-diol-3,11,20-trione. which comprises subjecting 9α-fluoro-4-pregnen-17α,21-diol-3,11,20-trione to the action of a member of the group consisting of *Corynebacterium simplex* and *Corynebacterium hoagii*.

19. Process for the manufacture of 9α-fluoro-1,4-pregnadien-11β,17α,triol-3,20-dione, which comprises subjecting 9α-fluoro-4-pregnen-11β,17α,21-triol-3,20-dione to the action of a member of the group consisting of *Corynebacterium simplex* and *Corynebacterium hoagii*.

References Cited in the file of this patent

UNITED STATES PATENTS

2,186,906	Mamoli	----------------	Jan. 9, 1940
2,280,828	Inhoffen	--------------	Apr. 28, 1942
2,341,110	Mamoli	----------------	Feb. 8, 1944
2,602,769	Murray	----------------	July 8, 1952
2,649,402	Murray	----------------	Aug. 18, 1953
2,658,023	Shull	------------------	Nov. 3, 1953
2,705,237	Djerassi	--------------	Mar. 29, 1955

OTHER REFERENCES

Vischer, Experientia IX, 10 (1953), pages 171–172.
Fried et al., J. A. C. S. 75 (1953), pages 5764. 5765.
Finch et al., Mfgrs. Chemist, June 1954, pages 247–251.

UNITED STATES PATENT OFFICE
Certificate of Correction

Patent No. 2,837,464

June 3, 1958

Arthur Nobile

It is hereby certified that error appears in the printed specification of the above numbered patent requiring correction and that the said Letters Patent should read as corrected below.

Column 19, lines 39 to 43, for that portion of the formula reading

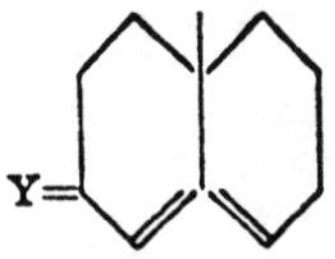

read

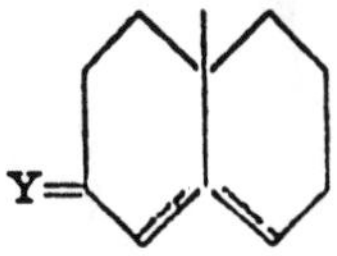

column 20, line 31, for "-11β,17α,triol-" read — -11β,17α,21-triol- —.

Signed and sealed this 14th day of April 1959.

[SEAL]

Attest:
KARL H. AXLINE,
Attesting Officer.

ROBERT C. WATSON,
Commissioner of Patents.

CHAPTER TWO

1

2,953,582

4-CHLORO-ADRENOSTERONE

Bruno Camerino, Milan, Italy, assignor to Società Farmaceutici Italia, a corporation of Italy

No Drawing. Filed Oct. 26, 1956, Ser. No. 618,441

Claims priority, application Italy Apr. 23, 1956

1 Claim. (Cl. 260—397.3)

This invention relates to a new class of steroids characterized by high anabolic activity coupled with low androgen activity.

The herein claimed compounds are prepared by a modification of the process disclosed in the copending application of July 19, 1956, Serial No. 598,754, now abandoned, entitled "New Steroid Hormone Derivatives Substituted in the 4-Position and Method of Preparing Same" of which this application is a continuation-in-part. The compounds disclosed in said copending application are prepared by reacting 4,5-epoxy-3-keto-steroids of the general formula

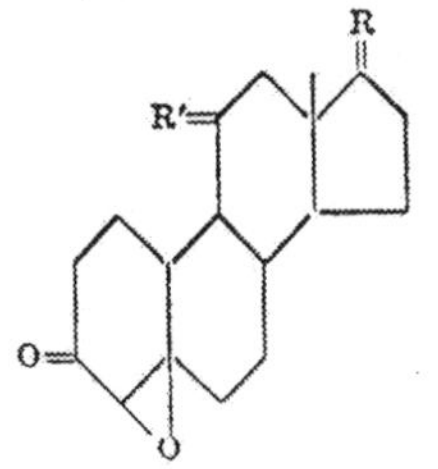

wherein R may represent =O, (H)OH and (CH₃)OH, and R′ represents H₂, =O and (H)OH with mineral acid in an organic solvent.

The compounds obtained according to this invention have the general formula

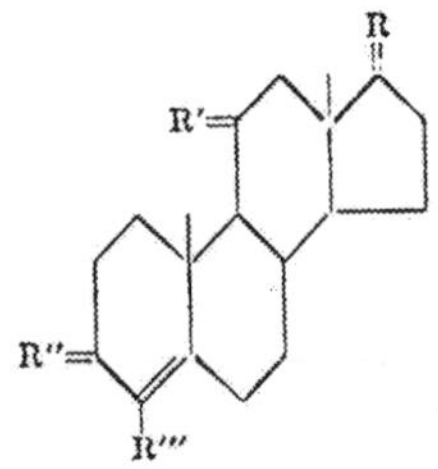

wherein R represents =O, (H)OH, (CH₃)OH and (H)OR^{IV}, R′ represents H₂, =O and (H) OH, R″ represents=O, (H)OH, (H)OR^{IV}, =NOH and

$$=NNHCSNH_2$$

R‴ represents F, Cl and R^{IV} represents acyl and alkoxy.

According to the aforementioned, copending patent application, steroids wherein R‴ represents F or Cl are prepared from only the β-form of 4.5-epoxides.

We have now found that steroids of this type can be also obtained from the α-form of 4,5-epoxides upon treating with halogenhydric acids in chloroform solution or in a chloroform solution containing 10% absolute ethanol. Moreover, if R‴ is to become Cl, it is sufficient to heat the epoxide with a chloroform solution of pyridinium chloride.

According to the present invention, it is therefore possible to prepare 4-chloro and the 4-fluoro-steroids directly from a mixture of 4,5β- and 4,5α-epoxides obtained by treating a 3-keto-Δ⁴-steroid with alkaline hydrogen peroxide. Consequently, the process results in a substantial

2

increase in yield, coupled with a simplification of the operations.

The compounds claimed in the present invention display strong anabolic activity on proteins, while being devoid of any substantial androgen activity. Therefore, they are of great importance in human and veterinary medicine. Anabolic as well as androgen activity are always jointly present in steroids that have been hitherto used in anabolitic therapy. Now we are able to provide products that do not produce any substantial androgen effect.

Therefore, it is possible to take advantage of the anabolic activity of these compounds without stimulating the sexual activity and this property is particularly useful for the treatment of decay, osteoporosis, emaciation, convalescences, premature newborns, underdevelopment, senility.

In addition, the products of the present invention also exhibit the other properties of previously known anabolic substances on the basis of which they have been used in treating certain ovary malfunctions, etc.

The following examples illustrate the present invention without limiting its scope.

EXAMPLE 1

4-chloro-testosterone

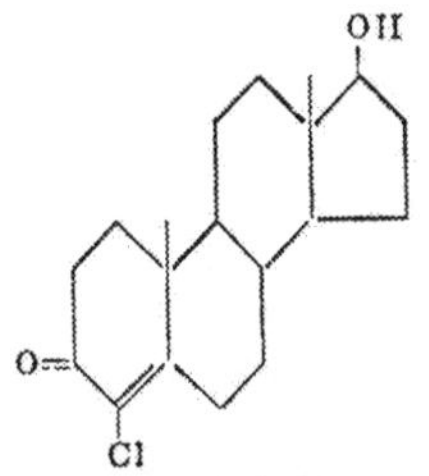

15 g. of a mixture of 4β,5-epoxy-etiocholane-17β-ol-3-one and 4α,5-epoxy-androstane-17β-ol-3-one, dissolved in 375 cc. chloroform, are treated with a stream of gaseous HCl at room temperature for about 2 hours.

The chloroform solution is neutralized with a sodium bicarbonate solution, washed with water and dried.

The residue is crystallized from benzene or aqueous methanol. 9 g. of needle-shaped crystals, M.P. 186–188° C., are obtained. Upon concentrating the mother-liquor, 3.2 g. of a product having a M.P. of 180–184° C. are recovered.

λ max. 256 mμ, ε=13.160

EXAMPLE 2

4-chloro-testosterone

Example 1 is repeated, except that the chloroform is substituted by methylene chloride containing 3% methanol.

EXAMPLE 3

4-chloro-testosterone

Example 1 is repeated except that the saturation with gaseous HCl is carried out at —10° C. for 2 hours.

EXAMPLE 4

4-chloro-testosterone-acetate

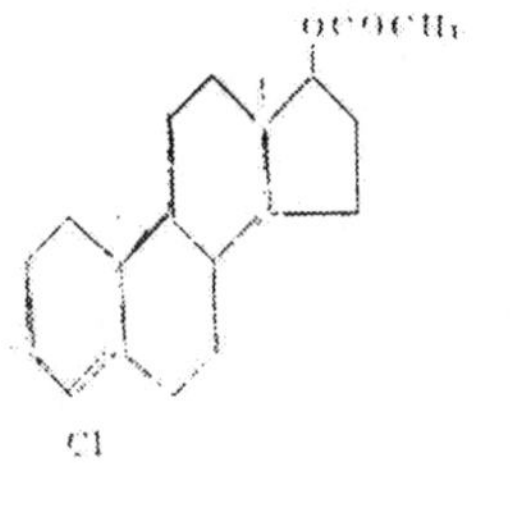

5 g. 4β,5-epoxy-etiocholane-17β-ol-3-one-acetate, M.P. 156° C., are dissolved in 125 cc. anhydrous chloroform and treated with a gaseous HCl stream at room temperature.

The solution becomes yellow-green and subsequently dark and turbid. After 2 hours the organic solution is washed first with a sodium bicarbonate solution and then with water, and is finally evaporated to dryness whereby the drying is completed under vacuum.

The residue is taken up with 400 cc. hot methanol, and the solution is cooled and filtrated. 3.3 g. 4-chloro-testosterone-acetate are obtained, M.P. 228–230° C., λ max. 255 mμ, ε=13,300, [α]$_D$=+118° ±4° (in chloroform).

0.5 g. of a product having a M.P. of 215–220° C. is recovered upon concentrating the filtrate.

EXAMPLE 5

4-chloro-testosterone-acetate

4 g. 4β,5-epoxy-etiocholane - 17β - ol - 3 - one - acetate, M.P. 156° C., are refluxed with 50 cc. of a 1.2/N solution of pyridinium chloride in chloroform for 5 hours. The organic solution is washed with diluted hydrochloric acid, sodium bicarbonate and water and is finally evaporated to dryness.

The crystalline residue, M.P. 220–228° C., consists of almost pure 4-chloro-testosterone-acetate. After a recrystallization the product melts at 228–230° C.

EXAMPLE 6

4-chloro-testosterone-acetate

2 g. 4α,5-epoxy-androstane-17β-ol-3-one-acetate M.P. 170–172° C., dissolved in 50 cc. anhydrous chloroform, are treated with anhydrous HCl for 2 hours at room temperature. The solution becomes pale-yellow without any further darkening. The solution is neutralized by washing and concentrated. The residue obtained upon evaporation is recrystallized from methanol and 1.5 g. 4-chloro-testosterone-acetate, M.P. 226–228° C., are obtained.

EXAMPLE 7

4-chloro-testosterone-acetate

1 g. 4α,5-epoxy-androstane-17β-ol-3-one-acetate are boiled for 8 hours in 15 cc. of a 1.2/N solution of pyridinium chloride in coloroform.

The resulting solution is washed with dil. hydrochloric acid, diluted alkali, water and is finally reduced to dryness. An almost quantitative yield of 4-chloro-testosterone-acetate is obtained.

EXAMPLE 8

4-chloro-testosterone-acetate

1 g. 4-chloro-testosterone are acetylated with 1 cc. acetic anhydride and 5 cc. pyridine at room temperature for 16 hours. Ice is added to the solution, and the precipitate is filtered off and recrystallized from chloroform-ethanol; 1 g. 4-chlorotestosterone-acetate, M.P. 228–230° C., is obtained.

EXAMPLE 9

4-chloro-testosterone-propionate

OCOCH₂CH₃

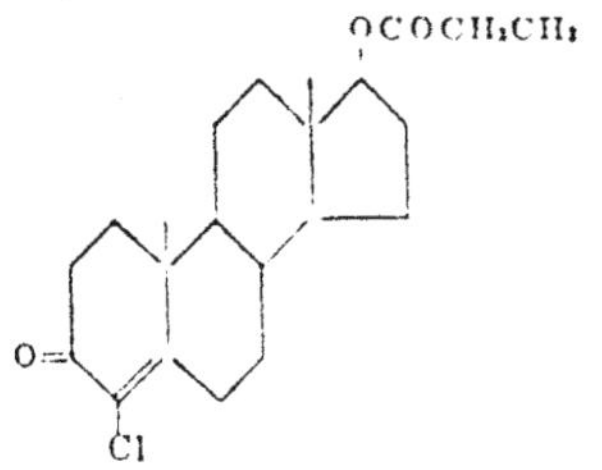

3 g. 4β-5-epoxy-etiocholane-17β-ol-3-one-propionate, M. P. 158–160° C., dissolved in 120 cc. chloroform, are treated with anhydrous HCl for 10 minutes. At the conclusion of the aforementioned operation steps, the residue is crystallized from methanol. 2 g. chloro-testosterone-propionate, M.P. 164–165° C., are obtained.

EXAMPLE 10

4-chloro-testosterone-emisuccinate

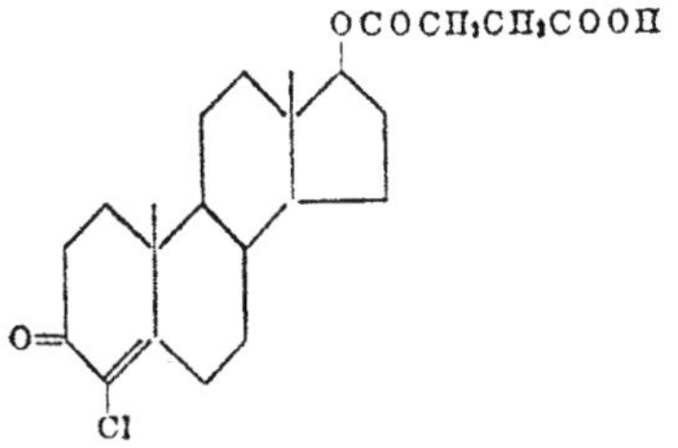

OCOCH₂CH₂COOH

0.7 g. 4-chloro-testosterone, M.P. 188° C., are treated with 7 cc. pyridine and 1.2 g. succinic anhydride at 70° C. for 5 hours. After pouring the solution into ice-cold water, extracting with benzene and treating the extract with diluted hydrochloric acid, washing with water and drying by evaporation, the residue is crystallized from aqueous methanol. 0.4 g. of crystals, M.P. 203–204° C., [α]$_D^{22}$=116° ±4, are obtained.

EXAMPLE 11

4-chloro-testosterone-palmitate

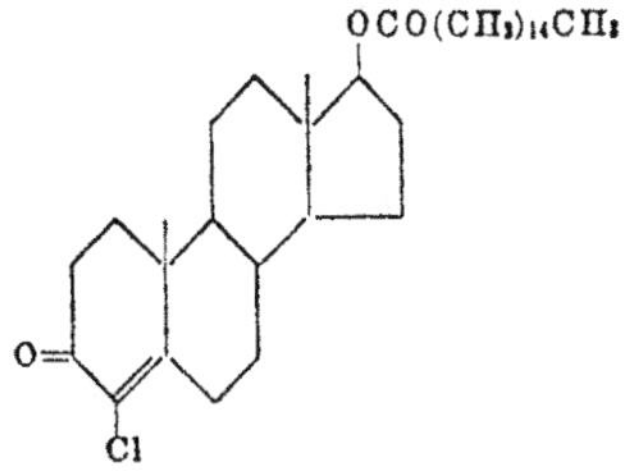

OCO(CH₂)₁₄CH₃

1 g. 4-chloro-testosterone, dissolved in 10 cc. benzene and 3 cc. pyridine, are treated with 1.3 g. palmityl chloride at −10° C. and left standing at room temperature for 12 hours. The solution is then diluted with benzene, and washed with diluted HCl, diluted NaOH and water. The benzene is evaporated and the residue is recrystallized from methanol. 0.8 g. 4-chloro-testosterone-palmitate, M.P. 56° C., are obtained.

EXAMPLE 12

4-chloro-17α-methyl-testosterone

OH
CH₃

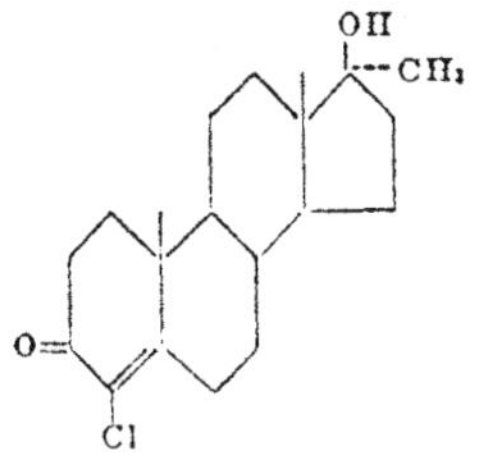

3 g. 4α,5 - epoxy - 17 - methyl-androstane-17β-ol-3-one, M.P. 80–82° C., [α]$_D$=+ 12° ±4°, dissolved in 90 cc. chloroform and 9 cc. ethanol, are treated with anhydrous HCl until the solution is saturated. After standing for 15 min., the solution is washed with water and dried by distilling off the solvent. The residue is chromatographically fractionated on 90 g. Florisil and the fractions eluted with ether are recrystallized from ether. 2.2 g. 4-chloro-17α-methyl-testosterone are obtained, M.P. 148–150° C., λ max. 256 mμ, ε=14,000.

5
EXAMPLE 13
4-chloro-Δ⁴-androstene-3,17-dione

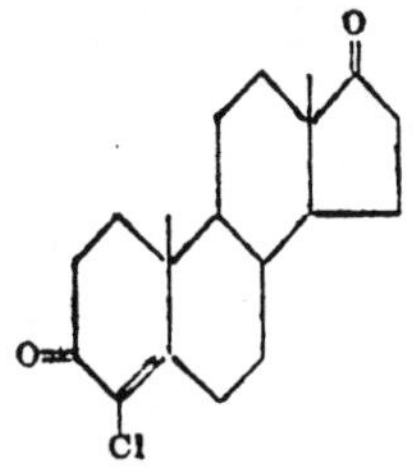

2 g. 4-chloro-testosterone dissolved in 20 cc. pyridine are treated, at room temperature, with a suspension of 1 g. CrO₃ in 20 cc. pyridine. After 24 hours the reaction mixture is diluted with benzene, washed with diluted hydrochloric acid, diluted NaOH and water and is finally dried.

The solvent is evaporated and the residue is crystallized from aqueous methanol. 0.7 g. 4-chloro-Δ⁴-androstene-3,17-dione are obtained, M.P. 175° C., [α]$_D^{22}$ =+218° ±4°.

EXAMPLE 14
4-chloro-adrenosterone

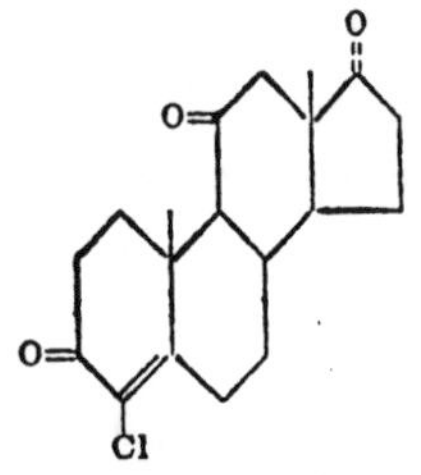

0.2 g. of a mixture of 4β,5-epoxy-etiocholane-3,11,17-trione and 4α,5-epoxy-androstane-3,11,17-trione (obtained by epoxidizing 0.2 g. adrenosterone with H₂O₂ and NaOH) are dissolved in 15 cc. chloroform and 1.5 cc. ethanol and for 30 minutes treated with anhydrous HCl. After recovery in the usual manner the residue is recrystallized from ether. 90 mg. 4-chloro-adrenosterone are obtained, M.P. 175–177° C., λ max. 255 mμ, ε=11.630.

EXAMPLE 15
4-chloro-Δ⁴-androstene-3β-17β-diol

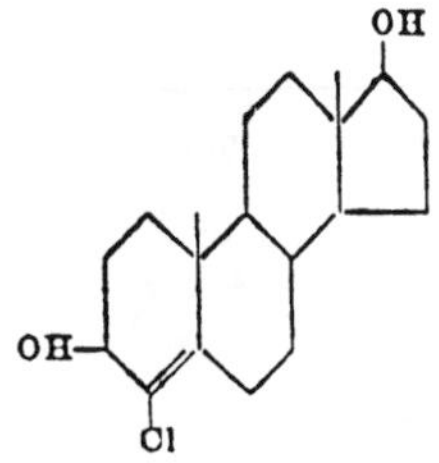

2 g. 4-chloro-testosterone, dissolved in 120 cc. pure methanol, are cooled to −5° C. and treated for 2 hours with 0.5 g. NaBH₄ at +5° C. After a short time, a voluminous crystalline precipitate appears in the solution. This precipitate is extracted with methylene chloride and washed with diluted hydrochloric acid and water. 1.7 g. residue, M.P. about 140° C., are obtained. After recrystallization from methanol, the melting point of the product is 252° C.; [α]$_D^{22}$=+114° ±4°. No ultraviolet absorption between 220 and 300 mμ.

By acetylation with a mixture of acetic anhydride and pyridine, the 4-chloro-Δ⁴-androstene-3β-17β-diol-diacetate is obtained which, when recrystallized from methanol, melts at 150° C., [α]$_D^{22}$=+56° ±4°.

6
EXAMPLE 16
4-fluoro-testosterone-acetate

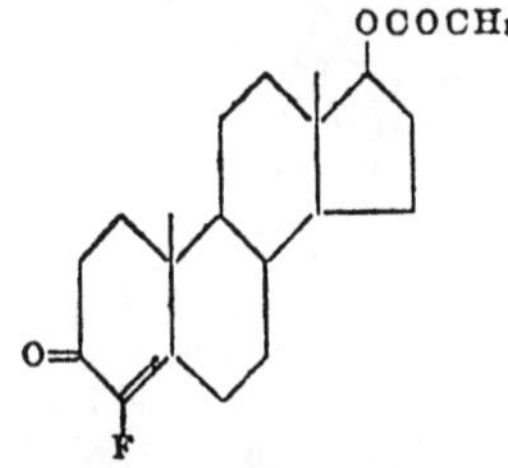

1 g. 4,5β-epoxy-etiocholane-17β-ol-3-one-acetate, dissolved in 30 cc. chloroform and 30 cc. absolute ethanol, are treated with anhydrous HF for 1 hour. A 2 N NaOH solution is then added until the solution is only slightly acid. The precipitate is separated, washed with H₂O, dried and the solvent contained therein is distilled off. Upon recrystallization from ether, 190 mg. 4-fluoro-testosterone-acetate are obtained; M.P. 178–180° C., λ max. 241 mμ, ε=11.670.

EXAMPLE 17
4-fluoro-testosterone-propionate

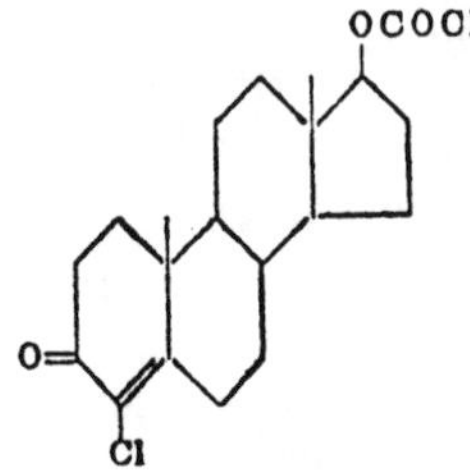

Proceeding as in Example 16, but starting with the 4β,5-epoxyetiocholane-17β-ol-3-one-propionate, 4-fluoro-testosterone-propionate is obtained by recrystallization from petroleum, M.P. 128–130° C., λ max. 243 mμ, ε=12.300.

EXAMPLE 18
4-chloro-testosterone-acetate-oxime

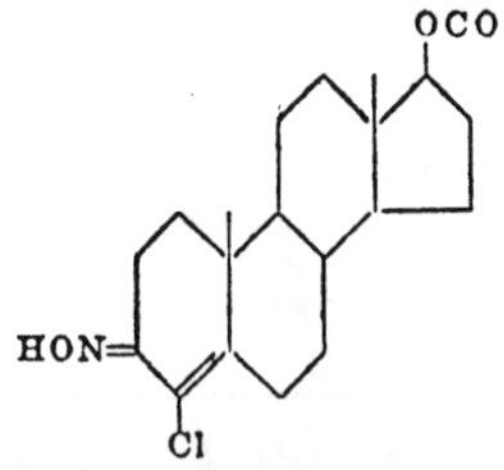

1 g. 4-chloro-testosterone-acetate are refluxed for 2 hours with 3 g. hydroxylamine hydrochloride, 250 cc. absolute ethanol, 1 cc. pyridine and 5 cc. acetic acid. The solution is then concentrated and the precipitate is recrystallized from ethyl alcohol. 0.7 g. of the oxime are obtained, M.P. 204–205° C. (decomposition).

EXAMPLE 19
4-chloro-testosterone-acetate-thiosemicarbazone

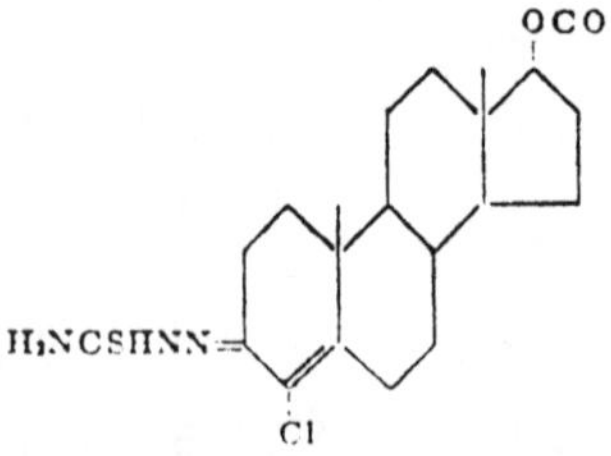

1 g. 4-chloro-testosterone-acetate are refluxed for 16 hours with 0.6 g. thiosemicarbazide and 90 cc. ethanol.

7

The solution is concentrated and the precipitate is filtered off and recrystallized from ethanol. 0.6 g. thiosemicarbazone are obtained, M.P. 197–204° C. (decomposition).

EXAMPLE 20

4-chloro-testosterone-trimethylacetate

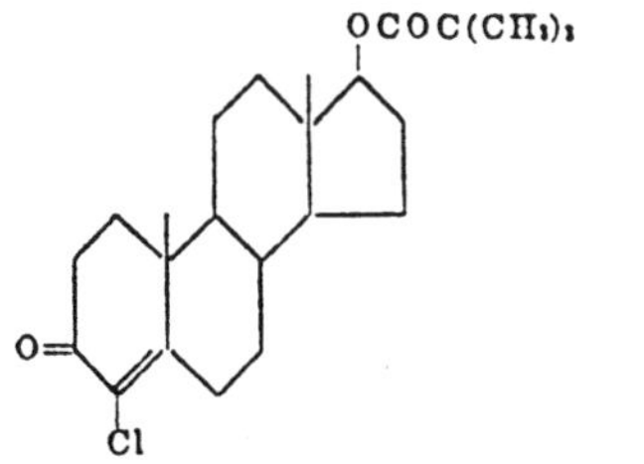

2 g. 4-chloro-testosterone are dissolved in 50 cc. anhydrous methylene chloride and 2 cc. pyridine, and are treated with 1.5 trimethylacetyl chloride dissolved in 50 cc. methylene chloride, first at —20° C. for 1 hour and then at room temperature for 15 hours. The solution is washed with ice-cold water, diluted hydrochloric acid, diluted NaOH solution and water until neutral. The solvent is then evaporated and the crystalline residue is taken up with methanol. 1.2 g. of the ester, M.P. 200–202° C., are obtained.

EXAMPLE 21

4-chloro-testosterone-phenylpropionate

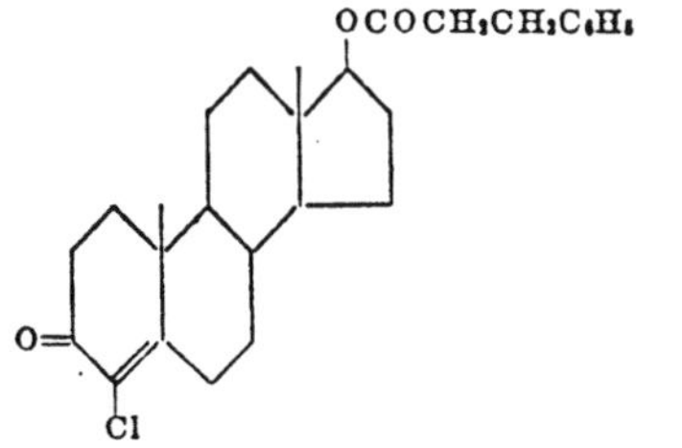

2 g. 4-chloro-testosterone are esterified with 2 g. phenylpropionyl acid chloride as described in Example 20. 1.7 g. of the phenylpropionate, M.P. 145° C., are obtained.

EXAMPLE 22

4-chloro-testosterone-enanthate

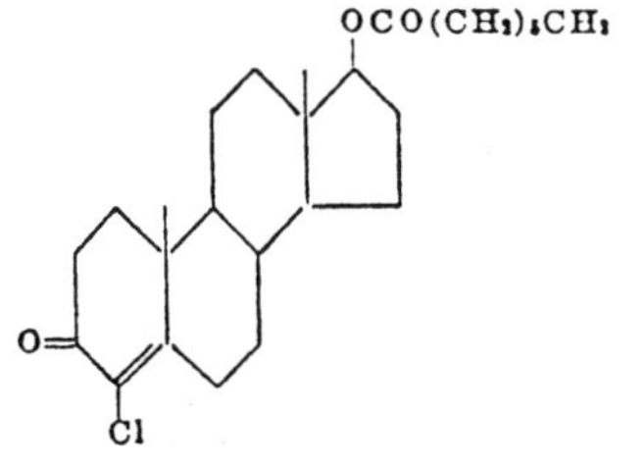

1 g. 4-chloro-testosterone dissolved in 5 cc. pyridine are heated for 5 hours to 90° C. with 2 g. enanthic anhydride. The solution is diluted with water, and extracted with benzene. The benzene extract is washed with diluted hydrochloric acid, diluted NaOH solution and water until neutral. The solvent is evaporated and the oily residue is purified chromatographically on silica gel. The fraction eluted with benzene-ether produces 1.1 g. of the enanthate, M.P. 59° C.

EXAMPLE 23

Pharmacological activity of the 4-chloro-testosterone-acetate

4-chloro-testosterone-acetate, injected into impuberal rats castrated according to the Hershberger et al. method

8

(Proc. Soc. Exp. Biol. and Med. 83, 175 (1953)), shows high anabolic activity coupled with poor androgen activity.

Thus, a daily dose of 500 γ of the afore-mentioned compound increases the weight of the "levator ani" muscle from 5 to 42 mg. while 500 γ testosterone propionate increase the weight of this muscle to 28.5 mg. Under similar condition 4-chloro-testosterone-acetate increases the prostate weight from 6.7 to 48 mg. while the testosterone-propionate increases this weight to 90 mg. The seminal bladders increase from 4.1 mg. to 36.5 mg. as a result of the action of the 4-chloro-testosterone-acetate and to 96 mg. as a result of the action of the testosterone-propionate.

Consequently, the ratio between the anabolic and the androgen activity, calculated according to Hershberger et al., is 0.88 for 4-chloro-testosterone-acetate and 0.28 for testosterone-propionate.

4-chloro-testosterone-acetate is still active in doses as little as 250 γ and 100 γ per day.

The toxicity of 4-chloro-testosterone-acetate is low: a dose of 1.5 g./kg. administered by one subcutaneous injection of the aqueous solution is readily tolerated by rats.

Doses of 50 mg./kg. a day for 10 days are also well tolerated by rats while a dose 10 times as great may be considered the maximum dose tolerated upon continuous administration.

EXAMPLE 24

Pharmacological activity of other derivatives

The 4 - chloro - testosterone - propionate increases the weight of the "levator ani" muscle from 5 to 27 mg.;

The 4-hydroxy-testosterone-17-acetate from 5 to 20.5 mg.;

The 4-chloro-testosterone from 5 to 19 mg.;

The 4-chloro-17α-methyl-testosterone from 9.8 to 24.5 mg.;

The 4-fluoro-testosterone-propionate from 7.9 to 20 mg.

The 4 - chloro - testosterone - propionate increases the weight of the prostate from 6.7 to 43 mg. (ratio between anabolic and androgen activity 0.61); the 4-hydroxy-testosterone-17-acetate from 6.7 to 32 mg. (ratio as above mentioned, 0.61);

The chloro-testosterone from 6.7 to 31.5 mg. (ratio, as above-mentioned, 0.57),

The 4-chloro-17α-methyl-testosterone from 4.2 to 48.7 mg. (ratio, as afore-mentioned, 0.35);

The 4-fluoro-testosterone-propionate from 5.2 to 39.2 mg. (ratio, as afore-mentioned, 0.35).

I claim:

4-chloro-adrenosterone.

References Cited in the file of this patent

UNITED STATES PATENTS

2,845,381   Tindall ----------------- July 29, 1958
2,933,510   Julian et al. ------------ Apr. 19, 1960

OTHER REFERENCES

Kochakian et al.: J. Biol. Chem. vol. 122 (1938), pages 433–438 (page 433 necessary).

Cavallini et al.: Boll., Soc. Ital. Biol. Sper., vol. 27 (1951), pages 629–30; abstracted in Chem. Abst., vol. 48 (1954), column 866 f.

Bremer: "Congress Handbook, XIVth Internat. Congr., Pure and Applied Chemistry" (Zurich, Switz.: Berichthaus Zurich, 1955) pages 162 and 163.

Kirk et al.: J. Chem. Soc. (March 1956), pages 627–629.

Kirk et al.: J. Chem. Soc. (May 1956), pages 1184–1186.

Camerino et al.: J. Am. Chem. Soc., vol. 78 (July 20, 1956), pages 3540 and 3541.

1

2,933,510

3-KETO-4-HALO-$\Delta^{4,5}$ STEROID

Percy L. Julian, Oak Park, and Helen C. Printy, Chicago, Ill., assignors to The Julian Laboratories, Inc., Franklin. Park, Ill., a corporation of Illinois

No Drawing. Application December 21, 1955
Serial No. 554,419

17 Claims. (Cl. 260—397.3)

This invention relates to new steroid compounds and the method of preparing them. More particularly, it relates to certain physiologically active 3-keto-4-halo-$\Delta^{4,5}$ compounds and the method of preparing them. The invention provides 4-halo derivatives of active androgenic, anabolic, progestational and corticoid hormones.

The components of this invention have hormone activity and, more specifically, variously have advantageous anabolic, androgenic, progestational and cortical activity with minimal side effects. It is well known that the active steroid hormones normally exhibit a plurality of physiological effects and that subsidiary effects limit the clinical use of the hormones. It has been found that the compounds of this invention have an advantageous ratio of desirable to undesirable activity.

In addition, this invention provides a novel and inexpensive method for producing halogen derivatives of important steroids.

The compounds of this invention are 3-keto-4-halo-$\Delta^{4,5}$ steroids derived from 4-estrenes, 4-androstenes or 4-pregnenes. Advantageously the compounds of this invention have the following structure:

FORMULA 1

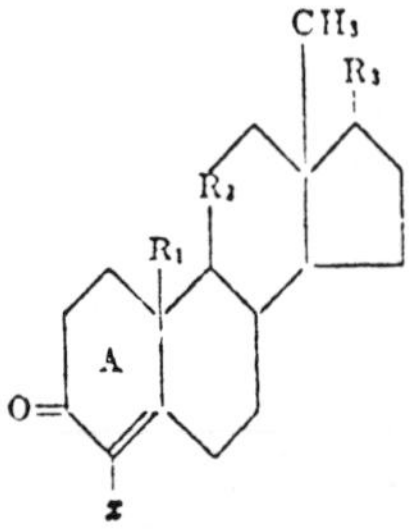

in which:

R_1 is hydrogen or methyl, R_2 is $C=O$, CH_2 or $OH-C-H$

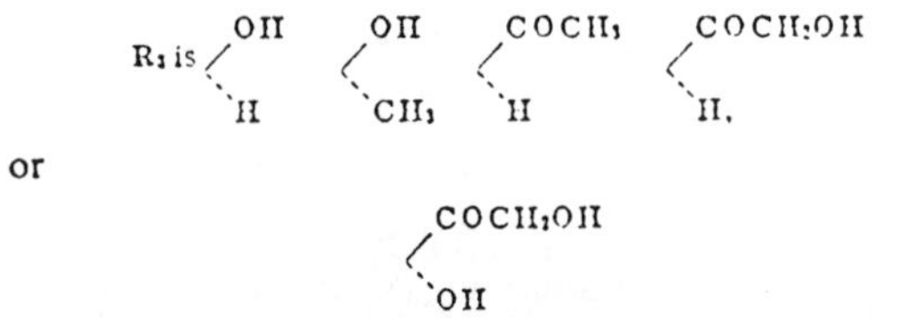

R_3 is

$$\begin{array}{cccc} OH & OH & COCH_3 & COCH_2OH \\ H & CH_3 & H & H. \end{array}$$

or

$$COCH_2OH \atop OH$$

and x is halogen, preferably chlorine or bromine.

Aliphatic, aryl and aralkyl esters of the above compounds such as, for example, acetate, benzoate, propionate, phenylacetate and half-succinate esters are also included within the scope of this invention. Such esters may be obtained by utilizing the desired ester of the epoxy starting material or by the preferred method of reacting the 4-halo derivative with the desired acyl halide or anhydride in a tertiary amine such as pyridine.

The method in accordance with this invention comprises treating a 3-keto-4,5-epoxysteroid with a hydrohalic

2

acid or the hydrohalic acid salt of a tertiary amine to obtain the corresponding 3-keto-4-halo-$\Delta^{4,5}$ steroid. The 3-keto-4,5-epoxysteroid has the following structural formula:

FORMULA 2

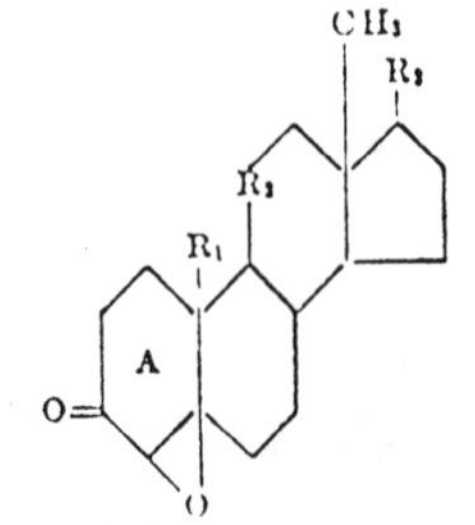

in which R_1, R_2 and R_3 are as given above. It will be understood that the above structure includes the $4\alpha,5\alpha$-epoxides and the $4\beta,5\beta$-epoxides, the bonds indicated by the solid lines in the 4 and 5 positions and connected to the oxygen not specifically indicating the isomeric form but rather being intended to include both the alpha and beta forms in the formula as given above and where used hereinafter, including in the claims. Since it is known to the art that epoxy compounds react with a hydrohalic acid to give the related halohydrins, it is surprising that the method in accordance with this invention produces halogen-containing olefins under comparable conditions.

More specifically, the desired 4-halo end product can be obtained by treating a solution or suspension of the 4,5-epoxysteroid in a halogenated or oxygenated water immiscible solvent such as carbon tetrachloride, methylene chloride, chloroform or ether with hydrohalic acid such as, for example, hydrogen chloride or hydrogen bromide either as a solution in a solvent miscible with the solvent for the epoxy compound or as a gas bubbled through the reaction mixture. The solvent for the hydrohalic acid may be, for example, a ketone solvent such as acetone or a lower aliphatic alcohol such as methanol, ethanol or propanol. Alternatively, the epoxy compound may be dissolved in a water miscible solvent such as, for example, dioxane, acetic acid, propionic acid, acetone or ethanol and reacted with an aqueous or acetic acid solution of the hydrohalic acid. In the case of both methods it is preferred to maintain the temperature of the reaction fluid from about 0° C. to about 35° C. for from about 10 minutes to several days.

Where the hydrohalic acid salt of a tertiary aromatic amine is employed, a solution of the 4,5 epoxysteroid in a suitable solvent is heated at from about 60° C. to about 100° C. and preferably at reflux temperature for from about 2 to about 20 hours with a solution of the amine hydrohalide in a solvent miscible with the solvent for the epoxy compound. Exemplary of suitable solvents for both the epoxy compound and the amine hydrohalide are ethanol, chloroform, methanol, carbon tetrachloride, dioxane and dimethylformamide. The hydrohalide of a tertiary amine may be, for example, pyridine hydrobromide, collidine hydrochloride or α-picoline hydrobromide.

The 3-keto-4-halo-$\Delta^{4,5}$ steroid of this invention is obtained from the reaction mixture by use of ordinary isolation procedures well known to the art. Thus, for example, the reaction mass may be diluted with water and the 3-keto-4-halo-$\Delta^{4,5}$ compound extracted with a suitable solvent such as, for example, methylene chloride, benzene, chloroform or ether. The solvent extract is washed with water, dried and concentrated to a crystalline mass. If desired, the end product can be recrystallized from an alcohol such as, for example, ethanol or from a mixture of solvents, such as methylene chloride-pentane.

The epoxy starting materials of Formula 2 are readily

3

prepared by treating a 3-keto-Δ⁴-steroid compound of the 4-estrene, 4-androstene, or 4-pregnene series in a water miscible solvent with an alkaline hydrogen peroxide aqueous solution. This reaction is shown in the following scheme, in which R_1, R_2 and R_3 are as given above:

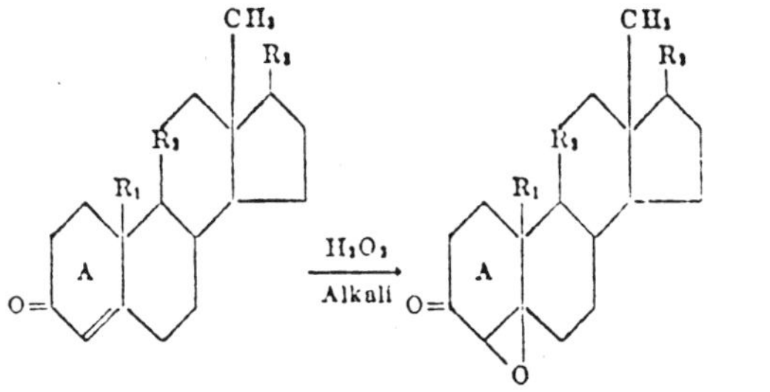

The alkali used may be any alkali metal hydroxide or carbonate, such as, for example, sodium hydroxide, potassium hydroxide, sodium carbonate or potassium carbonate.

The water miscible solvent may be, for example, a lower aliphatic alcohol such as methanol or ethanol, a ketone solvent such as acetone and methyl ethyl ketone or dioxane. By way of further example solvent mixtures such as benzene or a chlorinated methane such as chloroform, carbon tetrachloride or methylene chloride in admixture with a major proportion of a lower aliphatic alcohol such as methanol or ethanol are satisfactory.

The reaction will be carried out at a low temperature, preferably from about −20° C. to about 30° C. and advantageously from about −20° C. to +10° C.

The reaction is preferably carried out until the major proportion of the starting material has been expoxidized. Advantageously the course of the reaction will be checked spectrophotometrically and the reaction mixture quenched preferably with cold water immediately after the disappearance of unsaturation in ring A, which is indicated by the disappearance of the characteristic α,β-unsaturated ketone absorption in the 238 mμ–242 mμ region. The quenching at this state of the reaction insures the avoidance of further undesired oxidation to acidic products. The desired 4,5-epoxy compounds are obtained by filtration or by solvent extraction.

The epoxy starting materials of Formula 2 and the method of their preparation are fully set forth in our copending patent application, Serial No. 486,014, filed February 3, 1955, the disclosure of which is incorporated herewith. Reference may be made to said application, Serial No. 486,014, for specific examples of said epoxy starting materials as well as for specific detail as to the method of their preparation.

The compounds of this invention and the method of their preparation will be more specifically illustrated by the following examples. Our copending patent application, Serial No. 486,014, specifically illustrates the preparation of the starting material used in each of the following examples.

Example I.—4-bromotestosterone

A solution of 0.5 g. of 4,5-epoxytestosterone, M.P. 138–140° C., was dissolved in 5 ml. of glacial acetic acid and cooled to 15° C. One milliliter of 30% hydrogen bromide in acetic acid was added and the reaction kept at 10–15° C. for 30 minutes. The solution was poured with stirring into 200 ml. of water, and the precipitated solid was collected by filtration. The product, 4-bromotestosterone, M.P. 152–154° C. had an absorption maximum at 261 mμ=11,600, and weighed 590 mg.

Example II.—4-bromotestosterone

When 0.5 g. of the isomeric 4,5-epoxytestosterone, M.P. 152–155° C., was treated in the manner described in Example I, 0.58 g. of the identical 4-bromo-testosterone, M.P. 155–157° C., E_{261}=11,800 was obtained. This

4

gave no depression when melted with the 4-bromotestosterone described in Example I.

Example III.—4-chlorotestosterone

To a solution of 1.0 g. of 4,5-epoxytestosterone (stereoisomeric mixture) in 10 ml. of glacial acetic acid was added 2 ml. of an 8% hydrogen chloride in acetic acid solution. The reaction was kept for 12 hours at room temperature, then diluted cautiously with water to induce crystallization. The precipitate was removed by filtration and dried yielding 1.04 g. of 4-chlorotestosterone, M.P. 210–218° C. Recrystallization from methylene chloride-pentane afforded glistening prisms, M.P. 215–222° C., E_{253}=11,600.

Example IV.—4-bromoprogesterone

One gram of 4,5-epoxyprogesterone (stereoisomeric mixture) was dissolved in 10 ml. of glacial acetic acid and the solution cooled to 15° C. To the cooled solution, 1 ml. of a 30% hydrogen bromide in acetic acid solution was added, and the reaction kept at 15° C. for 20 minutes. The solution was poured into 200 ml. of water and the precipitated product collected by filtration. The product, 1.18 g. of 4-bromoprogesterone, was crystallized from methylene chloride-pentane to give glistening prisms, M.P. 170–172° C. dec., E_{262}=9,000.

Example V.—4-bromoprogesterone

One gram of 4,5-epoxyprogesterone (stereoisomeric mixture) was dissolved in 10 ml. of purified dioxane and 2 ml. of 48% hydrobromic acid were added. The reaction was kept at 25° C. for 36 hours with occasional swirling, then was diluted with 75 ml. of water. The precipitated solid was filtered and washed well with water. Crystallization from methylene chloride-ether afforded 0.7 g. of 4-bromoprogesterone, M.P. 178–180° C., E_{261}=10,000, which gave no depression on melting with that of Example IV.

Example VI.—4-chloroprogesterone

To one gram of 4,5-epoxyprogesterone (stereoisomeric mixture) dissolved in 10 ml. of glacial acetic acid, 1 ml. of a 25% solution of hydrogen chloride in acetic acid was added. The reaction mixture was kept at room temperature for 15 hours, during which time crystals of 4-chloroprogesterone came out. The crystals, 410 mg. were collected by filtration. They melted at 205–213° C., and had an absorption maximum at 255 mμ=13,000. A second crop of material, 540 mg. melting at 209–215° C., E_{255}=11,000 was obtained from the mother liquor.

Example VII.—4-bromodesoxycorticosterone

Three grams of 4,5-epoxydesoxycorticosterone (stereoisomeric mixture) and 5 g. of pyridine hydrobromide were refluxed for 2 hours in 50 ml. of anhydrous ethanol. The solution was then concentrated to remove the solvent, diluted with water and extracted with methylene chloride. The methylene chloride extract was washed with water, dried and concentrated to a crystalline mass. Upon recrystallization from ethanol, 4-bromodesoxycorticosterone, M.P. 173–175° C., E_{261} mμ=,200.

Example VIII.—4-bromocortisone

A solution of 1.0 g. of cortisone oxide (stereoisomeric mixture) in 10 ml. of methylene chloride was cooled to 5° C., and 2 ml. of 30% hydrogen bromide in acetic acid was added. The reaction was held at 5–10° C. for 30 minutes; then was poured into 100 ml. of water and extracted with additional methylene chloride. The methylene chloride extract was washed free of acid and dried. Removal of solvent afforded 4-bromocortisone as a pale yellow fluff, E_{263}=8,300.

Example IX.—4-bromohydrocortisone

A solution of 1 g. of 4,5-epoxyhydrocortisone (stereo-

5

isomeric mixture) in 10 ml. of chloroform was cooled to 5° C. and treated for 30 minutes at 5–10° C. with 2 ml. of 30% hydrogen bromide in acetic acid. Upon working up the reaction, 4-bromohydrocortisone was obtained as a yellow fluff, E_{263} mμ=9,000.

Example X.—4-bromo-19-nortestosterone

One gram of 4,5-epoxy-19-nortestosterone was dissolved in 10 ml. of glacial acetic acid and the solution cooled to 15° C. One ml. of a 30% hydrogen bromide in acetic acid solution was added and the solution kept at 15° C. for one hour. Dilution with water afforded a precipitate which was extracted with benzene, washed with water and dried. The benzene extract upon concentration yielded 100 mg. of 4-bromo-19-nortestosterone, M.P. 125–128° C., dec., E_{262}=8,000.

Example XI.—4-bromo-19-nortestosterone benzoate

A solution of 1.5 g. of 4,5-epoxy-19-nortestosterone benzoate (stereoisomeric mixture) in 20 ml. of acetic acid was cooled in an ice bath and treated with 2 ml. of 27% hydrogen bromide in acetic acid for 20 minutes. The reaction was diluted with water and the bromo compound extracted with methylene chloride. The methylene chloride extract was washed with water, sodium bicarbonate solution and water. The solution was concentrated in vacuo and the product crystallized from ether. The yield of product, M.P. 118–122° C. dec., E_{262}mμ=13,000 was 1.35 g.

Example XII.—4-bromo-19-nortestosterone benzoate

One gram of crude 4,5-epoxy-19-nortestosterone benzoate (stereoisomeric mixture) was dissolved in 15 ml. of anhydrous ether, cooled, and stirred for 20 minutes with 2 ml. of 27% hydrogen bromide in acetic acid. Upon working up as described in the previous example, 420 mg. of 4-bromo-19-nortestosterone benzoate, M.P. 118–120° C. dec., E_{262}mμ=12,000 was obtained.

Example XIII.—4-bromo-17α-methyltestosterone

A solution of 4 g. of 4,5-epoxy-17α-methyltestosterone (stereoisomeric mixture) in 50 ml. of glacial acetic acid was cooled in an ice bath. A saturated solution of hydrogen chloride in glacial acetic acid was added. The mixture was allowed to come to room temperature and to stand for 24 hours with occasional swirling. The desired 4-bromo-17α-methyltestosterone was isolated by quenching in water, filtering and washing well with water. A characteristic unsaturated ketone absorption on the crude product was observed spectrophotometrically.

Example XIV.—4-chlorotestosterone-17-acetate

A solution of 1.2 g. of 4,5-epoxytestosterone-17-acetate, M.P. 132–135° C., in 40 ml. of dimethylformamide was mixed with a solution of one equivalent of collidine hydrochloride in 5 ml. of dimethylformamide. The reaction mixture was heated at 80 to 90° C. for ten hours. After quenching in water, extracting with chloroform and washing with water and dilute acid, the desired crude compound as indicated by ultraviolet absorption was obtained.

Example XV

One gram of 4-bromotestosterone in 4 ml. of pyridine was reacted with 0.3 g. of succinic anhydride at room temperature for two days. The reaction mixture was quenched carefully with water to separate the desired 17-succinate half ester after washing well with water and air drying. A satisfactory E_1' was noted on the ultraviolet spectrum.

Example XVI.—4-bromotestosterone

A solution of 0.5 g. of 4,5-epoxytestosterone (stereoisomeric mixture) in dry ether was saturated with hydrogen bromide gas several times over a period of twelve hours at room temperature. The excess acid was removed from

6

the reaction mixture by washing with carbonate solution. The ether was dried and evaporated in vacuo, yielding 500 mg. of crude 4-bromotestosterone.

It is not desired to be limited except as set forth in the following claims.

This application is a continuation-in-part of our application, Serial No. 486,014, filed February 3, 1955, now abandoned.

What is claimed is:

1. A compound having the following basic structural formula:

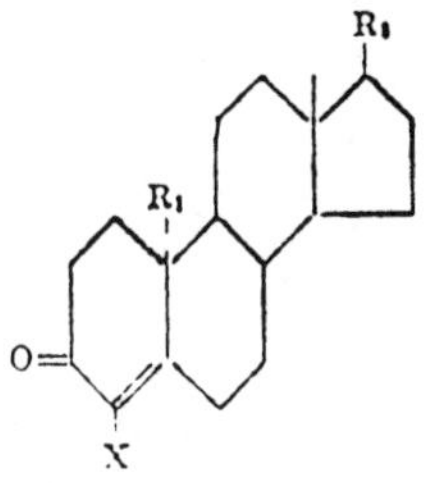

wherein X is a member selected from the group consisting of bromo and chloro; R_1 is a member selected from the group consisting of hydrogen and methyl; when R_1 is hydrogen R_3 is a member selected from the group consisting of

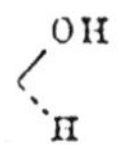

and

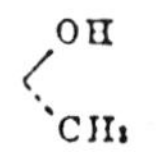

and when R_1 is methyl R_3 is a member selected from the group consisting of

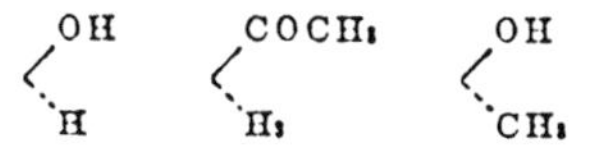

and

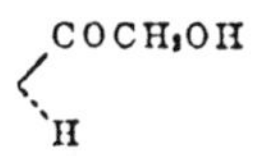

2. 4-chloroprogesterone.
3. A compound having the formula

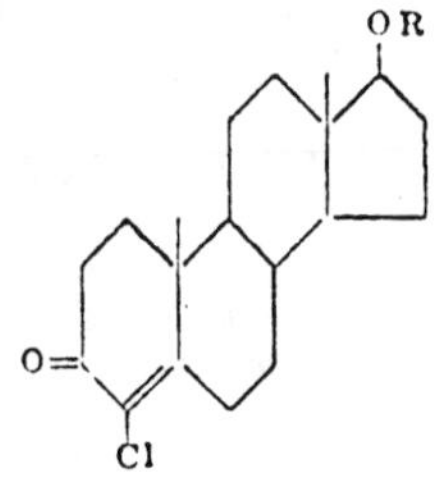

wherein R is selected from the group consisting of hydrogen and acyl.

4. 4-chlorotestosterone-17-acetate.
5. 4-chlorotestosterone.
6. 4-bromotestosterone.
7. A compound having the formula

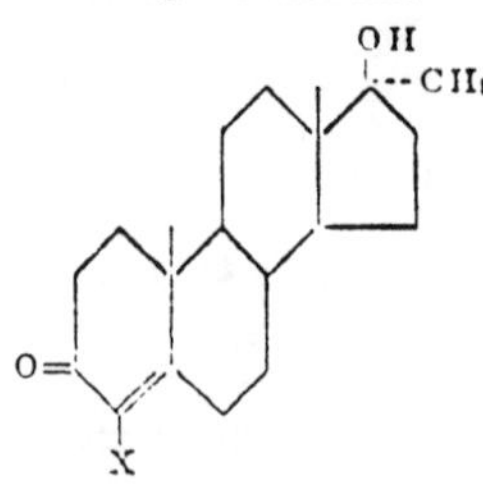

wherein X is a member selected from the group consisting of bromo and chloro.

7

8. 4-bromo-17α-methyltestosterone.
9. A compound having the formula

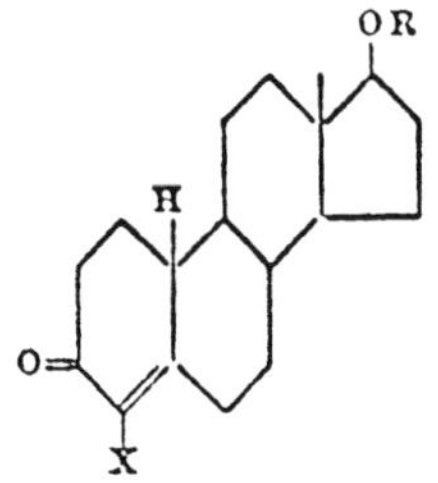

wherein X is a member selected from the group consisting of bromo and chloro and R is selected from the group consisting of hydrogen and acyl.

10. 4-bromo-19-nortestosterone.
11. 4-bromo-19-nortestosterone benzoate.
12. 4-bromocortisone.
13. 4-bromohydrocortisone.
14. 4-bromodesoxycorticosterone.
15. The process of preparing a steroid having the following structural formula:

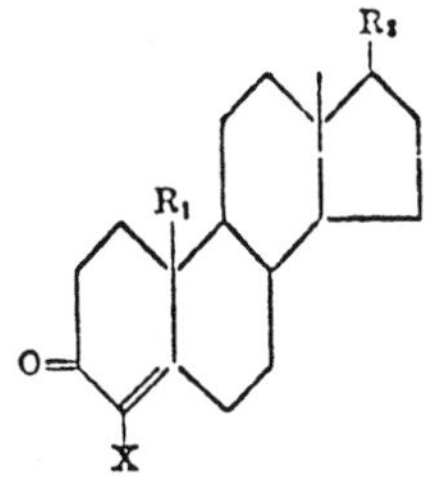

wherein X is a member selected from the group consisting of bromo and chloro; R_1 is a member selected from the group consisting of hydrogen and methyl; when R_1 is hydrogen R_3 is a member selected from the group consisting of

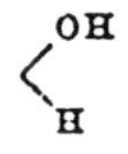

and

8

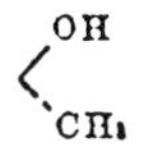

and when R_1 is methyl R_3 is a member selected from the group consisting of

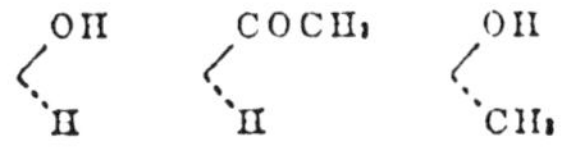

and

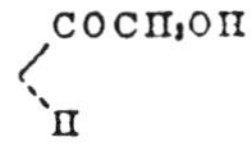

which comprises reacting a 3-keto-4,5-epoxy steroid having the following formula:

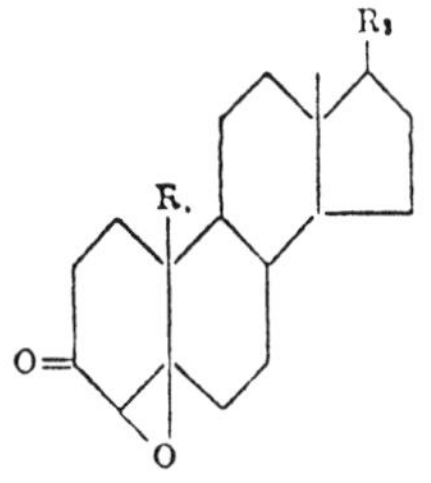

wherein R_1 and R_3 are as defined above, with a hydrohalic acid reagent selected from the group consisting of hydrobromic acid, hydrochloric acid, the hydrochloride of a tertiary aromatic amine and the hydrobromide of a tertiary aromatic amine.

16. The process of claim 15 in which the epoxy compound and the hydrohalic acid reagent are in mutually miscible solvents.

17. The process of claim 16 in which the reaction is carried out at a temperature in the range of from about 0° C. to about 35° C.

References Cited in the file of this patent

UNITED STATES PATENTS

2,280,828	Inhoffen	Apr. 28, 1942
2,681,353	Archer	June 15, 1954
2,727,912	Colton	Dec. 20, 1955

OTHER REFERENCES

Bremer: "Congress Handbook, XIVth Internat. Congr. Pure and Applied Chemistry," (Zurich, Switz.: Berichthaus Zurich, July 21, 1955), pages 162 and 163.

CHAPTER THREE

1

2

2,908,693

PROCESS FOR THE PRODUCTION OF 2-METHYL-DIHYDROTESTOSTERONES

Howard J. Ringold and George Rosenkranz, Mexico City, Mexico, assignors to Syntex S.A., Mexico City, Mexico, a corporation of Mexico

No Drawing. Application December 16, 1957
Serial No. 702,760

Claims priority, application Mexico December 17, 1956

4 Claims. (Cl. 260—397.4)

The present invention relates to a novel process for the production of cyclopentanophenanthrene derivatives.

More particularly the present invention relates to a process for the production of 2-methyl dihydrotestosterone derivatives and esters thereof as well as 2-methyl dihydrotestosterone derivatives having a C–17 lower alkyl group. The products of the process of the present invention have a useful high anabolic-androgenic ratio and are especially valuable for treatment of those ailments where an anabolic or antiestrogenic effect together with a lesser androgenic effect is desired.

In our U.S. application Serial No. 636,860, filed January 29, 1957, there is disclosed a process for the production of 2-methyl androstane compounds having a C–17 lower alkyl group involving preparing the corresponding 2-hydroxymethylene derivatives, transformation of these derivatives into 2-methyl-2'-formyl compounds and removal of carbon monoxide to prepare the 2-methyl product.

In accordance with the present invention it has been discovered that 2-methyl androstane compounds or dihydrotestosterone derivatives may be prepared by a simple one step process involving catalytic hydrogenation of the corresponding 2-hydroxymethylene starting material. In its more specific aspects the process therefore involves treating dihydrotestosterone or a 17-lower alkyl dihydrotestosterone as with ethyl formate and sodium hydride to form the corresponding 2-hydroxymethylene derivative and catalytically hydrogenating the 2-hydroxymethylene derivative. Further it has been discovered that catalytic hydrogenation of a 2-acyloxymethylene derivative also produces the desired 2-methyl compounds.

The process of the present invention may therefore be illustrated by the following equation:

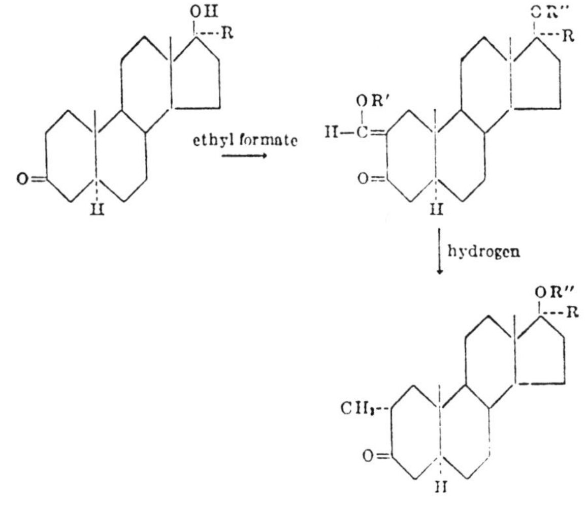

In the above equation R represents hydrogen or R represents a lower alkyl group of less than 7 carbon

atoms such as methyl, ethyl or propyl. R' represents an acyl group of a hydrocarbon carboxylic acid of 2 to 12 carbon atoms as conventional in esterified steroid alcohols such as acetoxy, propionoxy, benzoyloxy etc. or R' represents hydrogen. R'' represents hydrogen when R is a lower alkyl group and is either hydrogen or an acyl group similar to R' when R is hydrogen.

In practicing the process as outlined above, dihydrotestosterone, or a 17-lower alkyl dihydrotestosterone, such as 17-methyl dihydrotestosterone or 17-ethyl dihydrotestosterone (which may be prepared by treatment of the known testosterone, 17-methyl testosterone or 17-ethyl testosterone with an alkali metal in liquid ammonia for example) are suspended in an inert organic solvent such as benzene and then mixed with ethyl formate and sodium hydride. The mixture is then stirred for a period of time of the order of 5 hours at room temperature and under nitrogen atmosphere. The suspension is then filtered and the mixture of the sodium salt of the desired hydroxymethylene compound is then treated with acid such as hydrochloric acid to precipitate the hydroxymethylene compound.

The hydroxymethylene compound thus prepared may then be conventionally esterified to form a diester of a conventional type as previously set forth when the 17-hydroxy group of the starting compound is secondary or a monester if the 17-hydroxy group is tertiary (as in 17-lower alkyl derivatives). The hydroxymethylene compound or the ester thereof in organic solvent solution is then hydrogenated in the presence of a hydrogenation catalyst preferably at room temperature and atmospheric pressure until absorption of hydrogen ceased.

Suitable organic solvents for the hydrogenation step are for example lower aliphatic alcohols such as methanol, ethyl acetate, dioxane or acetic acid. Preferable hydrogenation catalysts are palladium or platinum catalysts such as palladium on charcoal or palladium on barium sulfate or platinum oxide. This hydrogenation step produces the corresponding 2-methyl compound from either the ester of or the free hydroxymethylene compound and leaves any 17-ester group intact. The resultant crude 2-methyl products were then purified by chromatography. Where the free hydroxymethylene derivatives were being treated or when a free 2α-methyl product was desired it was found desirable to treat the crude hydrogenation product with alkali prior to chromatography.

The following specific examples serve to illustrate but are not intended to limit the present invention.

Example I

A suspension of 10 g. of dihydrotestosterone in 500 cc. of anhydrous benzene free of thiophene was mixed with 10 cc. of ethyl formate and 3 g. of sodium hydride and the mixture was stirred for 5 hours under an atmosphere of nitrogen and at a temperature of approximately 25° C. The resulting suspension was filtered, the resulting mixture of the sodium salt of the hydroxymethylene compound and the excess of sodium hydride was washed with benzene and dried. This mixture was slowly added to a vigorously stirred solution of 20 cc. of concentrated hydrochloric acid in 500 cc. of water, and the stirring was continued for 30 minutes at the end of which the precipitate was collected and well washed with distilled water. After drying in vacuo, there was obtained 9.7 g. of 2-hydroxymethylene-dihydrotestosterone.

7 g. of 2-hydroxymethylene-dihydrotestosterone was dissolved in 300 cc. of methanol and mixed with 2.5% of a 10% palladium on charcoal catalyst. The mixture was hydrogenated at approximately 25° C. at atmospheric pressure until the absorption of hydrogen ceased. The catalyst was removed by filtration, 1 g. of potassium hydroxide in 5 cc. of water was added to the solution which

3

was then kept for 1 hour at room temperature. 2 cc. of acetic acid was added, the solvent was completely removed under reduced pressure, water was added to the residue and the product was extracted with methylene dichloride. The extract was washed with water, dried over anhydrous sodium sulfate and evaporated to dryness under vacuum. The residue was dissolved in benzene and transferred to a chromatographic column with 125 g. of alkaline alumina. The column was washed with successive fractions of 100 cc. of benzene, whereupon the desired product was eluted from fractions 2 to 6. After evaporating the solvent, the product was crystallized from a mixture acetone-hexane to yield 3.3 g. of pure 2α-methyl-dihydrotestosterone.

Example II

2 g. of 2-hydroxymethylene-dihydrotestosterone, obtained in accordance with Example I, dissolved in 80 cc. of acetic acid was hydrogenated with 1.0 g. of 10% palladium on charcoal catalyst under the conditions described in the previous example. After removing the catalyst by filtration, the solvent was evaporated to dryness under reduced pressure and the residue was mixed with 100 cc. of methanol and 1 g. of potassium hydroxide. The solution was refluxed for 30 minutes and then diluted with water and extracted with methylene dichloride. The extract was washed with water to neutral, dried over anhydrous sodium sulfate and evaporated to dryness under vacuum. The residue was dissolved in benzene and chromatographed under the conditions described in Example I. There was thus obtained 2α-methyl-dihydrotestosterone.

Example III

A mixture of 1 g. of 2-hydroxymethylene-dihydrotestosterone, obtained in accordance with the method described in Example I, 10 cc. of pyridine and 2 cc. of acetic anhydride was allowed to react at room temperature for 16 hours and then poured into water. The product was extracted with methylene dichloride and washed consecutively with dilute hydrochloric acid, sodium bicarbonate solution and water, dried and evaporated to dryness under reduced pressure. There was thus obtained the diacetate of 2-hydroxymethylene-dihydrotestosterone.

This diacetate was hydrogenated and then worked up by the methods described in the previous examples, thus producing 2α-methyl-dihydrotestosterone, identical to the one obtained in accordance with such examples.

Example IV

Following the method described in the previous examples, 17α-methyl-dihydrotestosterone was converted into 2α,17α-dimethyl-dihydrotestosterone.

4

Example V

Following the method described in Examples I, II, and III, 17α-ethyl-dihydrotestosterone was converted into 2α-methyl-17α-ethyl-dihydrotestosterone.

Example VI

A mixture of 1 g. of 2-hydroxymethylene-dihydrotestosterone, obtained in accordance with Example I, 10 cc. of pyridine and 2 cc. of propionic anhydride was allowed to react at room temperature for 16 hours and then poured into water. The resulting suspension was heated for 1 hour on the steam bath to hydrolyze the excess of propionic anhydride, cooled and extracted with methylene dichloride. The extract was consecutively washed with dilute hydrochloric acid, sodium bicarbonate solution and water, dried over anhydrous sodium sulfate and evaporated to dryness under vacuum. There was thus obtained the dipropionate of 2-hydroxymethylene-dihydrotestosterone which was treated with hydrogen, in methanol solution, under the conditions described in Example I. When the uptake of hydrogen ceased, the catalyst was filtered and the solution was evaporated to dryness under vacuum. The residue was dissolved in a mixture benzene-hexane, transferred to a chromatographic column with neutral alumina and the product was eluted with mixtures benzene-hexane, gradually increasing the proportion of benzene in the mixture. Crystallization of the eluates from acetone-hexane yielded the propionate of 2α-methyl-dihydrotestosterone.

We claim:

1. A process for the production of compounds selected from the class consisting of 2α-methyl dihydrotestosterone, 17-esters thereof of hydrocarbon carboxylic acids of 2 to 12 carbon atoms and 2α-methyl 17α-lower alkyl dihydrotestosterone comprising hydrogenating the corresponding 2-hydroxymethylene derivatives in the presence of a hydrogenation catalyst selected from the group consisting of palladium and platinum catalyst.

2. The process of claim 1 wherein the starting material is a diester of 2-hydroxymethylene dihydrotestosterone and the product is a 17-ester of 2α-methyl dihydrotestosterone.

3. The process of claim 1 wherein the starting material is 2-hydroxymethylene dihydrotestosterone and the product is 2α-methyl dihydrotestosterone.

4. The process of claim 1 wherein the starting material is a 17α-lower alkyl 2-hydroxymethylene dihydrotestosterone and the product is a 17α-lower alkyl 2α-methyl dihydrotestosterone.

References Cited in the file of this patent

Hogg: J. A. C. S., December 5, 1955, pages 6401–6402.

1

2,908,694

7-SUBSTITUTED THIO-4-ANDROSTENES

Robert E. Schaub, Paramus, and Martin J. Weiss, Oradell, N.J., assignors to American Cyanamid Company, New York, N.Y., a corporation of Maine

No Drawing. Application April 6, 1959
Serial No. 804,106

6 Claims. (Cl. 260—397.4)

This invention relates to new steroids of the androstene series. More particularly, it relates to 7-alkylthio-4-androstenes and 7-alkenylthio-4-androstenes and methods of preparing the same.

The use of steroids for their glucocorticoid activity in the treatment of collagen diseases is well known. Their use, however, as non- or low-virilizing anabolic agents is less well known. We have now found that the steroids described hereinafter possess these properties and are therefore useful as anabolic agents.

The compounds of the present invention may be illustrated by the general formula:

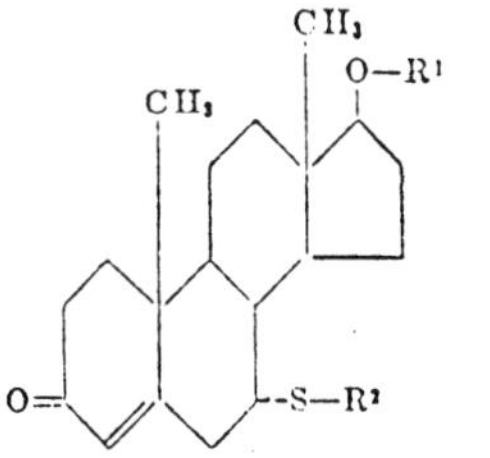

in which R^1 is a member of the group consisting of hydrogen, lower alkanoyl, cycloalkyl lower alkanoyl and aroyl radicals and R^2 is a member of the group consisting of lower alkyl and lower alkenyl radicals.

The compounds of the present invention are crystalline solids having relatively high melting points. They are relatively insoluble in water and somewhat soluble in the usual organic solvents. They are crystallizable from mixtures of ketones and hydrocarbon solvents.

The present compounds are prepared by reacting a 17β-lower alkanoyl-4,6-androstadiene-3-one with a lower alkyl or lower alkenyl mercaptan. The reaction is preferably carried out in a solvent such as glacial acetic acid in the presence of a mineral acid catalyst. The reaction takes place at a temperature between 0 and 50° C. and is usually complete in a matter of 2 or 3 hours to several days. The product is recovered by evaporation of the solvent used in the reaction followed by taking up the residue in a further organic solvent. Following removal of the latter solvent, the desired product is further purified by crystallization.

The process of this invention proceeds under steric influences and stereoisomers are formed, however, one is obtained in predominate amount. The isomer obtained in predominant amount has in each case been characterized herein as possessing the alpha configuration of the 7 lower alkylthio or lower alkenylthio group. This configuration has been designated in order to provide a more complete exposition of the present invention, and in order that the specification shall constitute a more useful contribution to the art. However, the designated configuration of the 7-lower alkylthio or lower alkenylthio group is based upon an analysis of molecular rotation data presently appearing in the chemical literature, and is therefore not to be interpreted except in relation to the state of the art presently known to organic chemists. It will be apparent that no part of the specification will be materially effective if it should later be established that the configuration is the opposite of that deducible from data presently available to workers in the field.

The compounds of the present invention can be used in the form of tablets, pills, powders, and so forth, which may also contain starch, excipients, and other ingredients necessary in the compounding of such dosage forms. They may be used singly or in combination with other steroids.

In the present application the term lower alkyl radical is intended to cover saturated hydrocarbon radicals having 1 to 6 carbon atoms. The term lower alkanoyl radical is intended to cover the acyl radicals obtained from alkanoic acids having 1 to 14 carbon atoms and the term cycloalkyl lower alkanoyl radical is intended to cover acyl radicals obtained from cycloalkyl substituted alkanoic acids having 7 to 11 carbon atoms with 5 or 6 carbon atoms in the cycloalkyl group.

The following examples illustrate in detail the preparation of the 7-alkylthio- and 7-alkenylthioandrostenes of the present invention.

EXAMPLE 1

Preparation of 17β-acetoxy-7α-methylthio-4-androsten-3-one

A solution of 0.6 g. of 17β-acetoxy-4,6-androstadien-3-one [C. Djerassi et al., J. Am. Chem. Soc., 72, 4538 (1950)], 1 ml. of concentrated hydrochloric acid and 5 ml. of methylmercaptan in 25 ml. of glacial acetic acid is allowed to stand at 5–8° C. for 48 hours. The reaction mixture is evaporated to dryness under reduced pressure and the concentrate is diluted with methylene chloride and washed with excess saturated sodium bicarbonate solution, and then with water. The organic phase is dried with anhydrous magnesium sulfate and evaporated to dryness under reduced pressure to give a glass. Crystallization from acetone-petroleum ether gives 17β-acetoxy - 7α - methylthio-4-androsten-3-one. Recrystallization from acetone-petroleum ether affords white crystals

$$\lambda_{max}^{MeOH} \ 240 \ m\mu$$

($\epsilon = 15,500$); ν 1730, 1675, 1620, 1240 cm.$^{-1}$.

EXAMPLE 2

Preparation of 17β-acetoxy - 7α - ethylthio-4-androsten-3-one

A solution of 0.865 g. of 17β-acetoxy-4,6-androstien-3-one, 2 ml. of concentrated hydrochloric acid and 10 ml. of ethylmercaptan in 75 ml. of glacial acetic acid is allowed to stand at 5–8° C. for 72 hours. The reaction mixture is evaporated to dryness under reduced pressure and the concentrate is diluted with methylene chloride and washed with excess saturated sodium bicarbonate solution, and then with water. The organic phase is dried with anhydrous magnesium sulfate and evaporated to dryness under reduced pressure to give a glass. Crystallization from acetone-petroleum ether gives 17β-acetoxy - 7α - ethylthio-4-androsten-3-one. Recrystallization from acetone-petroleum ether gives white crystals;

$$\lambda_{max}^{MeOH} \ 240 \ m\mu$$

($\epsilon = 15,800$); ν 1730, 1675, 1620, 1240 cm.$^{-1}$.

EXAMPLE 3

Preparation of 17β-acetoxy-7α-n-propylthio-4-androsten-3-one

A solution of 1.3 g. of 17β-acetoxy-4,6-androstadien-3-one, 2 ml. of concentrated hydrochloric acid and 10 ml. of n-propylmercaptan in 75 ml. of glacial acetic acid is treated according to the procedure described for the preparation of 17β-acetoxy-7α-methylthio-4-androsten-3-one

3

(Example 1) to give 17β-acetoxy-7α-n-propylthio-4-androsten-3-one as white crystals;

$$\lambda_{max}^{MeOH}\ 240\ m\mu$$

(ε15,100); ν1730, 1675, 1622, 1240 cm.⁻¹.

EXAMPLE 4

Preparation of 17β-acetoxy-7α-allylthio-4-androsten-3-one

A solution of 1 g. of 17β-acetoxy-4,6-androstadien-3-one, 2 ml. of concentrated hydrochloric acid and 10 ml. of allylmercaptin in 75 ml. of glacial acetic acid is treated according to the procedure described in Example 1 to give 17β-acetoxy-7α-allylthio-4-androsten-3-one;

$$\lambda_{max}^{MeOH}\ 241\ m\mu$$

(ε15,500); ν1730, 1675, 1619, 1241 cm.⁻¹.

EXAMPLE 5

Preparation of 17β-acetoxy-7α-n-propylthio-4-androsten-3-one

A solution of 0.6 g. of 17β-acetoxy-4,6-androstadien-one, 1 ml. of concentrated hydrochloric acid and 5 ml. of isopropylmercaptin in 25 ml. of glacial acetic acid is treated according to the procedure described in Example 1 to give 17β-acetoxy-7α-isopropylthio-4-androsten-3-one.

$$\lambda_{max}^{MeOH}\ 240\ m\mu$$

(ε15,300); ν1732, 1675, 1622, 1241 cm.⁻¹.

EXAMPLE 6

Preparation of 7α-methylthiotestosterone

To a solution of 1 g. of 17β-acetoxy-4,6-androstadien-3-one in 25 ml. of reagent methanol, through which nitrogen is bubbled, is added 6.1 ml. of 1 N methanolic sodium methoxide. The solution is allowed to stand in a stoppered flask, under nitrogen atmosphere, for 4 days. The solution is acidified with glacial acetic acid, concentrated to a small volume under reduced pressure and filtered to give 17β-hydroxy-4,6-androstadien-3-one as white crystals;

$$\lambda_{max}^{MeOH}\ 283\ m\mu$$

(ε26,000); ν3340, 1650, 1620, 1580 cm.⁻¹.

A solution containing 0.585 g. of 17β-hydroxy-4,6-androstadien-3-one, 1 ml. of concentrated hydrochloric acid and 5 ml. of methylmercaptin in 25 ml. of dioxane is treated according to the procedure described in Example 1, to give 7α-methylthiotestosterone;

$$\lambda_{max}^{MeOH}\ 240\ m\mu$$

(ε=15,200); ν3450, 1670, 1620 cm.⁻¹.

EXAMPLE 7

Preparation of 7α-methylthiotestosterone propionate

A solution of 1.0 g. of 7α-methylthiotestosterone in 10 ml. of reagent pyridine is treated with 5 ml. of propionic anhydride and allowed to stand overnight at room temperature. The mixture is poured into water, extracted with methylene chloride, the methylene chloride extract washed successively with saturated sodium bicarbonate solution and water, and finally evaporated to dryness under reduced pressure to furnish 7α-methylthiotestosterone propionate as white crystals;

$$\lambda_{max}^{MeOH}\ 240\ m\mu$$

(ε15,100); ν1732, 1670, 1621, 1220 cm.⁻¹.

EXAMPLE 8

Preparation of 7α-methylthiotestosterone isobutyrate

A solution of 0.5 g. of 7α-methylthiotestosterone in 5 ml. of reagent pyridine is treated with 3 g. of isobutyric anhydride according to the procedure described in Example 7 to give 7α-methylthiotestosterone isobutyrate;

$$\lambda_{max}^{MeOH}\ 239\ m\mu$$

(ε14,800); ν1730, 1670, 1625, 1195 cm.⁻¹.

4

EXAMPLE 9

Preparation of 7α-methylthiotestosterone benzoate

A solution of 0.6 g. of 7α-methylthiotestosterone in 15 ml. of dry benzene is treated with 2 ml. of dry pyridine and 2 g. of benzoyl chloride and allowed to stand overnight at room temperature. The mixture is poured into water, extracted with methylene chloride, the methylene chloride extracts washed successively with dilute hydrochloric acid, saturated sodium bicarbonate solution and water, and finally evaporated to dryness under reduced pressure to give 7α-methylthiotestosterone benzoate;

$$\lambda_{max}^{MeOH}\ 228\ m\mu$$

(ε12,000); 240mμ. (ε16,200); ν1710, 1670, 1622, 1270, 1100 cm.⁻¹.

EXAMPLE 10

Preparation of 7α-methylthiotestosterone β-cyclopentyl-propionate

A solution of 1 g. of 7α-methylthiotestosterone in 25 ml. of dry benzene is treated with 3 ml. of dry pyridine and 3 g. of β-cyclopentylpropionyl chloride according to the procedure described in Example 9, to give 7α-methyl-thiotestosterone β-cyclopentylpropionate;

$$\lambda_{max}^{MeOH}\ 240\ m\mu$$

(ε15,100); ν1735, 1668, 1620, 1190 cm.⁻¹.

EXAMPLE 11

Preparation of 7α-methylthiotestosterone decanoate

A solution containing 1 g. of 7α-methylthiotestosterone in 25 ml. of dry benzene is treated with 3 ml. of dry pyridine and 4 g. of decanoyl chloride according to the procedure described in Example 10 to give 7α-methylthio-testosterone decanoate;

$$\lambda_{max}^{MeOH}\ 241\ m\mu$$

(ε14,800); ν1733, 1670, 1620, 1190 cm.⁻¹.

We claim:

1. Compounds having the general formula:

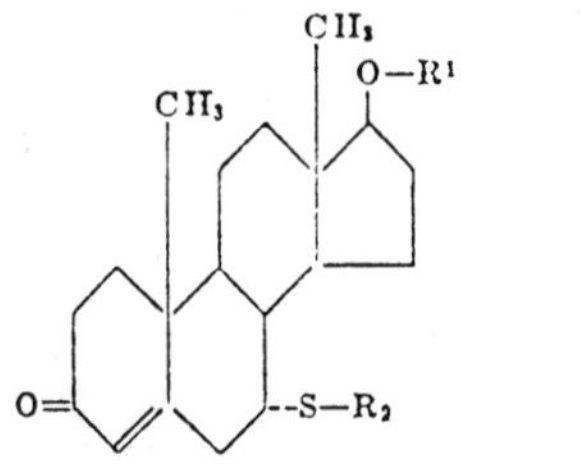

in which R^1 is a member of the group consisting of hydrogen, lower alkanoyl, cycloalkyl lower alkanoyl and aroyl radicals and R_2 is a member of the group consisting of lower alkyl and lower alkenyl radicals.

2. The compound 17β-acetoxy-7α-methylthio-4-androstene-3-one.

3. The compound 17β-acetoxy-7α-allylthio-4-androstene-3-one.

4. The compound 17β-hydroxy-7α-methylthio-4-androstene-3-one.

5. Compounds having the general formula:

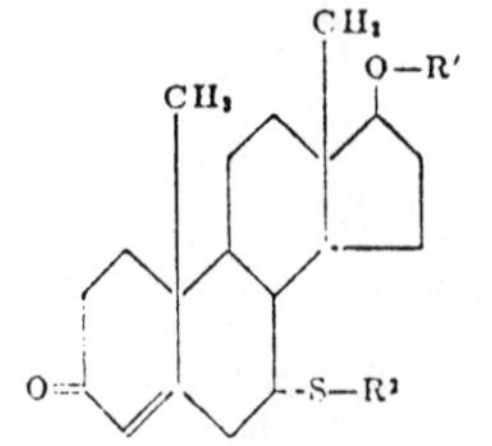

in which R′ is a lower alkanoyl radical and R^2 is a lower alkyl radical.

5

6. Compounds having the general formula

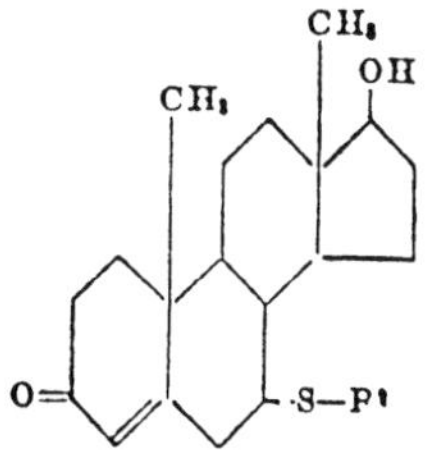

in which R^2 is a lower alkyl radical.

6

References Cited in the file of this patent

UNITED STATES PATENTS

2,837,543   Dodson et al. _____ June 3, 1958
2,859,222   Dodson et al. _____ Nov. 4, 1958

UNITED STATES PATENT OFFICE

Certificate of Correction

Patent No. 2,908,694   October 13, 1959

Robert E. Schaub et al.

It is hereby certified that error appears in the printed specification of the above numbered patent requiring correction and that the said Letters Patent should read as corrected below.

Column 3, line 19, Example 5, for the heading "*Preparation of 17β-acetoxy-7α-η-propylthio-4-androsten-3-one*" read —*Preparation of 17β-acetoxy-7α-isopropylthio-4-androsten-3-one*—.

Signed and sealed this 29th day of March 1960.

[SEAL]

Attest:
KARL H. AXLINE,
Attesting Officer.

ROBERT C. WATSON,
Commissioner of Patents.

CHAPTER FOUR

1

2,878,267

19-NOR-STEROID COMPOUNDS AND PROCESS
FOR THE PREPARATION THEREOF

Stefan Antoni Szpilfogel and Max Salomon de Winter,
Oss, Netherlands, assignors to Organon Inc., Orange,
N. J., a corporation of New Jersey

No Drawing. Application April 16, 1958
Serial No. 728,784

Claims priority, application Netherlands May 1, 1957

5 Claims. (Cl. 260—397.3)

The invention relates to new biologically active Δ^4-19-nor compounds of the androstane and pregnane series which are not oxygenated in 3-position and to a process for the preparation thereof.

More particularly it relates to novel 19-nor steroid compounds of the general formula:

$$\text{CH}_3$$
$$R_1 \cdots \cdots =R_2$$

in which R_1 is selected from the group consisting of H_2, (H)OH and $=O$ in case R_2 is selected from the group consisting of (H)COCH$_3$, (H)COCH$_2$OR$_3$ and (OH)COCH$_2$OR$_3$, in which R_3 is selected from the group consisting of hydrogen and acyl radicals derived from a carboxylic acid containing from 1 to 10 carbon atoms, and in which R_1 is selected from the group consisting of (H)OH and $=O$, in case R_2 is selected from the group consisting of (H)OR$_3$,(R$_4$)OR$_3$, and $=O$, in which R_3 is as indicated above and R_4 is selected from the group consisting of a methyl, ethyl, and vinyl group. These novel compounds exert strongly gonad-inhibiting effects.

These novel compounds also have anabolic, androgenic, and progestative properties.

The process according to the invention is characterized in that a Δ^4-3-hydroxy-19-nor steroid compound of the androstane or pregnane series etherified or esterified in 3-position is treated with an alkali metal in liquid ammonia or in a lower aliphatic primary amine, by which the substituent in 3-position is split off.

The Δ^4-3-hydroxy-19-nor steroid compounds to be applied as starting products can be obtained by reduction of the corresponding 3-keto compounds. This reduction may be carried out by means of one of the commonly used reduction agents, such as an alkali metal borohydride, an alkali metal aluminiumhydride, an alkali metal trialkoxyborohydride, or aluminium isopropoxide in isopropanol.

After the hydroxyl group in 3-position has been etherified or esterified, splitting off according to the invention may take place. This ether group may be an alkoxy, aryloxy, or aralkoxy group, e. g. a methoxy, ethoxy, isopropoxy, pentoxy, phenyloxy, benzoxy or triphenyl methoxy group.

The etherification may be carried out by treating the starting substance in a suitable organic solvent with an alcohol in the presence of an inorganic acid, e. g. hydrochloric acid. In some cases the alcohol may at the same time serve as a solvent. It is also possible to carry out the etherification by treating the 3-hydroxy compound with a hydro carbon halogenide, e. g. triphenylmethyl halogenide, in the presence of e. g. pyridine.

The esterification may be carried out by reacting the

2

Δ^4-3-hydroxy compound with an acid, preferably in the presence of a dehydrating agent, such as ethoxy acetylene, or by reacting the starting product with an acid anhydride, if desired in the presence of a suitable solvent, such as pyridine. It is also possible to carry out the esterification by means of the acid chloride, preferably in the presence of a tertiary base, such as pyridine or chinoline.

The splitting off of the substituent in 3-position takes place by treating the starting material, dissolved in a suitable solvent, with an alkali metal in the presence of liquid ammonia or of a lower aliphatic primary amine containing from 1 to 6 carbon atoms. As a solvent may e. g. be used a lower aliphatic ether, such as dimethyl ether, methyl ethyl ether, diethyl ether, further dioxane and tetrahydrofurane.

The alkali metal which is applied in this reaction may be e. g. lithium, sodium, or potassium. It has appeared of advantage to use lithium.

As examples of lower aliphatic primary amines to be used are mentioned methyl amine, ethyl amine, n-propylamine, isopropylamine, n-butylamine and n-amylamine.

If the present reduction is carried out in the presence of a lower aliphatic primary amine the reaction in question is e. g. carried out at the boiling-point of this amine. However, if the boiling-point of this amine exceeds 0° C., it is desirable to carry out the reduction at a temperature below 0° C.

If the 3-keto steroid compound to be reduced contains one or more keto groups in addition to the said 3-keto group, these groups may be protected, prior to the reduction, e. g. by ketalization. If these keto groups have not been protected, they are converted, in the course of the reduction reaction, into hydroxyl groups which can again be converted into keto groups by oxidation in the commonly used manner.

If the Δ^4-3-hydroxy steroid compound obtained after the reduction contains in addition a hydroxyl group in 17 or 21-position, the corresponding 17 or 21-acylate will, in most of the cases, be formed on esterifying the 3-hydroxyl group. If desired the 17 or 21-ester obtained after the splitting off of the 3-acyloxy group can then be saponified and, if necessary, again be esterified.

The etherification of the Δ^4-3-hydorxy steriod compound will only ocur at the 3-hydroxyl group, because this group is activated by the presence of the Δ^4-bond. After splitting off of the 3-ether group the thus obtained compound, if containing esterifiable hydroxyl groups, can be esterified, if desired.

The esterification is preferably carried out with an aliphatic, aromatic or araliphatic carboxylic acid containing from 1 to 10 carbon atoms or a functional derivative thereof, e. g. acetic acid, propionic acid, butyric acid, valeric acid, capronic acid, isocapronic acid, succinic acid, tartaric acid, cyclopentyl acetic acid, β-cyclopentyl propionic acid, cyclohexyl acetic acid, γ-cyclohexyl butyric acid, phenyl acetic acid, β-phenyl propionic acid, benzoic acid, glycine, alanine, and phenylalanine.

Example I

To a solution of 3.0 g. of Δ^4-11β,17β-dihydroxy-3-keto-17α-methyl-19-nor-androstene in 150 ml. of methanol are added 1.4 g. of sodium borohydride. After leaving to stand for 20 minutes the reaction mixture is neutralized with glacial acetic acid and then evaporated in vacuo to a volume of 25 ml. The residue is poured into 200 ml. of water, after which the Δ^4-3,11β,17β-trihydroxy-17α-methyl-19-nor-androstene crystallizes out.

The sucked off crystals are dissolved in 112 ml. of methanol, after which 1.6 ml. of 36% hydrochloric acid are added to this solution. The resulting solution is stirred at room temperature for 1 hour, after which the reaction mixture is neutralized with sodium bicarbonate and evaporated to 25 ml. The residue is poured into 200 ml. of water, after which the resulting crystals of Δ⁴-3-methoxy - 11β,17β - dihydroxy - 17α - methyl-19-nor-androstene are sucked off and subsequently recrystallized from acetone.

2.3 g. of this compound are dissolved in 25 ml. of dry ether, after which a solution of 2 g. of lithium in 90 g. of ethyl amine is added dropwise to this solution. After stirring for 10 minutes the excess of lithium is removed by slowly adding 15 ml. of methanol to the reaction mixture. After the reaction mixture has been discoloured the ethyl amine is evaporated in vacuo. The residue is taken up in ice water, after which the mixture is extracted some times with ether. The collected ether extracts are washed, after which the ether is evaporated in vacuo. The residue is distributed between 70% methanol and petroleum ether, the petroleum ether layer is separated, dried, and finally evaporated to dryness. On crystallization from petroleum ether the residue yields the Δ⁴-11β,17β-dihydroxy-17α-methyl-19-nor-androstene.

A solution of 1 g. of this compound in 3.2 g. of acetic anhydride and 4.0 g. of pyridine is heated on a steam-bath for one hour in nitrogen atmosphere and then poured into ice-water. The precipitate is separated and then crystallized from a mixture of methanol and petroleum ether, after which the Δ⁴-11β,17β-dihydroxy-17α-methyl-19-nor-androstene-17-acetate is obtained.

In a corresponding manner the esters of this compound have been prepared derived from capronic acid, succinic acid, cyclopentyl acetic acid, and β-phenyl propionic acid.

Example II

In an analogous manner as described in Example I the Δ⁴-3-keto - 11β,17β - dihydroxy - 17α - vinyl - 19 - nor-androstene is reduced to the corresponding 3-hydroxy compound, which is then converted, by means of isopropanol and hydrochloric acid, into the corresponding 3-isopropoxy compound.

Using the method of Example I this compound is treated with a solution of sodium in methylamine, after which the Δ⁴-11β,17β-dihydroxy-17α-vinyl-19-nor-androstene is obtained.

Esterification of this compound, in an analogous manner as described in Example I, yields the 17-esters, derived from propionic acid, t. butyl acetic acid, nonane carboxylic acid, and γ-cyclohexylbutyric acid.

In a corresponding manner and starting from Δ⁴-3,11-diketo-17β-hydroxy-17α-ethyl-19-nor-androstene, the Δ⁴-11-keto-17β-hydroxy - 17α - ethyl-19-nor-androstene has been obtained. Subsequently the 17-esters of this compound have been prepared, derived from acetic acid, nonane carboxylic acid, and cyclopentylpropionic acid.

Example III

3.04 g. of NaBH₄ are added to a solution of 2.9 g. of Δ⁴-21-hydroxy-3,20-diketo-19-nor pregnene in 400 ml. of methanol. The reaction mixture is stirred at room temperature for 1 hour, then adjusted to pH 5.4 with glacial acetic acid, subsequently evaporated in vacuo to about 30 ml., and finally diluted with 200 ml. of water. The solution is extracted with chloroform and the extract is washed with ice cold 1 N sodium hydroxide and subsequently with water till neutral. After drying and evaporating the solvent the crude Δ⁴-3,20,21-trihydroxy-19-nor-pregnene is obtained.

This is dissolved in 8 ml. of pyridine, after which 4.2 g. of propionic acid anhydride are added to this solution. The reaction mixture is stirred at room temperature for 20 hours, after which the solution is decomposed by the addition of water. The mixture is subsequently evaporated to dryness, after which the residue is recrystallized from methanol. Obtained is the Δ⁴-3,20,21-tripropionyloxy-19-nor pregnene.

The sucked off crystals are dissolved in 120 ml. of absolute ether, after which this solution is added to a solution

of 0.9 g. of sodium in 25 ml. of methylamine. The blue coloured solution is subsequently stirred at −15° C. for 2 hours, after which 18 ml. of absolute ethanol are added to the reaction mixture. Then the methylamine is evaporated, the residue is diluted with water, and the mixture is extracted a few times with ether. The collected ether extracts are washed with water, dried on sodium sulphate, and evaporated to dryness. The residue is crystallized from methanol and then from petroleum ether, after which the Δ⁴-20,21-dipropionyloxy-19-nor pregnene is obtained.

Saponification of this compound by treatment hereof with a 0.5% sodium hydroxide solution for 15 minutes at room temperature yields the Δ⁴-20,21-dihydroxy-19-nor pregnene.

3 g. of this compound are dissolved in 15 ml. of dioxane, after which 5 ml. of pyridine and 0.9 ml. of acetic acid anhydride are added. The reaction mixture is stirred at room temperature for 24 hours, after which it is evaporated to dryness in vacuo. The dry residue consisting of Δ⁴-20,21-dihydroxy-19-nor-pregnene-21-acetate is dissolved in 30 ml. of acetone. While stirring and at 0° C. a chromic acid solution is added dropwise to this solution. This chromic acid solution has been prepared by dissolving 84 g. of chromium trioxide in 120 ml. of water and 62 ml. of concentrated sulphuric acid, after which the solution is completed to 300 ml. with water. The chromic acid solution is added dropwise until constant yellow colouring has occurred. The reaction mixture is then evaporated to nearly dryness in vacuo, after which the residue is taken up in water. The aqueous mixture is extracted with chloroform, after which the chloroform layer is separated, washed with diluted sulphuric acid, then with a cold dilute sodium hydroxide solution, and subsequently with water till neutral. After evaporating the solvent the Δ⁴-21-hydroxy-20-keto-19-nor-pregnene-21-acetate is obtained. By saponification with a dilute sodium hydroxide solution the unesterified compound is obtained herefrom.

Acylation of this compound with butyric anhydride, β-cyclopentylpropionic anhydride or succinic anhydride in pyridine afford the 21-butyrate, 21β-cyclopentylpropionate, and 21-hemi succinate respectively.

Example IV

In accordance with the process described in Example III the Δ⁴-3,20-diketo-11β-17α-dihydroxy-19-nor-pregnene and the Δ⁴-3,20-diketo-17α,21-dihydroxy-19-nor-pregnene have been converted into Δ⁴-11β,17α-dihydroxy-20-keto-19-nor-pregnene, resp. into Δ⁴-17α,21-dihydroxy-20-keto-19-non-pregnene.

In accordance with the method described in Example III this latter compound has been converted into the corresponding 21-esters, derived from trimethyl acetic acid, benzoic acid, cyclohexyl acetic acid and β-phenylpropionic acid.

Example V

3.04 g. of NaBH₄ are added to a solution of 2.9 g. of Δ⁴-3,20-diketo-19-nor-pregnene in 400 ml. of methanol. The reaction mixture is stirred at room temperature for 1 hour, then adjusted to a pH of 5.4 with glacial acetic acid, subsequently evaporated in vacuo to about 30 ml., and finally diluted with 200 ml. of water. The solution is extracted with chloroform and the extract is washed with ice cold 1 N sodium hydroxide and subsequently with water till neutral. After drying and evaporating of the solvent the crude Δ⁴-3,20-dihydroxy-19-nor-pregnene is obtained.

This is dissolved in 65 ml. of methanol, after which 1.5 ml. of concentrated hydrochloric acid are added to this solution. The resulting solution is stirred at room temperature for 40 minutes, after which the mixture is neutralized with sodium bicarbonate and evaporated to 15 ml. The residue is poured into 200 ml. of water, when the Δ⁴-3-methoxy-20-hydroxy-19-nor-pregnene crystallizes out.

The sucked off crystals are dissolved in 120 ml. of absolute ether after which 120 ml. of liquid ammonia and subsequently 0.9 g. of sodium cut to small pieces are added to this solution. The blue coloured solution is subsequently stirred at −35° C. for 2 hours, after which 18 ml. of absolute ethanol are added to the reaction mixture. Then the ammonia is evaporated, the residue is diluted with water, and the mixture is extracted a few times with ether. The collected ether extracts are washed with water, dried on sodium sulphate, and evaporated to dryness. The residue is crystallized from methanol and then from petroleum ether, after which the Δ⁴-20-hydroxy-19-nor-pregnene is obtained.

0.5 g. of this compound is dissolved in 25 ml. of acetone. While stirring and at 0° C. a chromic acid solution is dropwise added to this solution. This chromic acid solution has been prepared by dissolving 70 g. of chromium trioxide in 100 ml. of water and 55 ml. of concentrated sulphuric acid, after which the solution is completed with water to 250 ml. The chromic acid solution is added dropwise for such a long time until remaining yellow coloration has occurred. Then the reaction mixture is evaporated in vacuo to nearly dryness, after which the residue is taken up in water. The aqueous mixture is extracted with chloroform, after which the chloroform layer is separated, washed with dilute sulphuric acid, then with a cold dilute sodium hydroxide solution and subsequently with water till neutral. After evaporating the solvent the Δ⁴-20-keto-19-nor-pregnene is obtained.

In a corresponding manner the Δ⁴-17α-hydroxy-3,20-diketo-19-nor-pregnene has been converted into the corresponding 3,17α,20-dihydroxy compound by means of sodium borohydride, and then, by treatment with triphenylchloromethane in the presence of pyridine converted into the Δ⁴-3-triphenyl methoxy-17α,20-dihydroxy-19-nor-pregnene.

Subsequently this compound has been converted into the Δ⁴-17α,20-dihydroxy-19-nor-pregnene, by means of sodium and isopropylamine, using the method of Example III. Oxidation of this compound by means of chromic acid in acetone afforded the Δ⁴-17α-hydroxy-20-keto-19-nor-pregnene.

Example VI

In accordance with the process described in Example III the Δ⁴-17α,21-dihydroxy-3,11,20-triketo-19-nor-pregnene has been converted into a Δ⁴-3-methoxy-17α,20β,21-trihydroxy-11-keto-19-nor-pregnene by reduction with sodium borohydride and a subsequent treatment with methanol and concentrated hydrochloric acid.

By a subsequent treatment with potassium and methylamine the Δ⁴-17α,20β,21-trihydroxy-11-keto-19-nor-pregnene has been obtained in accordance with the process described in Example I.

0.3 g. of this compound is dissolved in 1.5 ml. of dioxane, after which 75 ml. of pyridine and 70.5 ml. of acetic acid anhydride are added. The reaction mixture is stirred at room temperature for 24 hours, after which it is evaporated to dryness in vacuo. The dry residue consisting of Δ⁴-17α,20β,21-trihydroxy-11-keto-19-nor-pregnene-21-acetate is dissolved in 45 ml. of acetone and then oxidized in a manner as described in Example V.

Obtained is the Δ⁴-17α,21-dihydroxy-11,20-diketo-19-nor-pregnene-21-acetate. Saponification of this compound by treatment hereof with a 0.5% sodium hydroxide solution for 10 minutes at room temperature yields the Δ⁴-17α,21-dihydroxy-11,20-diketo-19-nor-pregnene.

By esterification with butyric anhydride, succinic anhydride, and β-phenyl propionic anhydride, this compound has been converted into the corresponding 21-esters thereof.

1. g. of Δ⁴-17α,21-dihydroxy-11,20-diketo-19-nor-preg-

nene-21-acetate is suspended in 27 ml. of methanol and 6.5 ml. of dimethyl formamide. To this mixture are added 0.7 g. of semicarbazide-HCl and a solution of 0.43 g. of sodium bicarbonate in 5 ml. of water. Then in nitrogen atmosphere the reaction mixture is refluxed for 3 hours and subsequently maintained at 45° C. for 24 hours. Then 35 ml. of water are added to the mixture, the mixture is cooled to 0° C., the 20-mono-semi-carbazone precipitated after some hours is filtered and dried in vacuo.

The resulting dry residue is suspended in 12 ml. of water and 50 ml. of tetrahydrofurane, after which the suspension is heated until a clear solution has been obtained. To the solution, cooled to room temperature, a solution of 220 mg. of sodium borohydride in 5 ml. of water is subsequently added in a nitrogen atmosphere and with stirring. Then the reaction mixture is stirred for 5 hours, after which it is brought to a pH of 6–7 with glacial acetic acid. The mixture is evaporated in vacuo to nearly dryness, after which the residue is taken up in a mixture of 15 ml. of chloroform and 15 ml. of 2 N sulphuric acid. It is refluxed for 5 minutes and then cooled. The chloroform layer is subsequently separated and the remaining aqueous layer is extracted with chloroform. The collected chloroform extracts are washed with a dilute sodium hydroxide solution and then with water till neutral. After drying and evaporating the solvent, the residue is crystallized from a mixture of methanol and acetone, after which the Δ⁴-11β,17α,21-trihydroxy-20-keto-19-nor-pregnene-21-acetate is obtained.

Saponification of this compound by treatment with a 0.5% sodium hydroxide solution for 15 minutes at room temperature yields the Δ⁴-11β,17α,21-trihydroxy-20-keto-19-nor-pregnene.

In accordance with the process described in Example III the 21-esters of this compound have been prepared derived from valeric acid, succinic acid, β-phenyl propionic acid, and glycine.

Example VII

2.75 g. of NaBH₄ are added to a solution of 5.5 g. of Δ⁴-17-hydroxy-3-keto-19-nor-androstene in 200 ml. of methanol at room temperature. After leaving to stand for 20 minutes the reaction mixture is neutralized with glacial acetic acid and then evaporated in vacuo to a volume of 25 ml. The residue is poured into 200 ml. of water, after which the Δ⁴-3,17-dihydroxy-19-nor-androstene crystallizes out.

The sucked off crystals are dissolved in 15 ml. of pyridine, after which 10.2 g. of acetic acid anhydride are added to this solution. The reaction mixture is kept at room temperature for 20 minutes, after which 20 ml. of water are added. The mixture is subsequently evaporated to dryness, after which the residue is recrystallized from methanol. Obtained is the Δ⁴-3,17-diacetoxy-19-nor-androstene.

2 g. of the thus prepared compound are dissolved in 25 ml. of dry ether, after which this solution is added dropwise to a solution of 2 g. of lithium in 90 g. of ethylamine. After stirring for 10 minutes the excess of lithium is removed by slowly adding 15 ml. of methanol to the reaction mixture. After the reaction mixture is discoloured, the ethylamine is evaporated in vacuo. The residue is taken up in ice-water, after which the mixture is extracted a few times with ether. The collected ether extracts are washed, after which the ether is evaporated in vacuo. The residue is distributed between 70% methanol and petroleum ether, the petroleum ether layer is separated, dried, and finally evaporated to dryness. On crystallization from petroleum ether the residue yields the Δ⁴-17β-acetoxy-19-nor-androstene. Saponification of this compound by treatment with a dilute methanolic sodium hydroxide solution yields the Δ⁴-17β-hydroxy-19-nor-androstene of melting-point 98° C.

Example VIII

To a solution of 5.8 g. of Δ⁴-3-keto-11β,17β-dihydroxy-19-nor-androstene in 200 ml. of methanol are added 2.79 g. of sodium borohydride at room temperature. After leaving to stand for 20 minutes the reaction mixture is neutralized with glacial acetic acid and then evaporated in vacuo to a volume of 25 ml. The residue is poured into 200 ml. of water, after which the Δ⁴-3,11β,17β-trihydroxy-19-nor-androstene crystallizes out.

The sucked off crystals are dissolved in 25 ml. of pyridine after which 30.3 g. of cyclopentyl propionic anhydride are added to this solution. The reaction mixture is refluxed for 30 minutes, after which 25 ml. of water are added. The mixture is subsequently evaporated to dryness, after which the residue is crystallized from methanol-petroleum ether. Obtained is the Δ⁴-3,11β,17β-trihydroxy-19-nor-androstene-3,17β-dicyclopentylpropionate.

2 g. of the thus prepared compound are dissolved in 25 ml. of dry ether, after which this solution is added dropwise to a solution of 2 g. of lithium in 90 g. of ethylamine. After stirring for 10 minutes the excess of lithium is removed by slowly adding 15 ml. of methanol to the reaction mixture. After the reaction mixture is discoloured, the ethylamine is evaporated in vacuo. The residue is taken up in ice-water, after which the mixture is extracted a few times with ether. The collected ether extracts are washed, after which the ether is evaporated in vacuo. The residue is distributed between 70% methanol and petroleum ether, the petroleum ether layer is separated, dried, and finally evaporated to dryness. On crystallization from petroleum ether the residue yields the Δ⁴-11β-17β-dihydroxy-19-nor-androstene-17β-cyclopentyl propionate. Saponification of this compound by treatment with a dilute methanol sodium hydroxide solution yields the Δ⁴-11β,17β-dihydroxy-19-nor-androstene.

According to the process described in example I this compound has been converted into the 17-esters derived from capronic acid, cyclohexyl acetic acid, and hexahydrobenzoic acid.

In addition, the above described Δ⁴-11β,17β-dihydroxy-19-nor-androstene has been oxidized to the corresponding Δ⁴-11,17-diketo-19-nor-androstene by means of a chromic acid solution in a mixture of water and acetic acid.

Example IX

In a corresponding manner as described in Example I the Δ⁴-17β-hydroxy-17α-methyl-3-keto-19-nor-androstene is reduced to the corresponding 3-hydroxy compound by means of sodium borohydride.

4.9 g. of this compound are then dissolved in 105 ml. of ethanol, after which 2.8 ml. of concentrated hydrochloric acid are added to this solution. The process of this reaction mixture is carried out as described in Example I, after which the Δ⁴-3-ethoxy-17β-hydroxy-17α-methyl-19-nor-androstene is obtained.

3 g. of this compound are dissolved in 125 ml. of absolute ether. To this solution are added 120 ml. of liquid ammonia and subsequently 0.9 g. of lithium cut to small pieces. The blue coloured solution is then stirred at —35° C. for 2 hours, after which 20 ml. of absolute ethanol are added at the same temperature as a result of which the blue colour disappears. The ammonia is evaporated, the residue is diluted with water and the resulting mixture is extracted a few times with ether. The collected ether extracts are washed with water, dried on sodium sulphate and evaporated to dryness. The residue is distributed between petroleum ether and 70% methanol (1:1), the petroleum ether layer is separated, the petroleum ether evaporated to half the original volume, after which crystallization of the Δ⁴-17β-hydroxy-17α-methyl-19-nor-androstene takes place. This compound has a melting-point of 147°–151° C.

Entirely in accordance with the process described in this example the Δ⁴-17β-hydroxy-17α-ethyl-3-keto-19-nor-

androstene is reduced to the Δ⁴-17β-hydroxy-17α-ethyl-19-nor-androstene via the 3-methoxy compound.

We claim:

1. Process for the preparation of new Δ⁴-19-nor-steroid compounds comprising reacting a compound of the formula:

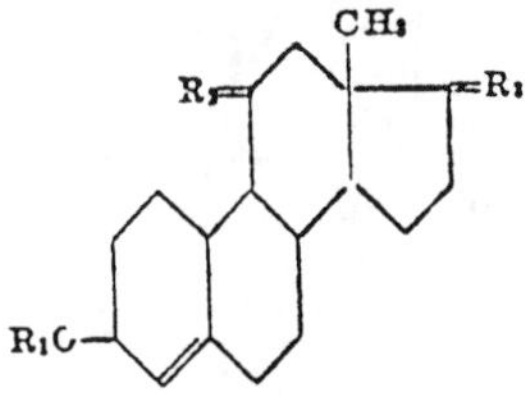

in which R₁ is selected from the group consisting of an acyl group derived from a carboxylic acid containing from 1 to 8 carbon atoms, and an alkyl group containing from 1 to 6 carbon atoms and the triphenyl methyl group, R₂ is selected from the group consisting of H₂, (H)OH and =O, and R₃ is selected from the group consisting of =O, (H)COCH₃, (H)COCH₂OR₄, (OH)COCH₂OR₄, (H)OR₄, and (R₅)OR₄, in which R₄ is selected from the group consisting of hydrogen and acyl radicals derived from a carboxylic acid containing from 1 to 10 carbon atoms, and R₅ is selected from the group consisting of a methyl, ethyl, and vinyl group, with an alkali metal in the presence of a compound selected from the group consisting of liquid ammonia and a lower aliphatic primary amine containing from 1 to 6 carbon atoms, and in the presence of an organic solvent selected from the group consisting of a lower aliphatic ether, dioxane and tetrahydrofurane, and at a temperature below 20° C., by which the substituent in 3-position is split off.

2. Process according to claim 1, wherein lithium is used as alkali metal.

3. Process according to claim 1, wherein the reaction is carried out below 0° C.

4. Steroid compounds of the formula:

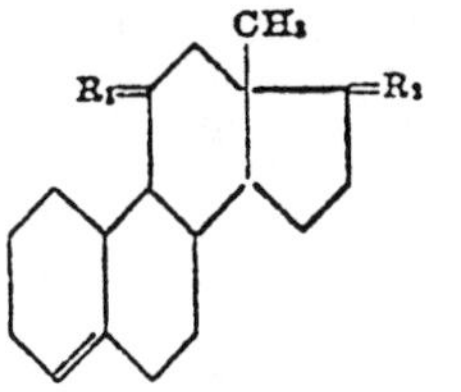

in which R₁ is selected from the group consisting of H₂, (H)OH and =O, and R₂ is selected from the group consisting of

(H)COCH₃, (H)COCH₂OR₃, and (OH)COCH₂OR₃

in which R₃ is selected from the group consisting of hydrogen and acyl radicals derived from a carboxylic acid containing from 1 to 10 carbon atoms.

5. Steroid compounds of the formula:

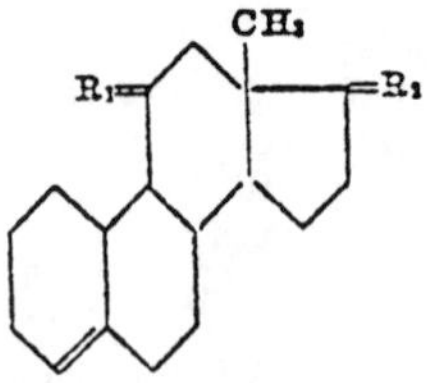

in which R₁ is selected from the group consisting of (H)OH, and =O, and R₂ is selected from the group consisting of =O, (H)OR₃, and (R₄)OR₃, in which R₃ is selected from the group consisting of hydrogen and acyl radicals derived from a carboxylic acid containing from 1 to 10 carbon atoms and R₄ is selected from the group consisting of a methyl, ethyl, and vinyl group.

References Cited in the file of this patent

UNITED STATES PATENTS

2,781,365   Djerassi et al. _____ Feb. 12, 1957

CHAPTER FIVE

1

2,813,881

9α-HALO-17α-METHYLANDROSTANE-3,11β,17β-TRIOL

Milton E. Herr, Kalamazoo, Mich., assignor to The Upjohn Company, Kalamazoo, Mich., a corporation of Michigan

No Drawing. Application March 19, 1956, Serial No. 572,231

7 Claims. (Cl. 260—397.5)

This invention pertains to organic compounds of the androstane series and is more particularly concerned with novel 9α-halo-17α-methylandrostane-3,11β,17β-triols of the formula

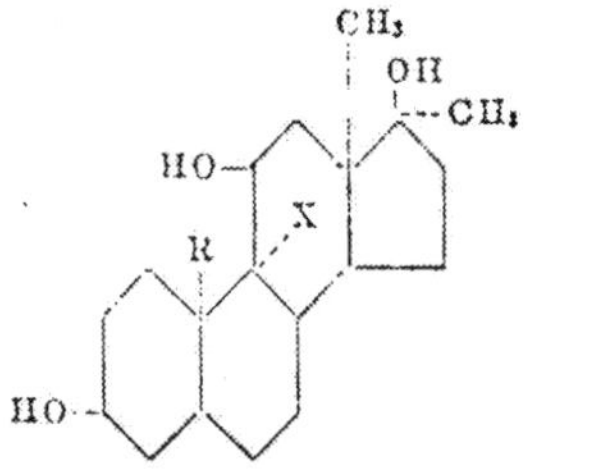

wherein R is selected from hydrogen and methyl and X is a halogen atom having an atomic weight from nineteen to 127, i. e. fluorine, chlorine, bromine, and iodine. Preferably X is a halogen atom having an atomic weight from nineteen to 36, i. e. fluorine and chlorine, fluorine being preferred. It is to be understood that the configuration of the 3-hydroxy group and the 5-hydrogen atom each can be α or β, and that compounds having both forms of the 3-hydroxy group and the 5-hydrogen atom are included within the scope of the present invention. This application is a continuation-in-part of copending application Serial No. 550,844, filed December 5, 1955, now abandoned.

It is an object of this invention to provide the 17α-methylandrostane-3,11β,17β-triols of the above formula. Said compounds are potent anabolic and androgenic agents and are used in place of prior anabolic and androgenic agents in known anabolic and androgenic pharmaceutical preparations. The compounds also have hypotensive, anti-pituitary, anti-estrogen, and central nervous system depressant activity, and are employed in place of known agents in pharmaceutical formulations used for such purposes. Other objects and uses will be apparent to one skilled in the art.

The 9α-halo-17α-methylandrostane-3,11β,17β-triols of the above formula are also useful in the form of their 17-monoacylate, 3,17-diacylate, 11,17-diacylate and 3,-11,17-triacylate. Their acylates. e. g., mono-, di-, or triacetate, propionate, trimethylacetate, α or β-cyclopentylpropionate, α or β-cyclohexylpropionate, benzoate, phenylacetate, cyclohexylacetate, α or β-phenylpropionate, or other hydrocarbon carboxylate, preferably containing from one to nine carbon atoms, inclusive, are useful for the same purposes as the parent compounds, and in addition these esters are useful for the purification of the parent 9α-halo-17α-methylandrostane-3,11β,17β-triols.

The 9α-halo-17α-methylandrostane-3,11β,17β-triols of the present invention can be prepared readily from the corresponding 9α-halo-11β,17β-dihydroxy-17α-methylandrostane-3-ones (starting compounds are described in copending applications Serial No. 550,846, filed December 5, 1955, now abandoned and Serial No. 572,232,

filed March 19, 1956) by hydrogenation of the 3-keto group to a 3-hydroxy group. The hydrogenation can be carried out by chemical reduction procedure, e. g., using a chemical reducing agent such as sodium borohydride, potassium borohydride, lithium aluminum hydride, or other dimetallic hydride, sodium and alcohol, etc. in a solvent which does not react readily with the reducing agent. The hydrogenation can also be carried out catalytically, e. g., employing hydrogen and a platinum catalyst employing an inert solvent such as ethyl alcohol. The 9α-halo-17α-alkylandrostane-3,11β,17β-triols and 9α-halo-17α-alkyl-19-norandrostane-3,11β,17β-triols wherein the alkyl radical is preferably a lower-alkyl radical containing from two to eight carbon atoms, inclusive, e. g. ethyl, propyl, isopropyl, butyl, secondary-butyl, amyl, hexyl, heptyl, octyl, etc., and wherein the halo atom is defined as above, are prepared by the same methods and have similar androgenic, hypotensive, anti-pituitary, central nervous system depressant, anti-estrogen, and anabolic activity.

The following examples are illustrative of certain preferred products and processes and are not to be construed as limiting.

Example 1.—A suspension of 9α-fluoro-11β,17β-dihydroxy-17α-methyl-5β-androstane-3-one in ethyl alcohol is stirred with a solution containing an excess of sodium borohydride in one-tenth normal aqueous sodium hydroxide. The starting steroid dissolves almost immediately and after ten minutes' stirring, the mixture is diluted with water and dilute aqueous acid is added to raise the pH of the mixture to pH 6. The product which precipitates is removed by filtration, washed with water, and dried in vacuo to provide 9α-fluoro-17α-methyl-5β-androstane-3α,11β,17β-triol. Recrystallization gave a melting point of 186–190 degrees centigrade (decomposes) and an $[\alpha]_D^{24}$ of plus 24 degrees in ethanol.

Anal.—Calcd. for $C_{20}H_{33}O_3F$: C, 70.54; H, 9.77; F, 5.58. Found: C, 70.85; H, 9.87; F, 5.70.

Example 2.—9α-fluoro-11β,17β-dihydroxy-17α-methyl-5α-androstane-3-one is converted to 9α-fluoro-17α-methyl-5α-androstane-3β,11β,17β-triol following the hydrogenation procedure of Example 1: A mixture of 0.5 gram of 9α-fluoro-11β,17β-dihydroxy-17α-methyl-5α-androstan-3-one and ten milliliters of 95 percent ethanol was treated with a solution of 250 milligrams of sodium borohydride in 2.5 milliliters of one-tenth normal aqueous sodium hydroxide and stirred at a temperature of about 25 degrees centigrade for ten minutes. The mixture was diluted with 25 milliliters of water and carefully neutralized with acetic acid. The 9α-fluoro-17α-methyl-5α-androstane-3β,11β,17β-triol which separated was recovered by filtration, washed with water and recrystallized from dilute acetone; yield 0.47 gram; melting point 260 degrees centigrade with decomposition; $[\alpha]_D^{24}$ plus seven degrees in ethanol.

Example 3.—Following the same hydrogenation procedure as shown in Examples 1 or 2, 9α-fluoro-11β,17β-dihydroxy-17α-methyl-19-nor-5α-androstane-3-one is converted to 9α-fluoro-17α-methyl-19-nor-5α-androstane-3β,11β,17β-triol and 9α-fluoro-11β,17β-dihydroxy-17α-methyl-19-nor-5β-androstane-3-one is converted to 9α-fluoro-17α-methyl-19-nor-5β-androstane-3α,11β,17β-triol. Also following the procedure of Examples 1 or 2, 9α-chloro-, 9α-bromo-, and 9α-iodo-11β,17β-dihydroxy-17α-methyl-5α(and 5β)-androstane-3-one are hydrogenated to provide 9α-chloro-, 9α-bromo-, and 9α-iodo-17α-methyl-5α(and 5β)-androstane-3β(and 3α),11β,17β-triol and 9α-chloro-, 9α-bromo-, and 9α-iodo-11β,17β-dihydroxy-17α-methyl-19-nor-5α(and 5β)-androstane-3-one are hydrogenated to provide 9α-chloro-, 9α-bromo-, and 9α-iodo-17α-methyl-

19 - nor - 5α(and 5β) - androstane-3β(and 3α),11β,17β-triol. Other 9α-halo-17α-alkyl-5α(and 5β)-androstane-3β(and 3α),11β,17β-triols and 9α-halo-17α-alkyl-19-nor-5α(and 5β)-androstane-3β(and 3α),11β,17β-triols, wherein the alkyl radical and halo atom are defined and illustrated above, are prepared by the same procedure from corresponding 9α - halo-11β,17β-dihydroxy-17α-alkyl-5α-(and 5β)-androstane-3-ones and 9α-halo-11β,17β-dihydroxy-17α-alkyl-19-nor-5α(and 5β)-androstane-3-ones.

Example 4.—A solution of 9α-fluoro-methyl-5α-androstane-3β,11β,17β-triol in dry pyridine is treated with acetic anhydride, the molar ratio of steroid to acetic anhydride being about two to four and the resulting mixture is heated under reflux for about five hours. The mixture is then cooled, diluted with water while stirring, and the solid precipitate obtained removed by filtration. The solid is washed with two percent aqueous hydrochloric acid solution and with water, and then dried under vacuum. Recrystallization of chromatographic separation provides purified 9α - fluoro-17α-methyl-5α-androstane-3β,11β,17β-triol 3,17-diacetate. In exactly the same manner 9α-fluoro-17α-methyl-5β-androstane-3α,11β,17β-triol 3,17-diacetate, 9α - fluoro - 17α-methyl-19-nor-5α-androstane-3β,11β,17β-triol 3,17-diacetate and 9α-fluoro-17α-methyl-19-nor-5β-androstane-3α,11β,17β-triol, 3,17-diacetate are obtained by using 9α-fluoro-17α-methyl-5β-androstane - 3α,11β,17β - triol, 9α-fluoro-17α-methyl-19-nor-5α - androstane-3β,11β,17β - triol and 9α-fluoro-17α-methyl-19-nor-5β-androstane-3α,11β,17β-triol, respectively, as the starting steroid in the foregoing procedure. Substituting the appropriate acylating agent, i. e., the appropriate acid, acid anhydride or acid chloride, for the acetic anhydride in the above process provides other 3,17-diacylates of 9α-fluoro-17α-methyl-5α(and 5β)-androstane - 3β(and 3α),11β,17β-triol and 9α-fluoro-17α-methyl-19-nor-5α(and 5β)-androstane-3β(and 3α),11β,-17β-triol including the 3,17-diformate, dipropionate, di-(trimethylacetate), difuroate, di-(α or β-cyclohexylpropionate), dibenzoate, di-(phenylacetate), di-(α or β-cyclopentylpropionate), di-(α or β-phenylpropionate), di-(methylbenzoate), di-(α or β-furylacrylate), divalerate, dimethacrylate, and the like. By following the foregoing acylation procedure 3,17-diacylates having acylate radicals as defined and illustrated above, are prepared from 9α-chloro-, 9α-bromo-, and 9α-iodo-17α-methyl-5α(and 5β)-androstane-3β(and 3α),11β,17β-triol and 9α-chloro-, 9α-bromo-, and 9α-iodo-17α-methyl-19-nor-5α-(and 5β)-androstane-3β(and 3α),11β,17β-triol.

Example 5.—A mixture of 9α-fluoro-17α-methyl-5α-androstane-3β,11β,17β-triol 3,17-diacetate, a large excess of acetic anhydride to serve as both acylating agent and solvent, and a trace of the strongly acidic catalyst sulfuric acid is heated at a temperature of about one hundred degrees centigrade for twelve hours. The hot solution then is poured over cracked ice and the resulting mixture stirred until hydrolysis of the excess acetic anhydride is complete. The solid product which precipitates is removed by filtration, washed with water and dried under vacuum. Purified 9α-fluoro-17α-methyl-5α-androstane-3β,11β,17β-triol 3,11,17-triacetate is obtained by recrystallization of chromatographic separation. 9α-fluoro - 17α - methyl - 5β - androstane - 3α,11β,17β - triol 3,11,17-triacetate is obtained in exactly the same manner by substituting 9α-fluoro-17α-methyl-5β-androstane-3α,11β,17β-triol for the above starting steroid. By sub-

stituting the appropriate acylating agent, i. e. the appropriate acid anhydride or isopropenyl acylate, in the above procedure other 3,11,17-triacylates of 9α-fluoro-, 9α-chloro-, 9α-bromo-, and 9α-iodo-17α-methyl-5α(and 5β)-androstane-3β(and 3α),11β,17β-triol and 9α-fluoro-, 9α-chloro-, 9α-bromo-, and 9α-iodo-17α-methyl-19-nor-5α(and 5β)-androstane-3β(and 3α),11β,17β-triol are obtained including the 3,11,17-tripropionate, triacetate, tri-(trimethylacetate), trifuorate, tri-(α or β-cyclohexylpropionate), tribenzoate, tri-(phenylacetate), tri-(α or β-cyclopentylpropionate), tri-(α or β-phenylpropionate), tri-methylbenzoates), tri-(α or β-furylacrylates), trivalerate, tri-(methacrylate), 11-acetate 3,17-diformate, 11-(β-cyclopentylpropionate) 3,17-diacetate, and the like. The foregoing 3,17-diacylates and 3,11,17-triacylates, and also 17-monoacylates and 11,17-diacylates as well as other 3,17-diacylates and other 3,11,17-triacylates, can be prepared by hydrogenation, according to the process of the present invention, of corresponding 17-acylates and 11,17-diacylates of 9α-fluoro-, 9α-chloro-, 9α-bromo-, and 9α-iodo-11β,17β-dihydroxy-17α-methyl-5α(and 5β)-androstane-3-one and 9α-fluoro-, 9α-chloro-, 9α-bromo-, and 9α - iodo - 11β,17β-dihydroxy-17α-methyl-19-nor-5α-(and 5β)-androstane-3-one, followed by acylation according to the procedure of Examples 4 and/or 5, when applicable, to obtain the desired acylated product. The 17-monoacylates, 3,17-diacylates, 11,17-diacylates and 3,11,17 - triacylates of other 9α-h lo-17α-alkyl-5α(and 5β)-androstane-3β(and 3α),11β,17β-triols and 9α-halo-17α - alkyl-19-nor-5α(and 5β)-androstane-3β(and 3α),-11β,17β-triols, wherein the alkyl and acylate radicals and the halo atom are as defined and illustrated above, also are prepared by the foregoing procedures.

I claim:

1. 9α - halo - 17α-methylandrostane-3,11β,17β-triol of the formula

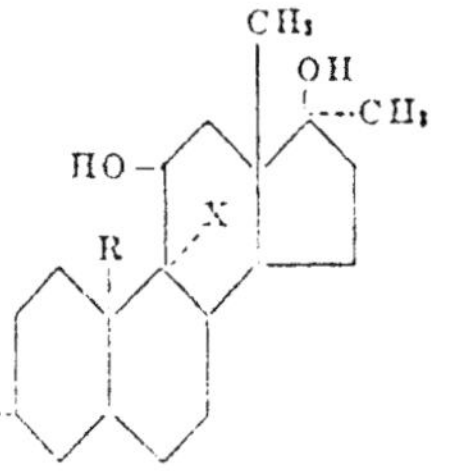

wherein R is selected from hydrogen and methyl and X is a halogen atom having an atomic weight from nineteen to 127.

2. 9α - halo - 17α - methylandrostane - 3,11β,17β-triol wherein the halo atom has an atomic weight from nineteen to 36.

3. 9α - halo - 17α - methyl - 19 - norandrostane - 3,-11β,17β-triol wherein the halo atom has an atomic weight from nineteen to 36.

4. 9α - fluoro - 17α - methyl - 5α - androstane - 3β,-11β,17β-triol.

5. 9α - fluoro - 17α - methyl - 5β - androstane - 3α,-11β,17β-triol.

6. 9α - fluoro - 17α - methyl - 19 - nor - 5α - androstane-3β,11β,17β-triol.

7. 9α - fluoro - 17α - methyl - 19 - nor - 5β - androstane-3α,11β,17β-triol.

No references cited.

CHAPTER SIX

1

3,361,773
1α-METHYL STEROIDS
Rudolf Wiechert, Berlin-Lichterfelde, Germany, assignor
to Schering A.G., Berlin, Germany
No Drawing. Filed Mar. 24, 1961, Ser. No. 98.026
Claims priority, application Germany, Apr. 6, 1960,
Sch 27,696; July 21, 1960, Sch 28,196; Dec. 23,
1960, Sch 28,955
12 Claims. (Cl. 260—397.4)

The present invention relates to 1α-methyl steroids, and more particularly to 1α-methyl-3-ketosteroids and to methods of producing the same.

German Patent No. 1,023,764 describes the hydrogenation of 1-methyl-Δ^1-3-ketosteroids produced by decomposition of diazomethane addition products of Δ^1-3-ketosteroids, the hydrogenation being carried out by normal methods. Since the hydrogen enters the steroid molecule by this hydrogenation due to steric influences at the back of the steroid molecule the resulting compound is a 1β-methyl-3-ketosteroid. Corresponding 1α-methyl-3-ketosteroids were not produced prior to the present invention.

It is accordingly a primary object of the present invention to provide for the production of 1α-methyl-3-ketosteroids.

It is another object of the present invention to provide a new series of compounds, namely 1α-methyl-3-ketosteroids which have valuable properties as intermediates in the production of other useful steroids, and which are themselves valuable for various pharmacological purposes, which are in general the same pharmacological purposes as for the corresponding steroids which do not contain a 1α-methyl group, however, the compounds of the present invention having improved activities in this respect.

The present invention also provides for various methods of producing not only the new 1α-methyl-steroids which are specifically claimed herein, but also methods which are generally applicable to the production of any 1α-methyl-3-ketosteroid.

Other objects and advantages of the present invention will be apparent from a further reading of the specification and of the appended claims.

With the above and other objects in view, the present invention mainly comprises a compound of the formula:

(I)

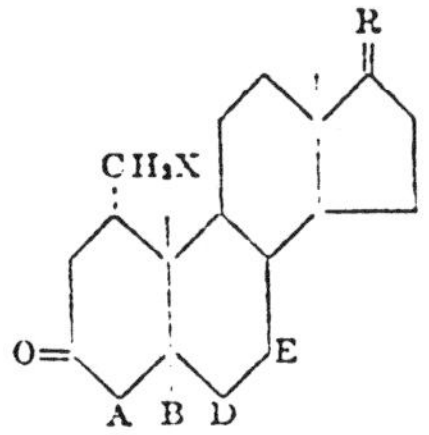

wherein X is selected from the group consisting of hydrogen and halogen, wherein

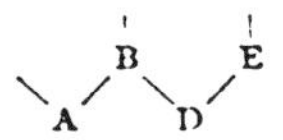

is selected from the group consisting of

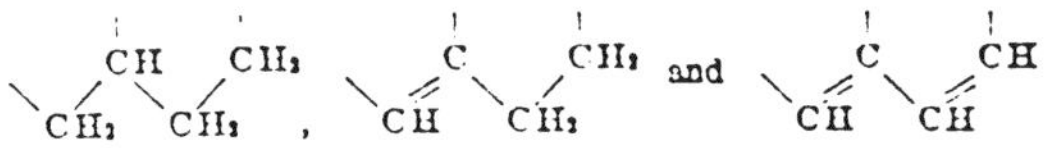

and wherein R is selected from the group consisting of

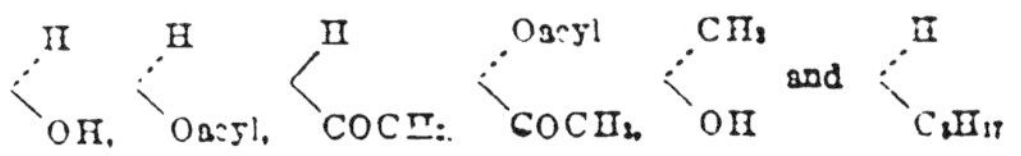

wherein acyl is derived from a lower aliphatic carboxylic acid.

As indicated above, one of the primary objects of the present invention is to provide for the production of the new 1α-methyl-3-ketosteroids which are set forth above.

It is still another object of the present invention to provide methods which can be used not only for the production of the particular 1α-methyl-3-ketosteroids set forth above, but which are actually generally applicable to the production of any 1α-methyl-3-ketosteroid. These methods will be further discussed below and it will be seen that although for purposes of convenience specific reference is had to the production of compounds of the above set forth general formula, that the methods are equally applicable to the production of other 1α-methyl-3-ketosteroids, and in fact to any 1α-methyl-3-ketosteroids.

In accordance with one method of embodiment of the present invention it has been found if the cyclopropane ring of a 1,2α-methylene-3-ketosteroid is opened with a hydrogen halide acid the resulting compound is a 1α-halomethyl-3-ketosteroid which can be dehalogenated by hydrogenation to produce the corresponding 1α-methyl-3-ketosteroid. The reaction proceeds in accordance with the following equations:

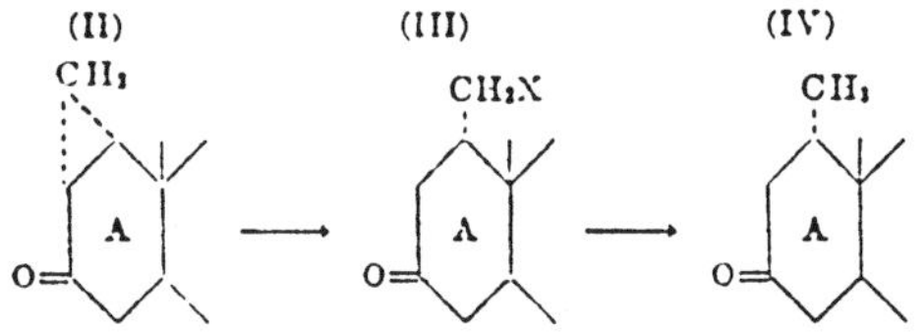

Suitable starting materials of this method are described in German Patent No. 1,072,991 and German Patent No. 1,096,353. Starting compounds for this method may also be produced according to the method of German Patent No. 1,023,764 and U.S. patent application Ser. No. 73,495 filed Dec. 5, 1960, now U.S. Patent No. 3,134,792, by Emanuel Kaspar et al. According to the method set forth therein 1,2-methylene-3-ketosteroids are obtained as side products along with the primarily produced products 1-methyl-Δ^1-3-ketosteroids, the 1,2-methylene-3-ketosteroids being obtained in relatively considerable amount. Accordingly, the method of the present invention which provides for the conversion of 1,2-methylene-3-ketosteroids into 1α-methyl-3-ketosteroids which are extremely valuable products, as will be further discussed below, is a technically valuable method in that it makes use of a side product.

According to another method embodiment of the present invention the desired 1α-methyl-3-ketosteroids are obtained in another manner starting from the same 1,2α-methylene-3-ketosteroids, not by treatment with a hydrohalic acid as described above, but by opening the cyclopropane ring of the mentioned 1,2-methylene-3-ketosteroids by catalytically directed hydrogen, preferably in the presence of a platinum catalyst in glacial acetic acid. This results in the production of the 1α-methyl-3-hydroxyl-steroid since the hydrogenation results simultaneously in the reduction of the 3-keto group to the corresponding secondary alcohol group, which latter may then be reconverted by oxidation into the keto group in known manner, for example by means of chromic acid or in accordance with the Oppenauer method, if the keto steroid is desired as the final product. This method of proceeding is summarized by the following reaction mechanism:

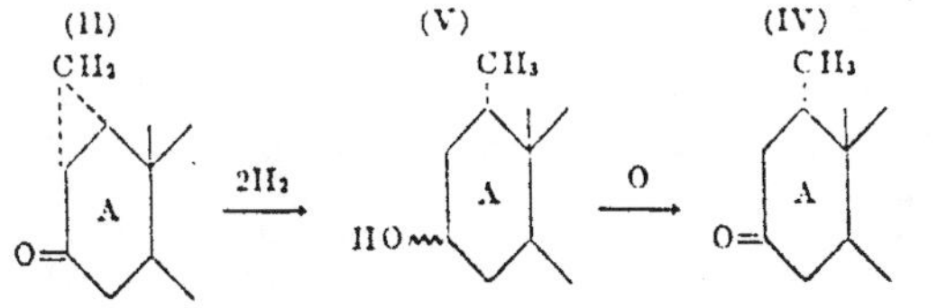

In accordance with still another embodiment of the present invention 1α-methyl-3-ketosteroids can be produced directly from the corresponding Δ^1-3-ketosteroids by reaction with methylmagnesiumhalide in the presence of cuprous chloride. It has been found that this Grignard reagent quite surprisingly does not react in the normal manner with the 3-keto group. Instead the reaction which occurs is a 1,4-addition of the Grignard reagent onto the Δ^1-3-keto group (the so-called anomalous Grignard reaction) and by further normal working up of the Grignardation mixture the desired 1α-methyl steroid is obtained. The reaction mechanism is as follows:

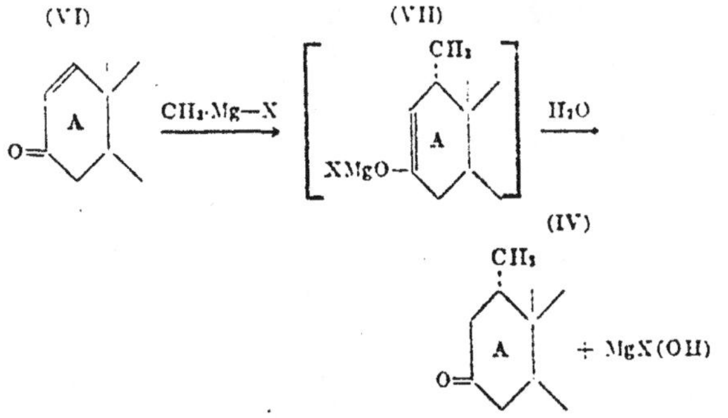

This last described method of proceeding is distinguished by its simplicity. This method saves an entire series of reaction stages, which becomes more clearly apparent, when it is remembered that in the first two methods variations set forth above the starting material i.e. 1,2α-methylene compounds are obtained in relatively moderate yields in multistage methods from the corresponding Δ^1-3-ketosteroids, in some cases even by a wide detour from the corresponding $\Delta^{1,4,6}$-3-ketosteroids.

The possibility of utilizing the anomalous Grignard reaction in accordance with the present invention could not certainly be predicted although it is known that Grignardation of α,β-unsaturated ketosteroids occasionally gives rise to an anomalous course of reaction. Comparison may be made for example with the conversion of Δ^{16}-20-ketosteroids to 16α-methyl-20-ketosteroids (Helv. Chimica Acta 42 [1959], page 2043). Since the Δ^{16}-20-ketosteroid in many reactions exhibits behavior which deviates from that of the α,β-unsaturated 3-ketosteroids (in the reaction with haloforms in the presence of potassium tertiary butylate the Δ^1-3-ketosteroid behaves in a different manner from the Δ^{16}-20-ketosteroid, and it has also been noted that the 18-Nor-Δ^{12}-11-ketosteroid in the presence of cuprous chloride does not give a 1,4-addition with methylmagnesium iodide) it could not be predicted that Δ^1-3-ketosteroids and Δ^{16}-20-ketosteroids would react in a comparable manner with Grignard reagents.

All three method variations have as a basis the treatment finally of Δ^1-3-ketosteroids with such agents which with saturation of the Δ^1-double bond are adapted to bind a methyl group or a group convertible to a methyl group with the carbon atom 1 standing β to the keto group, and if necessary the group convertible to the methyl group is subsequently converted to the methyl

group. All of this is illustrated by the following general reaction scheme:

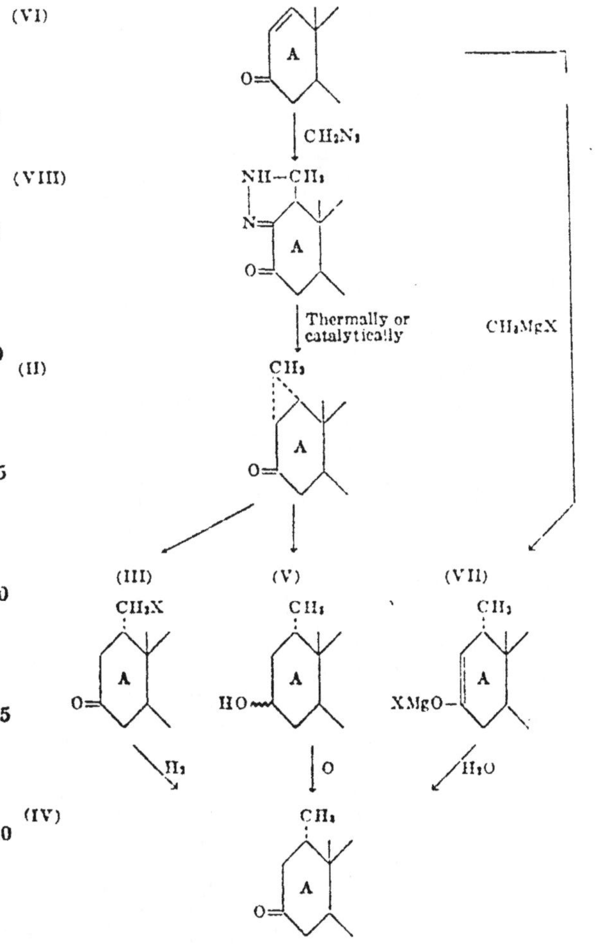

The method of the present invention is applicable, as indicated above, to all Δ^1-3-ketosteroids or their primary addition products, and these steroids can also contain various other substituents in various places of the molecule, for example substituents in 6,9,11,16 and 17-position of the molecule, such substituents being, for example, hydrocarbon radicals, halogens or hydroxyl groups either in free, esterified or etherified condition. Furthermore, in the 17-position there can be an acetyl group or a ketol side chain. In the case of the procedure with the Grignard reagent reactable groups such as a 20-keto group should first in known manner be blocked or protected, for example by prior acetalisation thereof.

A special discussion follows with respect to the presence of additional double bonds. The additional presence of a Δ^4-double bond practically prevents the addition of the diazomethane and the Grignard reagent onto the Δ^1-double bond, while this reaction proceeds normally as described above with the still further presence with the Δ^4-double bond of a Δ^6-double bond. The primary addition products of $\Delta^{1,4,6}$-3-ketosteroids have particular value for the method of the present invention since it is possible from its primary intermediate or end product, as illustrated in the following examples, in a smooth reaction to eliminate the Δ^6-double bond by selective hydrogenation. In this manner it is possible to arrive at the very valuable 1α-methyl-Δ⁴-3-ketosteroids. This is illustrated in the following reaction scheme:

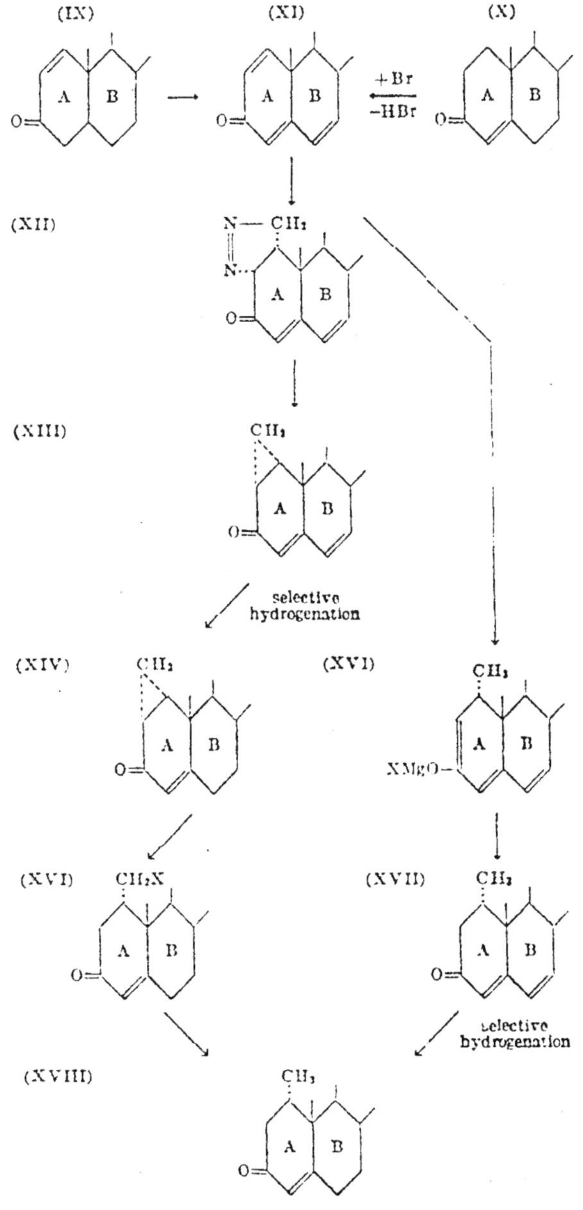

If it is desired in the final product (compound XVIII) to have any present hydroxyl group, for example in the 17-position, in esterified or etherified condition, it is naturally possible to start either with compounds in which the hydroxyl group is already in etherified or esterified condition, or to start with compounds which contain the free hydroxyl group and to esterify or etherify the resulting compound after carrying out the method of the invention.

The 1α-methyl-compounds produced by the method of the present invention are extremely valuable either themselves per se for therapeutic purposes or as intermediate products for the production of valuable steroids. In general these compounds have the same pharmacological properties as the corresponding compounds which do not contain a 1α-methyl group, however, the presence of the 1α-methyl group having the effect of improving the activity thereof.

Thus, for example, 1α-methyl-androstane-17β-ol-3-one-17-acetate (and even already the 1α-chloromethyl-androstane-17β-ol-3-one-17-acetate) exhibit a very strong androgenic and simultaneously a strong anabolic activity

upon subcutaneous administration to castrated male rats. The free 1α-methyl-androstane-17β-ol-3-one is in animal tests upon subcutaneous administration to rats stand to have an anabolic activity which is approximately 4.8 times as great as the same compound which is not methylated in the 1-position, which compound is sold commercially under the trade name of "Anaboleen."

Also the 1α-methyl-Δ⁴-androstene-17β-ol-3-one is anabolically active. Its 17 esters are still more active in this direction. Thus, its acetate in a dose of 12×1000γ (subcutaneously) in rats is anabolically as active as 1-methyl-Δ¹-androstene-17β-ol-3-one-17-acetate or 19-Nor-testosterone-phenyl propionate, however at the same time having only 45% of the undesired androgenic side action of the named comparison substances.

As an example of the use of the compounds produced according to the method of the present invention as intermediate products in the production of pharmaceutically valuable steroids there may be mentioned the conversion of the 1α-methyl-androstane-17β-ol-3-one, or its 17-acetate into the above named 1-methyl-Δ¹-androstene-17β-ol-3-one and its still more anabolically active ester.

The following examples are given to further illustrate the present invention. However, it is to be understood, particularly with respect to the methods of the present invention, that the invention is not meant to be limied to the specific details of the examples.

Example 1

1 g. of 1,2α-methylene-androstane-17β-ol-3-one-17-acetate having a melting point of 139–140° C.;

$$[\alpha]_D^{26} = +54° \text{ (CHCl}_3; \text{ c.}=1.00); \text{ U.V. } \epsilon_{208}=3{,}950$$

are dissolved in 10 cc. of methylene chloride. The solution is saturated with hydrogen chloride, after 16 hours of standing at room temperature it is diluted with methylene chloride, washed with water until neutral and dried over sodium sulfate. By evaporation of the solvent a residue remains of 1α-chloromethyl-androstane-17β-ol-3-one-17-acetate.

500 mg. of this residue in 20 cc. of ethyl alcohol are heated to boiling with 1 g. of Raney nickel for 4 hours in a reflux condenser. After filtering off the Raney nickel the alcoholic solution is diluted with methylene chloride, washed with water dried over sodium sulfate and evaporated in water to dryness. By recrystallization from hexane there is obtained 50 mg. of 1α-methyl-androstane-17β-ol-3-one-17-acetate having a melting point of 169–170° C. $[\alpha]_D^{26} = +16.7°$ (CHCl₃; c.=0.88).

Example 2

200 mg. of 1,2α-methylene-androstane-17β-ol-3-one-17-acetate are dissolved in 20 cc. of methylene chloride. The solution is saturated with hydrogen bromide, stored at room temperature for 30 minutes in a closed container, then washed with water until neutral, dried over sodium sulfate and concentrated under vacuum to dryness. The residue which remains is 1α-bromomethyl-androstane-17β-ol-3-one-17-acetate having a melting point of 135° C. The compound 1α-chloromethyl-androstadiene-17β-ol-3-one-17-acetate may be produced in an analogous manner.

By treatment with Raney nickel as described in Example 1 there is obtained from the residue 1α-methyl-androstane-17β-ol-3-one-17-acetate having a melting point of 169–170° C.

Example 3

930 mg. of 1,2α-methylene-androstane-17β-ol-3-one-17-acetate are stirred for 16 hours at 30° C. in 25 cc. of formic acid with 5 g. of potassium iodide. The solution is diluted with methylene chloride, washed with water until neutral, dried over sodium sulfate and evaporated to dryness under vacuum. By recrystallization of the residue from isopropyl ether there is obtained 1108 mg. of 1α-iodomethyl-androstane-17β-ol-3-one-17-acetate having a melting point of 155.5–157.5° C.

7

$[\alpha]_D^{25} = +27.9°$ (CHCl$_3$; c.=0.955)

790 mg. of 1α-iodomethyl-androstane-17β-ol-3-one-17-acetate are stirred for 4 hours at room temperature in 55 cc. of ethyl alcohol with 2.5 g. of Raney nickel, and then further worked up as described in Example 1. By recrystallization of the crude product from hexane there is obtained 510 mg. of 1α-methyl-androstane-17β-ol-3-one-17-acetate having a melting point of 169–170° C.

500 mg. of 1α-methyl-androstane-17β-ol-3-one-17-acetate are heated for 90 minutes under nitrogen and under refluxing in 5 cc. of 4% methanolic sodium hydroxide solution. It is then stirred into ice water, the precipitated product is filtered off under suction and recrystallized from isopropyl ether. The resulting 1α-methyl-androstane-17β-ol-3-one melts at 203.5–205° C.

$[\alpha]_D^{20} = +17.6°$ (CHCl$_3$; c.=0.875)

Example 4

200 mg. of 1,2α-methylene-Δ^{4,6}-androstadiene-17β-ol-3-one-17-acetate, 5 cc. of 98% formic acid and 1 g. of potassium iodide are treated and worked up as described in Example 3. There is recrystallized from is___ yl ether 230 mg. of 1α-iodomethyl-Δ^{4,6}-androstadiene-17β-ol-3-one-17-acetate having a melting point of 109.5–111.5° C. $[\alpha]_D^{25} = -17.9°$ (in chloroform c.=0.995).

200 mg. of 1α-iodomethyl-Δ^{4,6}-androstadiene-17β-ol-3-one-17-acetate in 15 cc. of ethanol with 600 mg. of Raney nickel are reacted and worked up as described in Example 1. There is recrystallized from isopropyl ether 130 mg. of 1α-methyl-Δ^{4,6}-androstadiene-17β-ol-3-one-17-acetate having a melting point of 156–157° C. UV.:ϵ_{285}=24.600.

Example 5

200 mg. of 1,2α-methylene-Δ^4-androstene-17β-ol-3-one in 5 cc. of 98% formic acid containing 1 g. of potassium iodide are reacted and worked up as described in Example 3. The resulting crude 1α-iodomethyl-Δ^4-androstene-17β-ol-3-one is treated and worked up in 15 cc. of ethanol containing 600 mg. of Raney nickel analogously to the method described in Example 3. There is recrystallized from isopropyl ether 1α-methyl-Δ^4-androstene-17β-ol-3-one having a melting point of 190–191° C. The yield is 125 mg. U.V.:ϵ_{243}=14.900.

500 mg. of 1α-methyl-Δ^4-androstene-17β-ol-3-one are allowed to stand at room temperature for 16 hours in 2 cc. of pyridine and 2 cc. of acetanhydride. After stirring into ice water there precipitates 1α-methyl-Δ^4-androstene-17β-ol-3-one-17-acetate which is filtered off under suction, dried and recrystallized from pentane. The compound melts at 140° C. $[\alpha]_D^{26} = +109°$ (CHCl$_3$; c.=1.00).

Example 6

90 mg. of 1.2α-methylene-Δ^{4,6}-pregnadiene-17α-ol-3.20-dione-17-acetate in 2 cc. of formic acid are treated with 450 mg. of potassium iodide as described in Example 3. further worked up, and rubbed with isopropyl ether. There is thus obtained 1α-iodomethyl-Δ^{4,6}-pregnadiene-17α-ol-3.20-dione-17-acetate having a melting point of 196–196.5° C. This compound is further treated in 6 cc. of ethanol with 250 mg. of Raney nickel as described in Example 3. and then isolated. There is thus obtained 1α-methyl-Δ^{4,6}-pregnadiene-17α-ol-3.20-dione-17-acetate having a melting point from ethyl acetate of 206–207° C. U.V.:ϵ_{281}=24.300.

Example 7

344 mg. of 1,2α-methylene-androstane-17β-ol-3-one-17-acetate are dissolved in 10 cc. of glacial acetic acid and then hydrogenated at room temperature with the addition of 100 mg. of platinum oxide until 2 mol equivalents of hydrogen has been taken up. The catalyst is then filtered off. the reaction mixture is stirred into ice water, extracted with methylene chloride and the methylene chloride phase is washed with sodium bicarbonate solution as

8

well as with water. After drying over sodium sulfate it is concentrated to dryness under vacuum.

The residue is mixed with 17 cc. of absolute toluene and 3.7 cc. of cyclohexanone. Several cc. of the solvent are then distilled off to remove any moisture present and then 186 mg. of aluminum isopropylate and 1.9 cc. of toluene are added thereto during a time period of 5 minutes. The reaction mixture is then heated for 45 minutes while slowly partially distilling off the solvent. It is then diluted with methylene chloride, with 2 normal sulfuric acid and washed with water. The methylene chloride phase is steam distilled off. The residue of the steam distillation is taken up in methylene chloride, the organic phase is dried over sodium sulfate, subsequently concentrated under vacuum after filtering off the drying agent. and the residue is recrystallized from hexane. There is thus obtained 1α - methylandrostane-17β-ol-3-one-17-acetate having a melting point of 169–170° C.

$[\alpha]_D^{25} = +16.7°$ (CHCl$_3$; c.=0.88)

Example 8

2 g. of 1.2α - methylene-androstane-17β-ol-3-one-17-acetate are dissolved in 58 cc. of glacial acetic acid and then hydrogenated at room temperature with the addition of 500 mg. of platinum oxide. When no more hydrogen is being taken up the the reaction mixture is filtered free of the catalyst. stirred into ice water and the precipitated product is filtered off. It is then dried under vacuum at 70° C. there is thus obtained 1.88 g. of crude 1α-methyl-androstane-3ξ.17β-diol-17-acetate which is reacted under stirring in 30 cc. of acetone with 1.3 cc. of chromic acid solution (chromic acid solution: 267 g. of chromium trioxide, 230 cc. of concentrated sulfuric acid, 400 cc. of water to dilute 1 liter). It is stirred into ice water. the precipitated product is filtered off under suction, washed, dried and recrystallized from hexane. There is thus obtained 1.27 g. of 1α-methyl-androstane-17β-ol-3-one-17-acetate having a melting point of 169–169.5° C.

Example 9

6.3 cc. of methyl iodide are slowly added dropwise to 2 g. of magnesium shavings and 70 cc. of absolute ether. at room temperature under stirring and under nitrogen atmosphere. After about 30 minutes 120 cc. of absolute tetrahydrofurane are slowly added thereto and subsequently liquid is distilled off until a boiling point of 62° C. is reached. After cooling to room temperature 400 mg. of cuprous chloride are added. 5.77 g. of Δ^1-androstene-17β-ol-3-one dissolved in 30 cc. of absolute tetrahydrofurane are then slowly added dropwise. The resulting precipitate is maintained in a stirrable condition by the addition of 120 cc. of absolute tetrahydrofurane. After 30 minutes of reaction time the reaction mixture is cooled to 0° C.. the excess Grignard reagent is reacted with saturated ammonium chloride solution. diluted with ether and the aqueous phase is separated. The ethereal phase is washed sequentially with aqueous sodium thiosulfate solution. saturated ammonium chloride solution and water. It is then dried over sodium sulfate and concentrated under vacuum to dryness. The residue is recrystallized from ethyl acetate. There is thus obtained 1α-methyl-androstane -17β-ol-3-one having a melting point of 203.5–205° C. $[\alpha]_D^{20} = +17.6$ (CHCl$_3$; c.=0.875). The yield corresponds to 65% of the theoretical (without working up the mother liquor).

Example 10

A Grignard solution is produced as described in Example 9 from 200 mg. of magnesium turnings. 7 cc. of absolute ether and 0.55 cc. of methyliodide. 12 cc. of absolute tetrahydrofurane are then added thereto and 11 cc. of liquid are distilled off. A solution of 661 mg. of Δ^1-androstene-17β-ol-3-one-17-acetate in 5 cc. of absolute tetrahydrofurane are then added dropwise to the Grignard reaction mixture. After the addition of 10 cc. of tetrahydrofurane the resulting slurry is maintained in stirrable condition. After 30 minutes the reaction mixture is worked up as described in Example 9.

The thus obtained 1α-methyl-androstane-17β-ol-3-one-17-acetate after recrystallization from isopropyl ether melts at 169–170° C.

$$[\alpha]_D^{26} = +16.7 \ (CHCl_3; \ c.=0.88)$$

The yield corresponds to 66% of the theoretical. Further amounts can be obtained from the mother liquor by subsequent acetylation thereof.

Example 11

12 cc. of absolute tetrahydrofurane are added to a Grignard solution prepared as described in Example 9 from 200 mg. of magnesium shavings, 7 cc. of absolute ether and 0.55 cc. of methyl iodide, and 11 cc. of liquid is then distilled off. 20 mg. of cuprous chloride are then added thereto at room temperature.

A solution of 605 mg. of 17α-methyl-Δ1-androstene-17β-ol-3-one in 5 cc. of absolute tetrahydrofurane are then added to the solution. After the addition of 10 cc. of absolute tetrahydrofurane the resulting slurry remains in stirrable condition. After 30 minutes of reaction time the working up proceeds as described in Example 9.

The thus obtained 1,17α-dimethyl-androstane-17β-ol-3-one after recrystallization from isopropyl ether melts at 177–178° C. $[\alpha]_D^{26} = +4.4°$ (CHCl₃; c.=0.997). The yield corresponds to 55% of the theoretical (without working up of the mother liquor).

Example 12

Methylbromide is added to 3.063 g. of magnesium shavings in 107 cc. of absolute ether until the metal goes into solution, the addition being made slowly at room temperature. After subsequent addition of 185 cc. of absolute tetrahydrofurane liquid is distilled off until a boiling point of 62° C. is attained. 613 mg. of cuprous chloride are then added thereto at room temperature and 10 g. of Δ1-androstene-17β-ol-3-one in 35 cc. of tetrahydrofurane are subsequently added. After the addition of 200 cc. the sediment remains in stirrable condition.

After 30 minutes the reaction mixture is further worked up as described in Example 9. The thus obtained residue is allowed to stand overnight in 40 cc. of pyridine and 40 cc. of acetanhydride at room temperature, and is then stirred into ice water. The resulting precipitate is filtered off under suction, dried and recrystallized from isopropyl ether. There is thus obtained 9 g. of 1α-methyl-androstane-17β-ol-3-one-17-acetate having a melting point of 169° C.

Example 13

769 mg. of Δ1-cholestene-3-one are reacted with methyl-magnesium iodide under the same molar relationships and under the same conditions described in Example 9, further worked up as described in Example 9 and then recrystallized from methanol. There is thus obtained 355 mg. of 1α-methyl-cholestane-3-one having a melting point of 130–131° C.

Example 14

8.42 cc. of methyl iodide are slowly added dropwise to 3.067 g. of magnesium shavings and 107 cc. of absolute ether at room temperature, under stirring and under a nitrogen atmosphere. After about 30 minutes 185 cc. of absolute tetrahydrofurane are added thereto and liquid is subsequently distilled off until a boiling point of 62° C. is reached. After cooling to room temperature 613 mg. of cuprous chloride are added thereto and thereafter 10 g. of Δ1.4.6-androstatriene-17β-ol-3-one-17-acetate in 110 cc. of tetrahydrofurane are slowly added. After 30 minutes of reaction time the reaction mixture is cooled to 0° C., the excess Grignard reagent is reacted with saturated ammonium chloride solution, diluted with ether and the aqueous phase is separated.

The ethereal phase is washed one after the other with aqueous sodium thiosulfate solution, saturated ammonium chloride solution and water. It is dried over sodium sulfate and evaporated to dryness under vacuum. The residue is dissolved in 40 cc. of pyridine and 20 cc. of acetic anhydride and allowed to stand at room temperature for 16 hours. It is stirred into ice water, the resulting precipitate is filtered off under suction, dried and recrystallized from isopropyl ether. There is thus obtained 1α-methyl-Δ4.6-androstadiene-17β-ol-3-one-17-acetate having a melting point of 156–157° C. $[\alpha]_D^{25} = -33.8°$ (in CHCl₃, c.=0.9). U.V.: $\epsilon_{286} = 25,800$. The yield corresponds to 65–70% of the theoretical.

4.67 g. of 1α-methyl-Δ4.6-androstadiene-17β-ol-3-one-17-acetate are dissolved in 273 cc. of methanol and after the addition of 350 mg. of 10% palladium on calcium carbonate as catalyst it is hydrogenated until 1 mol equivalent of hydrogen is taken up. After filtering off the catalyst the solution is reacted with 50 cc. of 2 normal hydrochloric acid and concentrated under vacuum to about one third its volume. It is then diluted with water and extracted with ether. The ethereal solution is washed with water until neutral, dried over sodium sulfate and concentrated. The crude product is heated on a steam bath for 90 minutes in 10 cc. of pyridine and 10 cc. of acetanhydride. The ether is then taken up and the ethereal phase washed with water until neutral. After drying and evaporation of the solution the obtained crude crystalline 1α-methyl-Δ4-androstene-17β-ol-3-one-17-acetate melts at 122–129° C. U.V.: $\epsilon_{244} = 13,500$. The yield corresponds to 98% of the theoretical.

The purified 1α-methyl-Δ4-androstene-17β-ol-3-one-17-acetate recrystallized from isopropyl ether melts at 138–139° C. U.V.: $\epsilon_{243} = 14,900$. $[\alpha]_D^{20} = +109°$ (in CHCl₃, c.=1.00).

Example 15

Δ1.4.6-androstatriene-17β-ol-3-one-17-propionate is reacted analogously to the method described in Example 14. Instead of acetanhydride propionic acid anhydride is utilized for the esterification. The esterification time amounts to 88 hours at room temperature. The obtained 1α-methyl-Δ4-androstene-17β-ol-3-one-17-propionate after recrystallization from pentane melts at 105–106° C.

Example 16

Δ1.4.6-androstatriene-17β-ol-3-one is reacted in the same manner and under the same molar ratios as described in Example 14 with methyl-magnesium iodide and then worked up. The obtained 1α-methyl-Δ4.6-androstadiene-17β-ol-3-one melts at 205–206° C. U.V.: $\epsilon_{286} = 26,300$.

By hydrogenation analogous to the manner described in Example 14 there is then obtained 1α-methyl-Δ4-androstene-17β-ol-3-one melting at 191° C. U.V.: $\epsilon_{244} = 14,600$.

Example 17

Methyl bromide is added to 3.067 g. of magnesium shavings and 107 cc. of absolute ether at room temperature until dissolution of the metal. This solution is reacted with 10 g. of Δ1.4.6-androstatriene-17β-ol-3-one-17-acetate as described in Example 14.

There is thus obtained 5.01 g. of 1α-methyl-Δ4.6-androstadiene-17β-ol-3-one-17-acetate having a melting point of 156–157° C.

Without further analysis, the foregoing will so fully reveal the gist of the present invention that others can by applying current knowledge readily adapt it for various applications without omitting features that, from the standpoint of prior art, fairly constitute essential characteristics of the generic or specific aspects of this invention and, therefore, such adaptations should and are intended to be comprehended within the meaning and range of equivalence of the following claims.

What is claimed as new and desired to be secured by Letters Patent is:

11

1. A compound of the formula:

wherein X is selected from the group consisting of hydrogen and halogen; wherein

is

and wherein R is selected from the group consisting of

wherein acyl is derived from a lower aliphatic carboxylic acid.

2. 1α-methyl-androstane-17β-ol-3-one.

3. Lower aliphatic carboxylic acid 17-esters of 1α-methyl-androstane-17β-ol-3-one.

4. 1α-iodomethyl-androstane-17β-ol-3-one-17-acetate.

5. 1α-bromomethyl-androstane-17β-ol-3- one - 17 -acetate.

6. 1α-chloromethyl - Δ4,6 - androstadiene-17β-ol-3-one-17-acetate.

7. 1α-iodomethyl-Δ4,6-androstadiene-17β-ol-3-one - 17-acetate.

8. 1α-iodomethyl-Δ4-androstene-17β-ol-3-one.

9. 1α - iodomethyl-Δ4,6-pregnadiene-17α-ol-3,20-dione-17-acetate.

12

10. The method which comprises reacting a 1,2α-methylene-3-ketosteroid with a hydrogen halide so as to open the cyclopropane ring and form the corresponding 1α-halomethyl-3-ketosteroid.

11. The method which comprises reacting a 1,2α-methylene-3-ketosteroid with a hydrogen halide so as to open the cyclopropane ring and form the corresponding 1α-halomethyl-3-ketosteroid; and hydrogenating said 1α-halomethyl-3-ketosteroid so as to dehalogenate the same and form the corresponding 1α-methyl-3-ketosteroid.

12. The method which comprises selectively hydrogenating the Δ6-double bond of a 1,2α-methylene-Δ4,6-3-ketosteroid by means of a palladium catalyst so as to form the corresponding 1,2α-methylene-Δ4-3-ketosteroid; reacting said 1,2α-methylene-Δ4-3-ketosteroid with a hydrogen halide so as to open the cyclopropane ring and form the corresponding 1α-halomethyl-Δ4-3-ketosteroid; and dehalogenating said 1α-halomethyl-Δ4-3-ketosteroid with hydrogen so as to form the corresponding 1α-methyl-Δ4-3-ketosteroid.

References Cited

UNITED STATES PATENTS

2,739,974	3/1956	Colton	260—397.3
2,908,693	10/1959	Ringold et al.	260—397.4
3,032,552	5/1962	Ringold et al.	260—239.55

OTHER REFERENCES

Bowers et al.: Journal of American Chemical Society, vol. 79 (1957), p. 4557 relied on.

Fieser et al.: "Steroids" (1959), Reinhold Publishing Corp., New York. p. 287 relied on.

Ringold et al.: Journal of American Chemical Society, vol. 78 (1956), p. 2477 relied on.

ELBERT L. ROBERTS, *Primary Examiner.*

L. H. GASTON, I. MARCUS, L. GOTTS, M. LIEBMAN.
Examiners.

CHAPTER SIX

1

2

3,361,774
1-METHYL-Δ¹-5α ANDROSTENE INCLUDING ESTERS AND PROCESS OF MAKING THE SAME

Josef Hader, Friedmund Neumann, and Rudolf Wiechert, Berlin, Germany, assignors to Schering Aktiengesellschaft, Berlin, Germany
No Drawing. Filed June 14, 1965, Ser. No. 463,852
Claims priority, application Germany, July 22, 1964, Sch 35,509
4 Claims. (Cl. 260—397.4)

ABSTRACT OF THE DISCLOSURE

1-methyl-Δ¹-5α-androstene-17β-ol-3-one 17-esters of the general formula

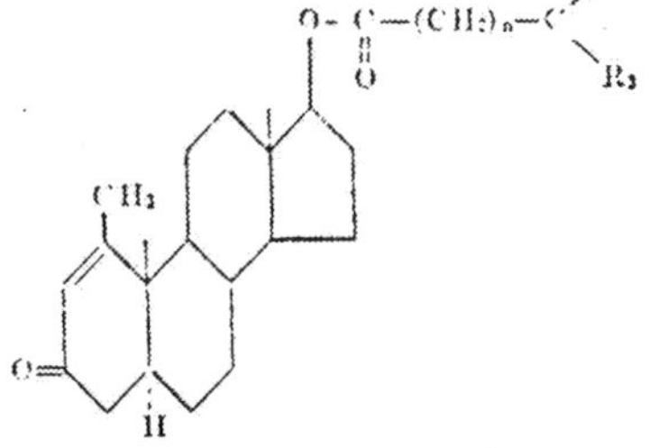

wherein R_1 is chlorine and R_2 and R_3 are members selected from the group consisting of hydrogen and chlorine and wherein n is 0 or 1.

1-methyl-Δ¹-5α-androstene 17β-ol-3-one is known. Likewise known are the 17-acetate and 17-propionate derivative of this compound. All of these compounds are useful as anabolics.

Surprisingly it was now found that the anabolic effect of the just mentioned compounds can be substantially increased by substituting the alkyl group of the ester residue and particularly of the acetate residue by halogen and preferably chlorine. The thus formed compounds of the invention have been tested in the conventional tests for anabolic and androgenic action using castrated male rats and administering them by subcutaneous application. Surprisingly there resulted not only greater weight increase of the levator ani, but the weight increase of the seminal vesicle was distinctly lower than in the case of the earlier mentioned known compounds. Thus the compounds of the invention provide opportunity for an unusually favorable differentiation of the ratio of activity (Q) between anabolic action and androgenic side effect. This favorable ratio was entirely unpredictable. It is more specifically illustrated by the following table which compares 17-dichloracetate of the invention with the 17-acetate of the prior art:

Substance	Dose mg./ Animal	Levator ani (mg.)	Seminal Vesicle (mg.)	Anabolic/ Q-androgenic
1-methyl-Δ¹-5α-androstene-17β-ol-3-one-dichloracetate	0.3	50	71	0.704
	0.1	45	23	1.958
	0.03	28	12	2.335
1-methyl-Δ¹-5α-androstene-17β-ol-3-one-acetate	0.3	50	121	0.414
	0.1	51	56	0.952
	0.03	19	15	1.255

The compounds of the invention may conveniently be made by esterifying the unsubstituted 17-alcohol with the desired halogenated fatty acid or a reactive derivative

thereof. The esterification may be carried out in any of the ways common in steriod chemistry as, for instance, by reacting the alcohol with the corresponding acid chloride or acid anhydride while using pyridine as a solvent or by reacting the alcohol with the unsubstituted acid in the presence of trifluoroaceticacidanhydride.

The principal utility of the esters of the invention is in the manufacture of anabolically active and in particular subcutaneously applicable medicaments.

The following examples shall illustrate the invention without being intended to limit the scope thereof.

Example 1

1.15 ml. dichloroacetylchloride were added to 3.024 g. of 1-methyl-Δ¹-5α-androstene-17β-ol-3-one dissolved in 70 ml. pyridine. The addition was made by dropping the acetylchloride into the solution upon stirring and under a nitrogen atmosphere at a temperature of 0° C. The reaction mixture was left overnight at the same temperature of 0°. Ice water was then stirred into the mixture followed by acidification with dilute hydrochloric acid and extraction with methylenechloride. The methylenechloride phase was washed out with dilute hydrochloride acid and thereafter with water, was dried over Na_2SO_4 and concentrated in vacuo by evaporation. The thus obtained crude reaction product was subjected to chromatography with 200 g. SiO_2+10+H_2O. By elution with a $CCl_4CH_2Cl_2$ mixture and combining of the different fractions one obtained 2.63 g. 1-methyl-Δ¹-5α-androstene-17β-ol-3-one-17-dichloracetate. This product after recrystallization from isopropylether had a melting point between 149 and 150 C.; UV: $\epsilon_{240}=13300$.

Example 2

302 mg. of 1-methyl-Δ¹-5α-androstene-17β-ol-3-one were heated together with 3 ml. dichloroacetic acid and 0.8 ml. trifluoroaceticacidanhydride in an argon atmosphere for 20 minutes in a steam bath. The reaction mixture was then permitted to cool, ice water was added and extraction effected with methylenechloride. The methylenechloride phase was washed out with a dilute $NaHCO_3$ solution and then with water and after drying was concentrated in vacuo over Na_2SO_4. The residue was subjected to recrystallization from isopropylether. There were obtained 250 mg. 1-methyl-Δ¹-5α-androstene-17β-ol-3-one-17-dichloracetate, melting point 148 to 150° C.

Example 3

5 g. of 1-methyl-Δ¹-5α-anstrostene-17β-ol-3-one were dissolved in 25 ml. pyridine and were reacted dropwise at a temperature between 0 and 5° C. upon stirring during a period of 20 minutes with a solution of 3.11 g. monochloraceticacidanhydride in 30 ml. abs. ether. Stirring was continued for four hours during which time the temperature of the reaction mixture slowly rose. Excess chloraceticanhydride was decomposed with 1 ml. water. The solution was drop added during one hour to 500 ml. water. The precipitated 1-methyl-Δ¹-5α-androstene-17β-ol-3-one-17-chloracetate was filtered off, then successively washed with 5% HCl, 2% sodium bicarbonate solution and water and was dried in vacuo at 50° C. The yield was 5.9 g. and the melting point 102 to 104° C.; UV: $\epsilon_{241}=13380$.

Example 4

500 mg. of 1-methyl-Δ¹-5α-androstene-17β-ol-3-one were dissolved in 5 ml. trichloracetic acid and 1 ml. trifluoraceticacidanhydride and were subjected to heating for 30 minutes over a steam bath under a nitrogen atmosphere. The mixture was permitted to cool, ice water was added and extraction was effected with methyleneachloride. The methylenechloride phase was washed with di-

lute $NaHCO_3$ solution and water. After drying over Na_2SO_4 and concentration in vacuo, recrystallization of the cooled product was effected with isopropylether. There were obtained 1-methyl-Δ^1-5α-androstene-17β-ol-3-one-17-trichloracetate melting point 134 to 135° C.; UV: $\epsilon_{241}=13800$.

Without further analysis, the foregoing will so fully reveal the gist of the present invention that others can by applying current knowledge readily adapt it for various applications without omitting features that, from the standpoint of prior art, fairly constitute essential characteristics of the generic or specific aspects of this invention and, therefore, such adaptations should and are intended to be comprehended within the meaning and range of equivalence of the following claims.

What is claimed as new and desired to be secured by Letters Patent is:

1. An androstene compound consisting of a member selected from the group consisting of

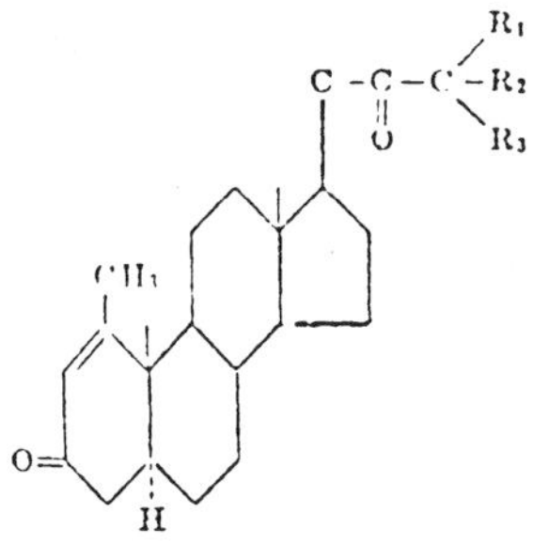

and

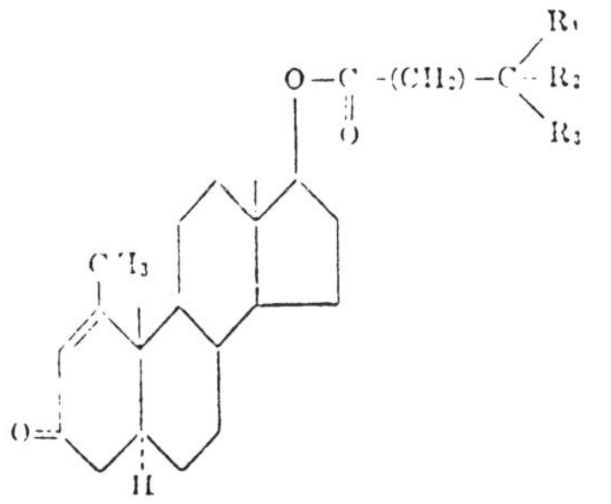

wherein R_1 is chlorine and R_2 and R_3 are members selected from the group consisting of hydrogen and chlorine.

2. 1-methyl-Δ^1-5α-androstene - 17β - ol - 3 - one-17-monochloracetate.

3. 1-methyl-Δ^1-5α-androstene-17β-ol - 3 - one-17-dichloracetate.

4. 1-methyl-Δ^1-5α-androstene-17β-ol - 3 - one-17-trichloracetate.

References Cited

UNITED STATES PATENTS

3,236,867	2/1966	Ringold et al.	260—397.4
3,249,628	5/1966	Wiechert	260—397.4
3,258,473	6/1966	Kincl	260—397.4

LEWIS GOTTS, *Primary Examiner.*

J. R. BROWN, *Assistant Examiner.*

UNITED STATES PATENT OFFICE
CERTIFICATE OF CORRECTION

Patent No. 3,361,774   January 2, 1968

Josef Hader et al.

It is certified that error appears in the above identified patent and that said Letters Patent are hereby corrected as shown below:

Column 3, lines 20 to 31, for that portion of the formula reading

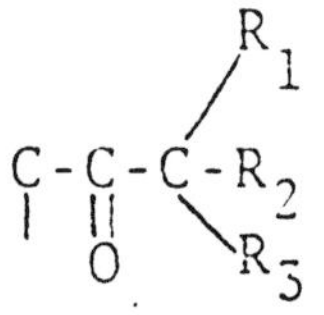

$$C-C-C\begin{matrix} -R_1 \\ -R_2 \\ -R_3 \end{matrix} \quad \text{read} \quad O-C-C\begin{matrix} -R_1 \\ -R_2 \\ -R_3 \end{matrix}$$

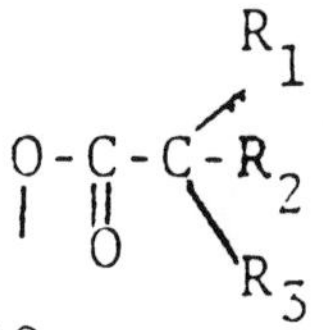

Signed and sealed this 22nd day of July 1969.

(SEAL)
Attest:

Edward M. Fletcher, Jr.

Attesting Officer

WILLIAM E. SCHUYLER, JR.

Commissioner of Patents

CHAPTER SEVEN

1

2

2,900,398

PROCESS FOR THE MANUFACTURE OF STEROID
DEHYDROGENATION PRODUCTS

Albert Wettstein and Alfred Hunger, Basel, Charles Meystre, Arlesheim, and Ludwig Ehmann, Basel, Switzerland, assignors to Ciba Pharmaceutical Products Inc.,
Summit, N.J.

No Drawing. Application June 11, 1957
Serial No. 664,920

Claims priority, application Switzerland June 15, 1956

10 Claims. (Cl. 260—397.4)

This invention relates to an improvement in the manufacture of steroid dehydrogenation products, especially
of $\Delta^{1.4}$-3-oxo-steroids of the pregnane—or androstane
series, such as the well known highly active hormone compounds 1-dehydro-cortisone and 1-dehydro-hydrocorti-
sone.

It is known that $\Delta^{1.4}$-3-oxo-steroids are obtained when
3-oxo-steroids are treated with selenium compounds having a dehydrogenating action. In individual cases, especially with certain 3-oxo-steroids saturated in the ring A,
this process is not entirely satisfactory since the yield
of $\Delta^{1.4}$-3-oxo-compound leave something to be desired.

The present invention is based on the observation that
the yields in the above dehydrogenation can be improved
when the dehydrogenation reaction is carried out in the
presence of a metal of the second or eighth group of the
periodic system. A further feature of the invention is
based on the observation that from the mother liquors
obtained by the recrystallization of the crude $\Delta^{1.4}$-3-oxo-
steroids formed by the known or by the new process,
further quantities of the desired final product can be obtained when the residues of these mother liquors, obtained after separation of the purified crystalline $\Delta^{1.4}$-3-
oxo-steroids and evaporation of the solvent are treated
with nickel or iron and, if desired, subsequently again
with the selenium compound of dehydrogenating activity
in the presence of a metal of the second or eighth group
of the periodic system.

The process of the present application for the dehydrogenation of 3-oxo-steroids to $\Delta^{1.4}$-3-oxo-steroids by means
of selenium compounds of dehydrogenating activity is
thus characterised in that the dehydrogenation is carried
out in the presence of a metal of the second or eighth
group of the periodic system. A special feature of this
process consists in treating the selenium-containing fraction obtained after separation of the crystallized $\Delta^{1.4}$-3-
oxo-steroids obtained by the dehydrogenation of a 3-oxo-
steroid by means of a selenium compound having a dehydrogenating action with nickel or iron, and if desired,
subjecting the reaction products again to a treatment with
a selenium compound of dehydrogenating action in the
presence of metals of the second or eighth groups of the
periodic system.

Especially suitable metals are magnesium, zinc, cadmi-
um, mercury and manganese, iron, cobalt, nickel, which
are used in finely divided form, care being taken during
the dehydrogenation reaction that a thorough mixing of
the reacting materials takes place. The reaction products
obtained according to the present process, compared with
the reaction products obtained without the addition of
metal, are less deeply coloured and can be purified in a
simpler manner.

From the selenium containing fraction of the reaction
prod.... obtained after separation of the crystallized
$\Delta^{1.4}$-3-oxo-steroids, further quantities of 1-dehydro-ster-
oids can be obtained by treatment with nickel or iron

in a suitable solvent; deactivated Raney nickel is primarily suitable such as is obtained for example by boiling
active Raney nickel in a ketone such as acetone or methyl-ethyl ketone, and iron powder. A suitable solvent is
for example an alcohol or ketone. When nickel is used
the crystallized fractions obtained from the reaction
product constitute a mixture of 3-oxo-steroids which are
completely or partially dehydrogenated in the ring A,
since under the conditions used the deactivated nickel is
capable of partial reduction of the $\Delta^{1.4}$-3-oxo-grouping.
For working up to the desired $\Delta^{1.4}$-3-oxo-steroids, the
resulting reaction products are therefore again treated
with the selenium compound of dehydrogenating action,
especially with selenium dioxide or selenious acid,
in the presence of a tertiary alcohol such as tertiary butanol or tertiary amyl alcohol and of a metal of the
second or eighth group of the periodic system.

The advantages that the new process offers can be
seen from the examples below. When, for example, 3,11,
20-trioxo-17α-hydroxy-21-acetoxy-pregnane is dehydrogenated by the known method with selenium dioxide, a
reaction product is obtained from which about 40% of
1-dehydro-cortisone acetate can be isolated. When the
dehydrogenation is carried out in the presence of mercury
or zinc, the yield is increased to above 60%. On the
other hand it was not hitherto possible to recover further
crystallized fractions from the mother liquors of 1-de-
hydro-cortisone or its 21-esters (obtained by dehydrogenation of cortisone, 3,11,20-trioxo-17α-21-dihydroxy-
pregnane, 3,11,20-trioxo-17α.21-dihydroxy-allopregnane,
or its 21-esters by the known selenium dioxide process).
By treatment of the residues of these mother liquors with
deactivated Raney nickel and renewed dehydrogenation
of the reaction product with selenium dioxide, it is now
possible by the present process to obtain a further quantity of about 4–10% of 1-dehydro-compound. Similar
yield improvements may be achieved when using as starting materials 3-oxo-steroids of the androstane or testane
series, which represents a remarkable progress for instance in the manufacture of certain 17α-substituted 1-
dehydro-testosterones with anabolic action, such as 1-
dehydro-17α-methyl-testosterone.

The following examples illustrate the invention:

Example 1

To 1.21 grams of 3,11,20-trioxo-17α-hydroxy-21-acet-
oxy-pregnane in 20 ml. of tertiary amyl alcohol and 1.0
ml. of glacial acetic acid, after the addition of 1.2 grams
of mercury, at reflux temperature and with brisk stirring,
0.74 gram of selenium dioxide in 33 ml. of tertiary amyl
alcohol is added dropwise and the whole is boiled under
reflux for 14 hours. Separated selenium, mercury selenide and mercury are filtered off, the filtrate is diluted
with ethyl acetate and the ethyl acetate solution is shaken
with ammonium sulphide and sodium carbonate solution,
dried and evaporated. From the residue, by crystallisation from acetone-ether, 0.73 gram of 1-dehydro-cor-
tisone acetate is obtained. 0.5 gram remains of a non-
crystallising mother liquor product.

The 0.5 gram of mother liquor product is stirred for 5
hours under reflux with 5 grams of a deactivated Raney
nickel suspension prepared by boiling of active Raney
nickel in methyl-ethyl ketone, and 50 cc. of methly-ethyl
ketone. After removal of the nickel by filtration and
evaporation of the solvent, 0.37 gram is obtained of crystalline residue which, as above described, is dissolved in
10 cc. of tertiary amyl alcohol and 0.5 cc. of glacial
acetic acid, and dehydrogenated with 0.23 gram of selenium dioxide in 10 cc. of tertiary amyl alcohol in the
presence of 0.5 gram of mercury. Working up by the
method described above yields a further 0.12 gram of

3

1-dehydro-cortisone acetate. The total yield thus amounts to 0.85 gram of 1-dehydro-cortisone acetate.

When the dehydrogenation is carried out without the addition of mercury and the mother liquors are not further treated according to the present process, from 1.21 grams of the above starting material 0.43 gram of 1-dehydro-cortisone acetate is obtained:

To 1.21 gram of 3,11,20-trioxo-17α-hydroxy-21-acetoxy-pregnane in 20 ml. of tertiary amyl alcohol and 10 ml. of glacial acetic acid, at reflux temperature and with stirring, 0.74 gram of selenium dioxide in 33 ml. of tertiary amyl alcohol is added dropwise and the whole is stirred under reflux for 14 hours. The separated selenium is filtered off and the filtrate diluted with ethyl acetate and the ethyl acetate solution is washed with ammonium sulphide and sodium carbonate solution, dried and evaporated. From the residue, by crystallization from acetone, 0.43 gram of 1-dehydro-cortisone acetate is obtained.

Example 2

When 10 grams of cortisone acetate are dehydrogenated with selenium dioxide, as described in Helv. Chim. Acta 39, 734 (1956), 8.0 grams of crystalline 1-dehydro-cortisone acetate and 2.0 grams of a mother liquor product are obtained, from the latter of which neither by crystallisation nor by other purification methods can further 1-dehydro-cortisone acetate be obtained.

The 2.0 grams of mother liquor product are boiled for 5 hours under reflux in 50 ml. of methyl-ethyl ketone with 20 grams of deactivated Raney nickel and the product is filtered from nickel and evaporated. 1.0 gram of a crystalline residue is obtained, consisting for the most part of cortisone acetate and 1-dehydro-cortisone acetate.

This residue, as described in Example 1, is dehydrogenated in 30 ml. of tertiary amyl alcohol and 1 ml. of glacial acetic acid in the presence of 1 gram of mercury with 0.6 gram of selenium dioxide dissolved in 15 ml. of tertiary amyl alcohol and the product is worked up. In this manner a further 0.4 gram of 1-dehydro-cortisone acetate is obtained.

Example 3

A suspension of 30 grams of 17α-methyl-testosterone and 10 grams of selenium dioxide in 600 cc. of tertiary amyl alcohol is treated with 60 grams of magnesium powder and 6 cc. of glacial acetic acid. The mixture is refluxed for 24 hours with good stirring in an atmosphere of nitrogen, another 10 grams of selenium dioxide being added after 10 hours. After some cooling, the suspension is filtered through some "hyflo" and washed thoroughly with ethyl acetate. The resulting brown solution is evaporated in vacuo and the residue dissolved in ethyl acetate. The ethyl acetate solution is then washed with water, dried and evaporated. To remove any selenium still present, the residue is dissolved in 200 cc. of methanol and mixed with 100 grams of iron powder and 2 grams of active carbon. The mixture is heated for 30 minutes with stirring under reflux, then filtered with suction, washed with methanol and the solution evaporated in vacuo. The residue is then chromatographed on 900 grams of aluminum oxide. The residues of the evaporated benzene and ether fractions are treated with active carbon in methanol or acetone, evaporated again, and the residue recrystallized from a mixture of acetone and ether. There are obtained 17.5 grams of pure 1-dehydro-17α-methyl-testosterone which melts at 163–164° C. From the mother liquors there can be obtained a small quantity of the same 1-dehydro-compound having a somewhat lower melting point. The further eluates of the chromatography, obtained with ethyl acetate and acetone, when recrystallized from acetone, give 4.2 grams of a mono-selenium derivative of 1-dehydro-testosterone of melting point 232–284° C.

When in the dehydrogenation there are added 130 grams of iron powder instead of the magnesium, there is ob-

4

tained the same yield of 1-dehydro-17α-methyl-testosterone and of mono-selenium derivative. However, if the same reaction is made without magnesium or iron there are obtained on working up in the same manner only 4.5 grams of 1-dehydro-17α-methyl-testosterone of melting point 163–164° C. and 19.5 grams of the mono-selenium derivative of melting point 282–284° C.

Example 4

A suspension of 5 grams of 17α-ethinyl-testosterone, 3 grams of selenium dioxide and 40 grams of iron powder in 400 cc. of tertiary amyl alcohol and 4 cc. of glacial acetic acid is refluxed with stirring in an atmosphere of nitrogen for 48 hours, another 3 grams of selenium dioxide being added after 24 hours. The reaction mixture is worked up as described in Example 3. The residue which is obtained is chromatographed over 150 grams of alumina. The benzene and ether eluates are treated together with some active carbon in methanol or acetone and then recrystallized from acetone or a mixture of acetone and isopropyl ether. There are obtained 2.8 grams of 1-dehydro-17α-ethinyl-testosterone of melting point 228–233° C. From the mother liquors there can be isolated small quantities of the same 1-dehydro compound having a somewhat lower melting point. From the further ethyl acetate and acetone eluates of the chromatography selenium-containing derivatives are obtained.

When in this reaction the iron powder is replaced by 20 grams of magnesium powder there is obtained under otherwise identical conditions the same yield of 1-dehydro-17α-ethinyl-testosterone.

However, if the reaction is carried out in the absence of iron or magnesium under otherwise identical conditions, only 550 mg. of the pure 1-dehydro-17α-ethinyl-testosterone of melting point 228–233° C. can be isolated.

Example 5

To 5.0 grams of 3,11,20-trioxo-17-hydroxy-21-acetoxy-allopregnane in 120 ml. of tertiary amyl alcohol and 2.5 ml. of glacial acetic acid there are added dropwise after the addition of 1.2 grams of mercury, at reflux temperature and with brisk stirring 6.9 grams of selenium dioxide in 70 ml. of tertiary amyl alcohol, and the whole is boiled under reflux for 14 hours. Separated selenium mercury selenide and mercury are filtered off, the filtrate is diluted with ethyl acetate and the ethyl acetate solution is shaken with ammonium sulfide and sodium carbonate solution, dried and evaporated. From the residue there are obtained by crystallization from acetone-ether 3.1 grams of 1-dehydro-cortisone acetate.

When the dehydrogenation is carried out in the same manner, but without the addition of mercury, there are obtained from 5 grams of the above starting material 2.2 grams of 1-dehydro-cortisone-acetate.

What is claimed is:

1. In a process for the dehydrogenation of steroids of the pregnane, androstane and testane series substituted in 3-position by an oxo group and which are at most unsaturated in ring A in the 4,5-position by means of selenium dioxide, the improvement wherein the dehydrogenation is carried out in the presence of mercury.

2. Process according to claim 1, wherein the selenium-containing fraction obtained after separation of the crystallized $\Delta^{1,4}$-steroid substituted by an oxo group in 3-position obtained by the dehydrogenation of a steroid substituted in 3-position by an oxo group and saturated at least in one of the positions 1,2 and 4,5 by means of a selenium dioxide is treated with a member selected from the group consisting of nickel and iron.

3. Process according to claim 2, wherein the treatment with a member selected from the group consisting of nickel and iron is carried out in the presence of a member selected from the group consisting of an alcohol and a ketone.

4. Process according to claim 2, wherein the reaction

5

products obtained are again subjected to a treatment with selenium dioxide in the presence of mercury.

5. Process according to claim 1, wherein there is used as starting material a member selected from the group consisting of a 3-oxo-steroid of the pregnane and the allopregnane series.

6. Process according to claim 5, wherein 3,11,20-trioxo-17α-hydroxy-21-acetoxy-pregnane is used as starting material.

7. Process according to claim 5, wherein 3,11,20-trioxo-17α-hydroxy-21-acetoxy-allopregnane is used as starting material.

8. Process according to claim 1, wherein there is used as starting material a member selected from the group

6

consisting of a 3-oxo-steroid of the androstane and the testane series.

9. Process according to claim 8, wherein there is used as starting material 17α-methyl-testosterone.

10. Process according to claim 8, wherein there is used as starting material 17α-ethinyl-testosterone.

References Cited in the file of this patent

Helv. Chem. Acta., vol. 39, 1956, 734–742, Meystre et al.

J. Org. Chem., vol. 21, 1956, 239–240, Ringold et al.

Rec. Trav. Chim Des-Pays Bas, 1956, vol. 75, pages 475–480, Szpelfogel et al.

1

2,900,399

ANDROSTAN-3,17-DIOL-4-ONE DERIVATIVES

Percy L. Julian, Oak Park, and Helen C. Printy, Chicago, Ill., assignors to The Julian Laboratories, Inc., Franklin Park, Ill., a corporation of Illinois

No Drawing. Application July 7, 1958
Serial No. 746,609

12 Claims. (Cl. 260—397.4)

This invention relates to novel androstan-4-one derivatives and to processes for utilizing them. More particularly, this invention relates to androstan-3-ol-4-ones and the process for converting these compounds into the corresponding anabolic 4-hydroxytestosterone congeners.

While the compounds of this invention are particularly important as intermediates in the preparation of anabolically active testosterones, they also have substantial anabolic activity in their own right. The term "anabolic activity" is used to connote tissue building activity at a level which results in a favorable therapeutic ratio to the virilizing or androgenic activity.

These novel androstan-4-one derivatives are represented by the following structural formula:

FORMULA I

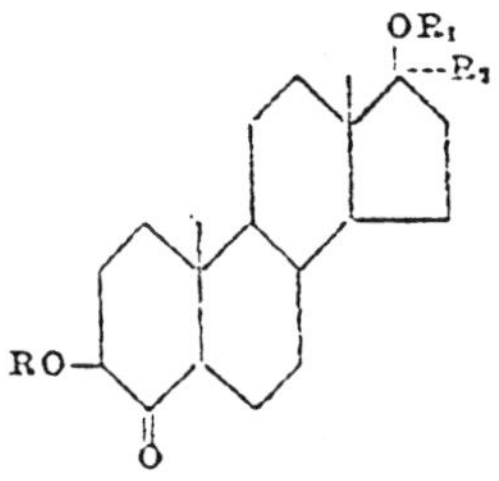

when:

R represents hydrogen or an acyl moiety derived from a hydrocarbon carboxylic acid which preferably contains fewer than 8 carbon atoms, for instance lower alkanoyl of 1 to 7 carbons, benzoyl or hexahydrobenzoyl;

R_1 represents hydrogen or an acyl moiety derived from a hydrocarbon carboxylic acid which preferably contains fewer than 8 carbon atoms, for instance lower alkanoyl of 2 to 7 carbons, benzoyl or hexahydrobenzoyl; and

R_2 represents hydrogen or lower alkyl. The term "lower alkyl" is used to define methyl or ethyl. Preferred and advantageous compounds are represented by Formula I when R and R_1 are hydrogen or acetyl and R_2 is hydrogen or methyl.

In practice, R and R_1 may represent any acyl derivative which possesses anabolic activity as such or upon hydrolysis in vivo to the hydroxylated parent structure. Illustrative of such active compounds are those in which one or both of R and R_1 are isobutyryl, cyclopentylpropionyl, phenylacetyl, chloroacetyl, 3,3-dimethylpentanoyl, 4-methylcyclohexanecarboxyl, 4-chlorophenoxyacetyl, 4-tert-butylphenoxyacetyl, palmityl, etc. Such acyl moieties advantageously will have less than 8 carbon atoms.

Many of these esters have prolonged anabolic activity. The acyl moieties must be derived from nontoxic, stable, pharmaceutically acceptable carboxylic acids.

The compounds of this invention are prepared by hydrogenation of the corresponding 2,5-androstadienes of the following structure:

2

FORMULA II

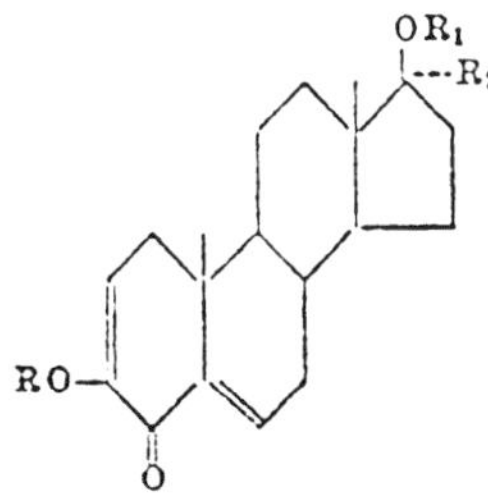

when R and R_1 represent an acyl moiety as described hereabove for Formula I, and R_2 represents hydrogen or lower alkyl.

The hydrogenation reaction is carried out in a suitable organic solvent unreactive under the reaction conditions described in which the androstadiene starting material is at least partially soluble. Exemplary of such solvents are ethers such as dioxane or ethyl ether, tertiary amines such as pyridine or lutidine, lower esters such as ethyl acetate, aromatic solvents such as toluene or benzene, and lower alcohols such as butanol or isopropanol. Preferably the hydrogenation solvent will be a water miscible alkanol, such as methanol, ethanol, isopropanol or aqueous mixtures thereof. The reaction is run at any convenient temperature, such as from about 20° C. up to the boiling point of the solvent used, such as up to about 75° C. Preferably, temperatures at about room temperature are used, for instance, about 25–30° C. The hydrogenation catalyst is preferably a palladium catalyst, such as palladium-on-calcium carbonate, palladium-on-charcoal, palladium-on-barium sulfate, palladium-silica gel, palladium-kieselguhr and the like. In order to limit the course of the hydrogenation as much as possible to the 2,5-unsaturated positions, the reaction conditions are preferably maintained substantially neutral, and the reaction is interrupted when about 2 molar equivalents of hydrogen are absorbed, usually within one-half to five hours. The reaction product is isolated by removing the spent catalyst and evaporating the solvent.

If the hydrogenation reaction is run under acid conditions, preferably in glacial acetic acid, until about 2.5 molar equivalents of hydrogen are absorbed, the corresponding androstan-4-one of Formula III, in which R_1 and R_2 are as described above for Formula I, is obtained as the major product:

FORMULA III

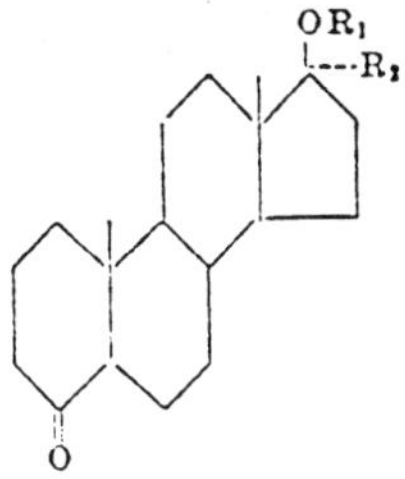

The androstane derivatives of Formula III are useful anabolic agents and intermediates.

The starting material androstadienes of Formula II are prepared by treating the 2,6-dibromotestosterone congeners with an excess of an alkali carboxylate at reflux in a low boiling solvent, thereby causing a rearrangement into the desired 2,5-androstadien-4-one derivative.

The novel compounds of this invention represented by Formula I when R and R_1 are hydrogen are obtained from the acylated congeners described above by hydrolysis, preferably using mild alkali, such as an aqueous solution of an alkali metal carbonate or bicarbonate, for instance potassium or sodium bicarbonate, in aqueous organic solvent mixture preferably an aqueous lower alcohol at about room temperature for from one-half to three hours.

The solvent for the hydrolysis is comprised of a mixture of water and a water miscible organic solvent which is not reactive under the hydrolysis conditions employed, such as a lower alcohol, for example methanol or ethanol, dioxane, acetone, dimethylacetamide, dimethylformamide, etc. Alternatively, alkali metal hydroxides such as dilute sodium or potassium hydroxide, or alkali metal alcoholates such as sodium methoxide, or potassium ethoxide can be used. In using the latter alkaline agents, the reaction is complete in from one to three minutes to as long as 15 minutes at room temperature. With mild hydrolysis conditions, such as with carbonates or bicarbonates, the 3-esters are preferentially hydrolyzed before the 17-esters. More vigorous conditions, such as with the hydroxides, remove ester moieties at both positions.

If varied acyl groups are desired for R and R_1 in the compounds of Formula I, for instance to prolong the anabolic activity of the compounds, acylation of the 3,7 diols alternatively can be carried out by conventional methods.

The compounds of this invention have unique utility as intermediates in the preparation of the biologically active 4-hydroxytestosterone congeners. The compounds of Formula I in which R and R_1 are acyl are hydrolyzed under mild alkaline conditions with alkali metal carbonates and bicarbonates in aqueous alcoholic solution as described above. The resulting 3-ol-4-ones, either crude or after purification, are then oxidized with an excess of bismuth trioxide in acid solution, preferably in glacial acetic acid, by stirring and gentle heating, for instance at about 85° C. to about 120° C. for from about five minutes to three hours. The formation of dark free bismuth during the reaction can be used as a rough guide of the extent of oxidation. The end products are isolated by filtering the reaction mixture to remove the free bismuth. The filtrate is concentrated in vacuo, washed with water and extracted with an immiscible-with-water organic solvent, preferably ether. The organic layer is extracted with alkali solution then concentrated and cooled to give the desired anabolic agent, for instance, 4-hydroxy - 17α - methyltestosterone or 4 - hydroxy - 17α-ethyltestosterone.

Alternatively, the oxidation can be carried out with copper acetate in alcohol or with mild chromic acid conditions, such as chromic oxide in pyridine or chromic acid in acetone at about room temperature. The bismuth oxide oxidation is, however, preferred.

The following examples will serve to illustrate the preparation of the novel compounds as well as variations of the processes of this invention. The scope of this invention is not to be limited by these examples since it will be obvious to one skilled in the art that these examples are merely illustrative of this invention and that modifications thereof are opssible.

Example 1

A solution of 3.3 g. (0.01 mole) of testosterone acetate in 110 ml. of anhydrous ether is cooled in an ice bath of 0–2° C. Two drops of 30% HBr in acetic acid are added, followed by a solution of 3.2 g. (0.02 mole) of bromine in 25 ml. of acetic acid, added over a seven minute period. The colorless brominated solution is kept at 0–2° C. for an additional ten minutes, then is concentrated in vacuo with gentle warming to a volume of 20 ml. The voluminous white crystalline precipitate, which is obtained, is filtered, washed with cold ethanol, and dried at room temperature. A first crop of 2,6-dibromotestosterone acetate, M.P. 170–172° C., is obtained.

A suspension of 1.0 g. of the dibromide and 4.0 g. of dry potassium acetate in 40 ml. of distilled acetone is stirred and refluxed for one hour. The reaction mixture

is concentrated to a thick slush, water added to dissolve the potassium salts, and the organic material extracted with methylene chloride. The methylene chloride is washed with water and concentrated to a solid, halogen-free crystalline mass. The residue crystallized from ether in glistening prisms gives 3,17β-diacetoxy-2,5-androstadien-4-one, M.P. 173–174° C., $[α]_D^{22}$—11.9° (ethanol).

A solution of 3.42 g. of 3,17β-diacetoxy-2,5-androstadien-4-one in 100 ml. of methanol is shaken with 0.6 g. of 10% palladium-on-charcoal catalyst at 3 atmospheres of hydrogen and room temperature for one hour at which time two molar equivalents of hydrogen are absorbed. The solution is filtered and concentrated to dryness. The residue, mainly 3β,17β-diacetoxyandrostan-4-one, is recrystallized from ether-petroleum ether to give white crystals of the 4-one, M.P. 138–139° C.

Example 2

A solution of 3.42 g. of 3-17β-diacetoxy-2,5-androstadien-4-one in 100 ml. of ethanol is hydrogenated at one atmosphere with 1.0 g. of 5% palladium-on-calcium carbonate. The reaction mixture is worked up as in Example 1 to give 3β,17β-diacetoxyandrostan-4-one, M.P. 136–139° C.

Example 3

A solution of 6.0 g. of 3β,17β-diacetoxyandrostan-4-one in 75 ml. of methanol is stirred under a stream of nitrogen at 30° C. for two hours with a solution of 2.5 g. of sodium bicarbonate in 25 ml. of water. The reaction mixture is neutralized with acetic acid and poured into water. After extraction with methylene chloride, drying and evaporating the solvent, 17β-acetoxy-3β-hydroxyandrostan-4-one is obtained. This crude product is dissolved in 50 ml. of glacial acetic acid, then heated at 100° C. with 3.5 g. of bismuth trioxide with stirring for 15 minutes. The mixture is filtered and concentrated in vacuo. The residue is washed with water and extracted with ether. After washing the ether extract with alkali, concentration and cooling gives 4-hydroxytestosterone, M.P. 216–218° C.

Example 4

A mixture of 2.3 g. of 3-acetoxy-17β-benzoyloxy-2,5-androstadien-4-one and 0.5 g. of 10% palladium-on-charcoal in 100 ml. of methanol is hydrogenated at three atmospheres and room temperature until two molar equivalents of hydrogen are absorbed. The filtered mixture is concentrated in vacuo to give crude 3-acetoxy-17β-benzoyloxy-androstan-4-one.

Example 5

A solution of 3.42 g. of 3,17β-diacetoxy-2,5-androstadien-4-one in 100 ml. of glacial acetic acid is shaken with 1.0 g. of 10% palladium-on-charcoal and is hydrogenated at four to five atmospheres until 2.5 molar equivalents of hydrogen are absorbed. After the catalyst is removed, the filtrate is evaporated in vacuo. The residue is taken up in ether which is washed with dilute bicarbonate solution, water and then dried. Low boiling petroleum ether is added to separate 17β-acetoxyandrostan-4-one, M.P. 175–178° C.

Example 6

A mixture of 100 mg. of 3,17β-dihydroxyandrostan-4-one (as prepared in Example 3), 0.5 g. of heptanoic anhydride and 1 ml. of anhydrous pyridine is agitated at ambient temperature overnight. The resulting mixture is quenched in ice water, then extracted with ether. The dried ether-extract is concentrated and mixed with petroleum ether to separate 3,17β-diheptanoyloxyandrostan-4-one.

Example 7

A solution of 9.5 g. of 3-acetoxy-17α-ethyl-17β-hydroxy-2,5-androstadien-4-one in 400 ml. of methanol with 4.0 g. of palladium-on-charcoal is hydrogenated and

5

worked up as in Example 1 to give 3-acetoxy-17α-ethyl-17β-hydroxyandrostan-4-one.

A portion (3.0 g.) of the crude 4-one is hydrolyzed with potassium bicarbonate solution and then, in turn, oxidized with bismuth trioxide as in Example 3 to give 17α-ethyl-4-hydroxytestosterone.

Example 8

A solution of 18.0 g. of 3-acetoxy-17β-hydroxy-17α-methyl-2,5-androstadien-4-one in 500 ml. of 95% methanol with 6.0 g. of 10% palladium-on-charcoal is hydrogenated at low pressure and room temperature until two molar equivalents of hydrogen are absorbed. The catalyst is removed by filtration and the filtrate concentrated and extracted into methylene chloride. The residue from the organic extracts is in part crystallized from ether to give 3-acetoxy-17β-hydroxy-17α-methylandrostan-4-one, M.P. 174–176° C.

The remaining crude residue is dissolved in 150 ml. of methanol and hydrolyzed under nitrogen for 90 minutes at 30° C. with a solution of 7.0 g. of potassium bicarbonate in 25 ml. of water.

The reaction mixture is neutralized with acetic acid and poured into water. Extraction with methylene chloride yields crude 3,17β-dihydroxy-17α-methylandrostan-4-one, a portion of which is recrystallized from ether, M.P. 150–155° C.

The crude hydrolysis product is dissolved in 100 ml. of glacial acetic acid. Bismuth trioxide (10.0 g.) is added. The mixture is stirred and heated at 100° C. for 15 minutes. The filtered reaction mixture is concentrated in vacuo, washed with water and extracted with ether. After extraction with alkali, concentration of the ether solution affords 4-hydroxy-17α-methyltestosterone. M.P. 215–218° C., $E_{280}=9,000$.

A mixture of 150 mg. of 4-hydroxy-17α-methyltestosterone, 1 ml. of acetic anhydride and 5 ml. of pyridine is allowed to stand overnight. Quenching in water gives the crude acetate derivative of the compound.

Example 9

A solution of 3.3 g. of 17β-acetoxy-4-formoxy-2,5-androstadien-4-one, M.P. 195–205° C., in 100 ml. of methanol with 0.8 g. of 10% palladium-on-charcoal is hydrogenated until two molar equivalents of hydrogen are absorbed. After working up as in Example 1, 17β-acetoxy-3-formoxyandrostan-4-one is recovered.

Example 10

A mixture of 200 mg. of 3,17β-dihydroxy-17α-methylandrostan-4-one, 0.5 g. of hexahydrobenzoyl chloride and 5 ml. of pyridine is reacted and worked up as in Example 6 to give the hexahydrobenzoate derivative.

In similar fashion, but using 0.5 g. of 3,3-dimethylpentanoyl chloride the 3-dimethylpentanoate derivative of 3,17β-dihydroxy-17α-methylandrostan-4-one is obtained.

What is claimed is:

1. A chemical compound having the structural formula:

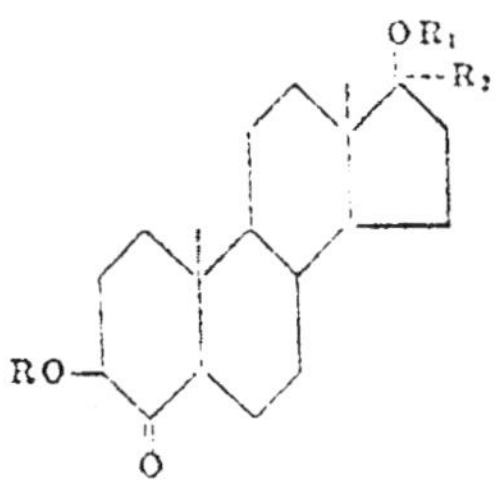

in which R is a member selected from the group consisting of hydrogen and an acyl moiety derived from a nontoxic, stable, pharmaceutically-acceptable carboxylic acid having from 1 to 7 carbon atoms; R₁ is a member selected from the group consisting of hydrogen and an acyl moiety derived from a nontoxic, stable, pharmaceutically-accept-

6

able carboxylic acid having from 2 to 7 carbon atoms; and R₂ is a member selected from the group consisting of hydrogen, methyl and ethyl.

2. 3β,17β-diacetoxyandrostan-4-one.
3. 3β-acetoxy-17β-hydroxy-17α-methylandrostan-4-one.
4. 3β,17β-dihydroxy-17α-methylandrostan-4-one.
5. 17β-acetoxy-3β-hydroxyandrostan-4-one.
6. 3β,17β-dihyrdroxyandrostan-4-one.

7. The method of forming a compound having the structural formula:

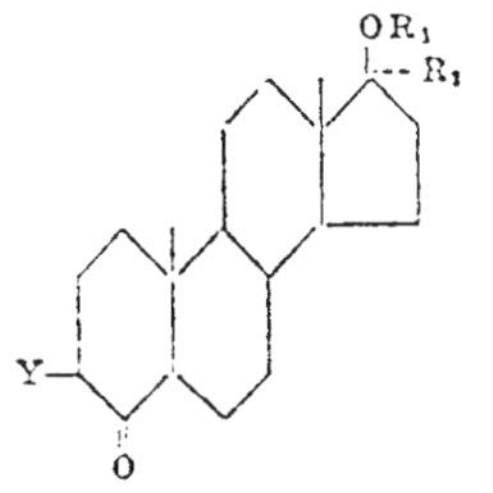

in which Y is a member selected from the group consisting of hydrogen and —OR in which R is an acyl moiety derived from a nontoxic, stable, pharmaceutically-acceptable carboxylic acid having from 1 to 7 carbon atoms; R₁ is a member selected from the group consisting of hydrogen and an acyl moiety derived from a nontoxic, stable, pharmaceutically-acceptable carboxylic acid having from 2 to 7 carbon atoms; and R₂ is a member selected from the group consisting of hydrogen, methyl and ethyl, which comprises hydrogenating with about two molar equivalents of hydrogen in the presence of a palladium catalyst over a period of one-half to five hours a compound having the structural formula:

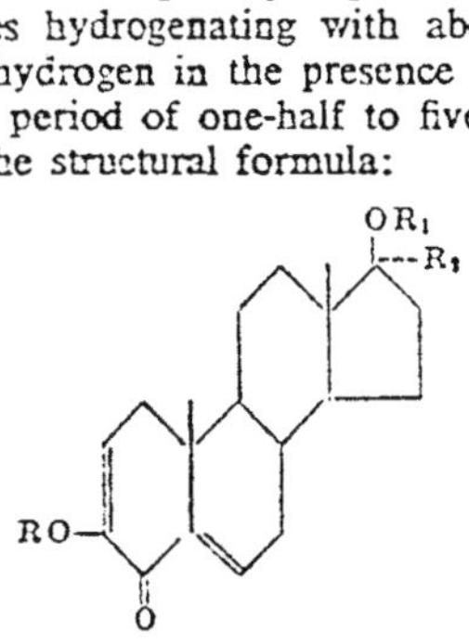

in which R is an acyl moiety derived from a nontoxic, stable, pharmaceutically-acceptable carboxylic acid having from 1 to 7 carbon atoms; R₁ is a member selected from the group consisting of hydrogen and an acyl moiety derived from a nontoxic, stable, pharmaceutically-acceptable carboxylic acid having from 2 to 7 carbon atoms; and R₂ is a member selected from the group consisting of hydrogen, methyl and ethyl.

8. The method of claim 7 characterized in that Y is —OR in which R is an acyl moiety derived from a nontoxic, stable, pharmaceutically-acceptable carboxylic acid having from 1 to 7 carbon atoms and the hydrogenation is carried out under substantially neutral conditions.

9. The method of claim 7 characterized in that Y is acetoxy; R is acetyl; R₁ is hydrogen and R₂ is methyl.

10. The method of claim 7 characterized in that Y is acetoxy; R is acetyl; R₁ is hydrogen and R₂ is ethyl.

11. The method of forming a compound having the structural formula:

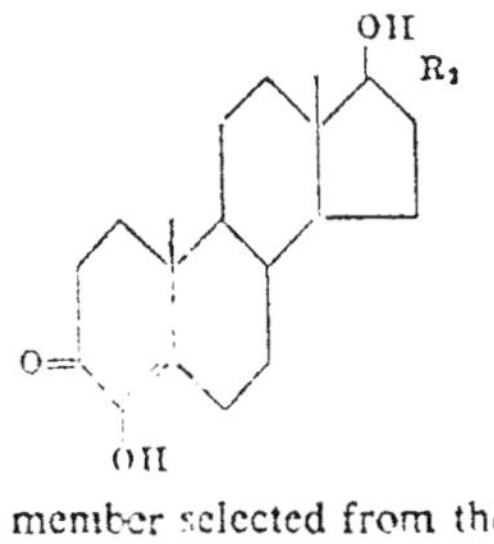

in which R₂ is a member selected from the group consist-

7

ing of hydrogen, methyl and ethyl, comprising hydrolyz-ing with alkaline hydrolyzing agents a compound having the structural formula:

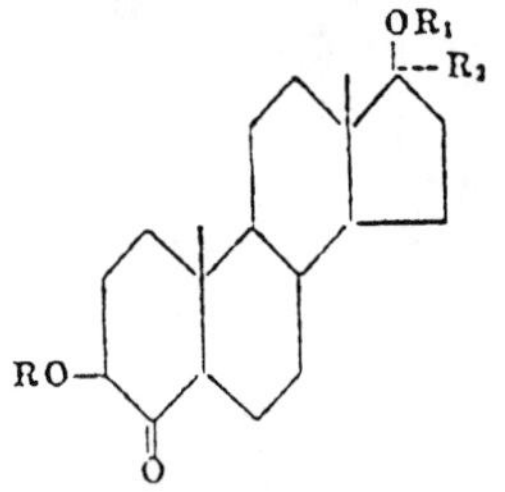

in which R is an acyl moiety derived from a hydrocarbon carboxylic acid having from 1 to 7 carbon atoms; R_1 is a member selected from the group consisting of hydrogen and an acyl moiety derived from a nontoxic, stable,

8

pharmaceutically-acceptable carboxylic acid having from 2 to 7 carbon atoms; and R_2 is a member selected from the group consisting of hydrogen, methyl and ethyl to form the corresponding 3,17-diol, and oxidizing the 3,17-diol product in acid solution at about 85° to about 120° C. with bismuth trioxide.

12. The method of claim 11 characterized in that R is acetyl; R_1 is hydrogen and R_2 is methyl.

References Cited in the file of this patent

UNITED STATES PATENTS

2,374,370 Miescher et al. _____ Apr. 24, 1945
2,762,818 Levy et al. _____ Sept. 11, 1956

OTHER REFERENCES

Camerino et al.: J. Am. Chem. Soc., vol. 78 (July 20, 1956), pages 3540 and 3541.

CHAPTER EIGHT

1

3,341,557
7-METHYLTESTOSTERONES
John C. Babcock, Kalamazoo, and J. Allan Campbell,
Kalamazoo Township, Kalamazoo County, Mich., assignors to The Upjohn Company, Kalamazoo, Mich.,
a corporation of Delaware
No Drawing. Filed June 5, 1961, Ser. No. 114,621
8 Claims. (Cl. 260—397.3)

The present invention relates to certain novel steroid compounds, more particularly to certain 7-methyltestosterones and the corresponding Δ^1-derivatives thereof, to certain 7-methyl-19-nortestosterones, and to processes for the production of the aforesaid compounds.

This application is a continuation-in-part of application Ser. No. 740,194, filed June 6, 1958, now abandoned, and application Ser. No. 69,557, filed Nov. 6, 1960, now abandoned.

The 7-methyltestosterones and the corresponding Δ^1-derivatives thereof, which compounds form part of the present invention, and processes for the production thereof, are illustratively represented by the following formulae in Reaction Scheme A wherein the dotted line between carbon atoms 1 and 2 indicates that these atoms can be joined by a single or double bond, R is a 17-substituent selected from the group consisting of β-hydroxy, β-hydroxy-17α-methyl, β-acyloxy-17α-methyl and β-acyloxy, R' is an 11-substituent selected from the group consisting of hydroxy (α and β), α-acyloxy, hydrogen, a 9(11)-double bond, and keto, the acyl radical of the acyloxy group in each instance being that of an organic carboxylic acid, preferably a hydrocarbon carboxylic and containing from one to twelve carbon atoms, inclusive, X is a halogen of atomic weight 35 to 127, inclusive, and X' is a halogen of atomic weight 19 to 127, inclusive. In the following formulae, the 7-methyl group represents both the alpha and beta stereoisomers and the mixture thereof.

The process of the instant invention as set forth in Reaction Scheme A below comprises: treating a 6-dehydrotestosterone (I) with a methyl Grignard reagent in the presence of a 1,6-addition-promoting agent, e.g., cuprous chloride, to produce a 7-methyltestosterone (II, III). The corresponding 1-dehydro-7-methyltestosterones [IIa and III (1,2-unsaturated)] can be prepared from the 7-methyltestosterones (II) or (III: 1,2-saturated) by methods well-known in the art, for example, by treatment with selenium dioxide using the procedure described by Meystre et al., Helv. Chim. Acta. 39, 734 (1956), or by treatment with a 1-dehydrogenating microorganism, for example, of the genus Septomyxa, using, for example, the procedure described in U.S. Patent 2,897,218. The 7-methyltestosterones (II) and the corresponding 1-dehydro derivatives (IIa) can then be converted to other 7-methyltestosterones and 1-dehydro-7-methyltestosterones, e.g., by dehydrating 7-methyl-11β-hydroxytestosterone or 17-acylate and 7,17-dimethyl-11β-hydroxytestosterone or 17-acylate and the corresponding 1-dehydro derivatives to produce 7-methyl-9(11)-dehydrotestosterone or 17-acylate and 7,17-dimethyl-9(11)-dehydrotestosterone or 17-acylate, and the corresponding 1-dehydro derivatives respectively (III); treating 7-methyl-9(11)-dehydrotestosterone, a 17-ester thereof, 7,17-dimethyl-9(11)-dehydrotestosterone or a 17-ester thereof, or the corresponding 1-dehydro derivatives thereof with a hypohalous acid to obtain a 7-methyl-9α-halo-11β-hydroxytestosterone, 17-ester, and 7,17-dimethyl-9α-halo-11β-hydroxytestosterone or 17-ester, and the corresponding 1-dehydro derivatives thereof, respectively (IV); treating the thus-produced 7-methyl-9α-halo-11β-hydroxytestosterone, 17-ester thereof, 7,17-dimethyl-9α-halo-11β-hydroxytestosterone, or 17-ester thereof or the corresponding 1-dehydro derivatives thereof, with a weak base, e.g., potassium or sodium hydroxide in slight excess so as

2

Reaction Scheme A

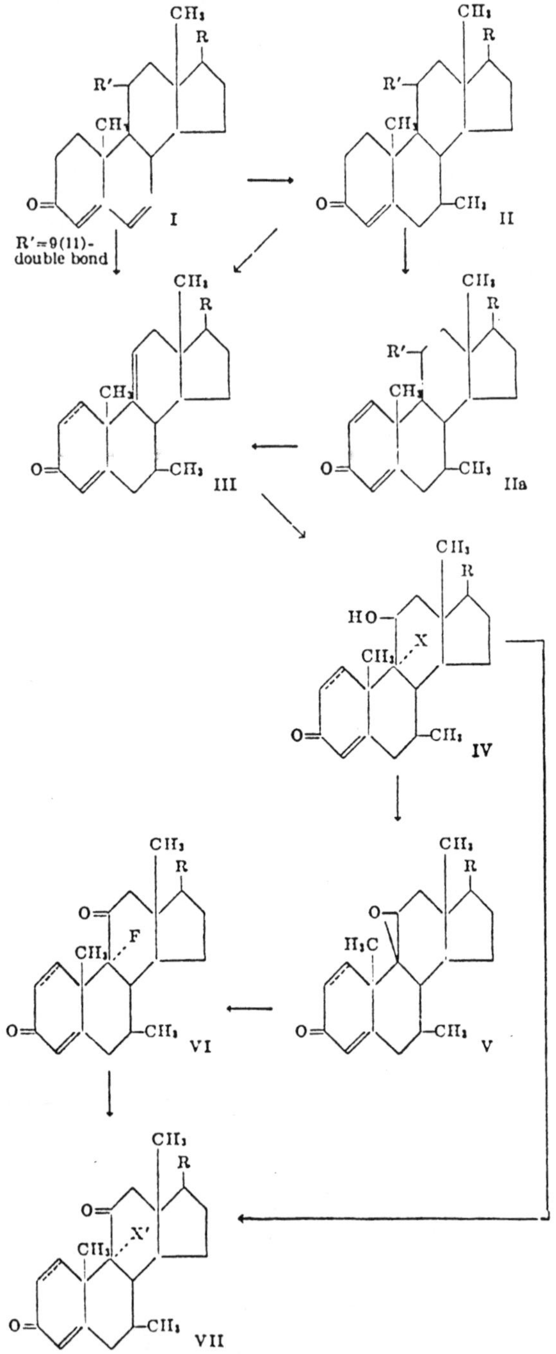

R'=9(11)-double bond

to produce a medium of pH 8 to 10, or potassium or sodium acetate, to obtain 7-methyl-9β,11β-epoxytestosterone, a 17-ester thereof, 7,17-dimethyl-9β,11β-epoxytestosterone, and 17-ester thereof, and the corresponding 1-dehydro derivatives thereof, respectively (V); and reacting the thus-produced 7-methyl-9β,11β-epoxytestosterone, 17-ester thereof, 7,17-dimethyl-9β,11β-epoxytestosterone, or 17-ester thereof or the corresponding 1-dehydro derivatives thereof, with hydrofluoric acid to obtain 7-methyl-9α-fluoro-11β-hydroxytestosterone, 17-ester thereof, 7,17-dimethyl-9α-fluoro-11β-hydroxytestosterone, and 17-ester thereof, and the corresponding 1-dehydro derivatives thereof respectively (VI). After each of the above steps, the 17-ester group, when present, can be hydrolyzed with acid in the case of IV or with base, if desired, to produce the corresponding free 17-hydroxy compound. Oxidation of a 7-methyl-9α-halo-11β-hydroxytestosterone or the 1-dehydro derivative thereof (IV or VI) with chromic acid produces the corresponding 7-methyl-9α-halo-11-ketotestosterone and 1-dehydro derivative thereof (VII). The 17-acylate group, when present, can be hydrolyzed with alkali-metal base to produce the corresponding 7-methyl-9α-halo-11-ketotestosterone or 1-dehydro derivative thereof. 7-methyl-9α-halo-11-ketotestosterone 17-acylates or 1-dehydro derivatives thereof can also be hydrolyzed in alcoholic acid solutions to give the corresponding 7-methyl-9α-halo-11-ketotestosterone or 1-dehydro derivative thereof.

A 17-acylate group can be introduced into any of the above compounds having a 17-hydroxy group, by techniques well known in the art. If there is also present a 17-methyl group, more vigorous esterification techniques are required, as is known in the art.

The 7-methyl-19-nortestosterones, which form part of the present invention, and processes for the production thereof, are illustratively represented by the following formulae in Reaction Scheme B:

Reaction Scheme B

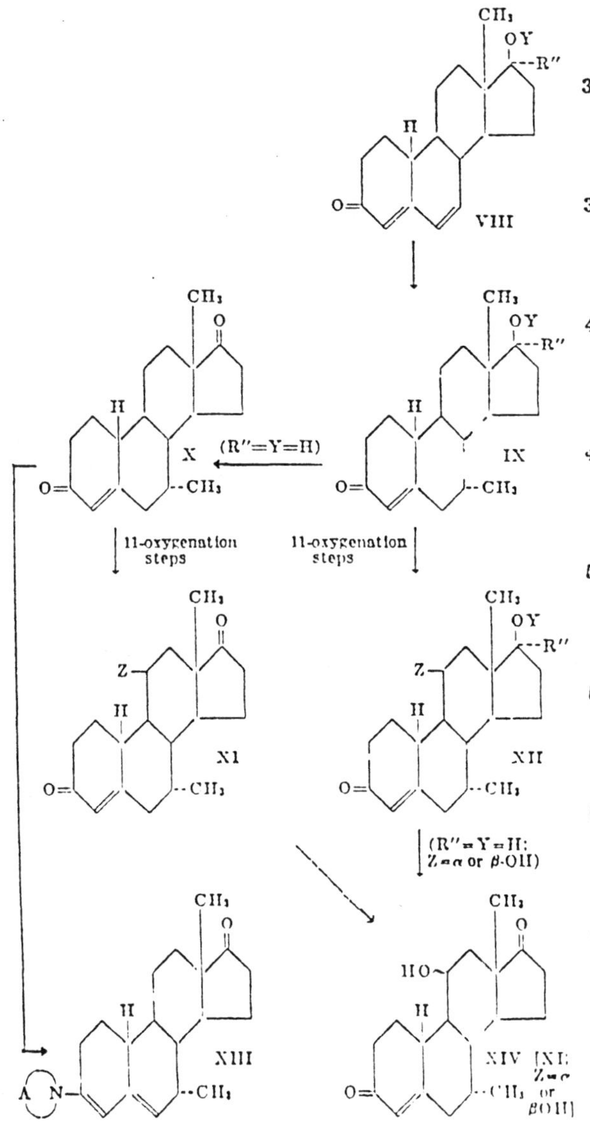

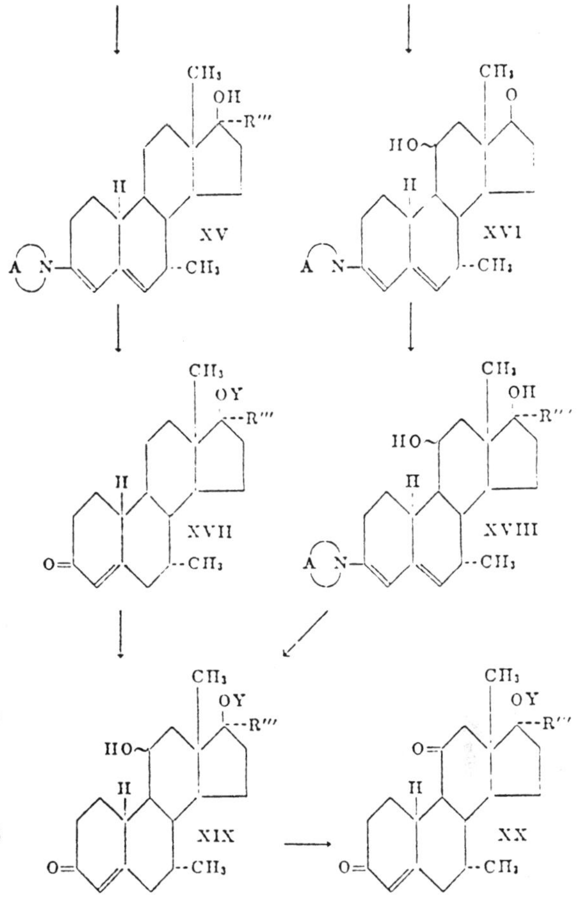

wherein R″ is selected from the class consisting of hydrogen and lower-alkyl containing from 1 to 4 carbon atoms, inclusive, R‴ is a lower aliphatic hydrocarbon radical containing from 1 to 4 carbon atoms, inclusive, Z is an 11-substituent selected from the class consisting of hydrogen, keto, hydroxy (α and β), and α-acyloxy, wherein the acyl of the acyloxy radical is that of an organic carboxylic acid preferably a hydrocarbon carboxylic acid as hereinbefore defined, Y is selected from the class consisting of hydrogen and the acyl radical of an organic carboxylic acid, preferably a hydrocarbon carboxylic acid as hereinbefore defined, and A is an alkylene group which, together with the attached nitrogen atom, forms a ring containing from 5 to 6 members, inclusive, and which preferably contains less than 9 carbon atoms.

The term "lower aliphatic hydrocarbon radical containing from 1 to 4 carbon atoms, inclusive" means a saturated or unsaturated 1 to 4 carbon atom aliphatic hydrocarbon radical such as alkyl, for example, methyl, ethyl, propyl, butyl, and isomeric forms thereof, alkenyl, for example, vinyl, propenyl, butenyl and isomeric forms thereof, and alkynyl, for example, ethynyl, propynyl, butynyl, and isomeric forms thereof.

The organic carboxylic acids, from which the acylates of the present invention are derived, include saturated and unsaturated aliphatic acids and aromatic acids such as acetic, propionic, butyric, isobutyric, tert-butylacetic, valeric, isovaleric, caproic, caprylic, decanoic, dodecanoic, acrylic, crotonic, hexynoic, heptynoic, actynoic, cyclobutanecarboxylic, cyclopentanecarboxylic, cyclopentenecarboxylic, cyclohexanecarboxylic, dimethylcyclohexanecarboxylic, benzoic, toluic, naphthoic, ethylbenzoic, phenylacetic, naphthaleneacetic, phenylvaleric, cinnamic, phenylpropiolic, phenylpropionic, p-hexyloxyphenylpropionic acid, p-butyloxyphenylpropionic acid, and like p-alkoxyphenylalkanoic acids.

The process of the invention as set forth in Reaction

5

Scheme B above comprises: treating a 6-heydro-9-nor-testosterone (VIII) with a methyl Grignard reagent in the presence of a 1,6-addition-promoting agent, for example, cuprous chloride, to produce a 7α-methyl-9-nortestoster-one (IX). The 7α-methyl-9-nortestosterone (IX) so produced can then be converted to other 7α-methyl-19-nor-testosterones. For example, the compound (IX) can be hydroxylated in the 11-position, illustratively by treatment with an 11α-hydroxylating microorganism using the procedures described in U.S. Patents 2,602,769, 2,649,400, 2,649,401, and 2,649,402 to yield the corresponding 11α-hydroxy compound (XII: Z=α-OH), or by treatment with an 11β-hydroxylating microorganism using procedures such as that described in U.S. Patent 2,602,769 to yield the corresponding 11β-hydroxy compound (XII: Z=β-hydrxoy). The 11-hydroxy compounds so obtained can be oxidized, for example, using chromic acid, sodium dichromate, potassium dichromate and the like, to yield the corresponding 11-keto compounds (XII: Z=keto). In the case where R'' and Y=H in the 11-hydroxy compound (XII; Z=α or β-OH) such oxidation will also result in oxidation at the 17-position to give the corresponding 11, 17-diketo compound.

The compound (IX; R''=Y=H) can also be oxidized, for example, with chromic acid or like oxidizing agents using procedures known in the art, to obtain the corresponding 17-keto compound (X). Compound (X) so obtained can be converted to the corresponding 11α- or 11β-hydroxy compounds (XI; Z=α or β-OH) using the procedures described above, and the resulting 11-hydroxy compounds can be oxidized to the corresponding 11-keto compound (XI; Z=keto) using the oxidation procedures described above.

The compound (X) can also be converted to the 3-enamine (XIII), the 3-enamine (XIII) treated with an appropriate alkylating agent such as the appropriate Grignard reagent, alkyl or alkenyl lithium compound or alkali metal alkyne derivative to obtain the compound XV, and the latter compound hydrolyzed using neutral, acidic or alkaline aqueous reaction conditions, to the corresponding 17-alkylated-7-methyl-19-nortestosterone (XVII; Y=H). The 17-hydroxy group in the compound (XVII; Y=H) so obtained can be acylated, if desired, using acylating conditions known in the art, to yield the corresponding 17-acyloxy compound (XVII; Y=Ac). The compound (XVII; Y=H or Ac) can then be subjected to 11-hydroxylation using the procedures described above to obtain the corresponding 11α- and 11β-hydroxy compounds (XIX; Y=H) which can then be converted to the corresponding 11α,17-diacyloxy compounds or 11β-hydroxy-17-acyloxy compounds by acylation using procedures well-known in the art. The 11-hydroxy compounds (XIX) can also be oxidized to the corresponding 11-keto compounds (XX) using oxidation procedures such as those described above.

In an alternative synthesis of the compounds (XIX), the compounds (XIV) obtained by Oppenauer oxidation of the compound (XII; R''=Y=H, Z=α- or β-OH) or the compound (XI; Z=α or β-OH) is converted to the corresponding 3-enamine (XVI) and the latter is treated with an alkylating agent such as those described above to obtain the 3-enamine of the corresponding 17-alkylated-11-hydroxy-7α-methyl-19-nortestosterone (XVIII). The latter compound is then hydrolyzed using the conditions hereinbefore described to obtain the compound (XIX; Y=H).

It is an object of this invention to provide 7-methyl-testosterones and the corresponding 1-dehydro derivatives (II–VII) and a process for their production. It is a particular object of this invention to provide

7-methyl-testosterone,
1-dehydro-7-methyltestosterone,
7-methyl-11β-hydroxytestosterone,
1-dehydro-7-methyl-11β-hydroxytestosterone,
7,17-dimethyltestosterone,

6

1-dehydro-7,17-dimethyltestosterone,
7,17-dimethyl-11β-hydroxytestosterone,
1-dehydro-7,17-dimethyl-11β-hydroxytestosterone,
7-methyl-9α-fluoro-11β-hydroxytestosterone,
1-dehydro-7-methyl-9α-fluoro-11β-hydroxytestosterone,
7,17-dimethyl-9α-fluoro-11β-hydroxytestosterone, and
1-dehydro-7,17-dimethyl-9α-fluoro-11β-hydroxytestoster-one,

and the 17-esters thereof, especially those of hydrocarbon carboxylic acids containing from one to twelve carbon atoms, inclusive.

It is a further object of this invention to provide 7-methyl-19-nortestosterones (IX, X, XI, XII, XIV, XVII, XIX and XX) and a process for their production. It is a particular object of this invention to provide 7-methyl-19-nortestosterone and the 17-esters thereof, 7-methyl-19-nor-Δ⁴-androstene-3,17-dione, 7-methyl-17-ethynyl-19-nortestosterone and the 17-esters thereof, 17-ethyl-7-methyl-19-nortestosterone and the 17-esters thereof, and 7,17-dimethyl-19-nortestosterone and the 17-esters thereof.

The 7-methyltestosterones and the 1-dehydro-7-methyl-testosterones of the present invention (II, IIA-VII) have androgenic and anabolic activity of improved therapeutic ratio. Compounds II, IIA, and VI, wherein R' is hydrogen and R is β-hydroxy, β-acyloxy or β-hydroxy-α-methyl, are particularly valuable in this respect. The compounds (II, IIA-VII) also possesses antiestrogenic, gonadotropin inhibiting activity, progestational, growth-promoting, and central nervous system regulating activities making them of value in medical and veterinary practice.

The 7-methyl-19-nortestosterones of the present invention (IX, X, XI, XII, XIV, XVII, XIX and XX) possess anabolic and androgenic activity with an improved potency and improved therapeutic ratio of anabolic to androgenic activity. They also possess antiestrogenic, gonadotropin inhibiting, progestational, growth-promoting, antifertility and central nervous system depressant activity. The compound 7α-methyl-17α-ethinyl-19-nortestosterone is of particular interest since it possess greater activity as an antifertility agent but lower activity as a progestational agent than the closely related known compound 17α-ethinyl-19-nortestosterone.

In addition, the 7α-methyl-19-nortestosterones (IX–XX) of the invention are intermediates in the preparation of the corresponding 7α-methylestrones and 7α-methylestradiols which latter compounds possess activity as gonadotropin inhibitors, antifertility agents, and blood cholesterol lowering agents of improved therapeutic ratio. Thus the 7α-methyl-19-nortestosterones of the invention can be dehydrogenated, for example, using *Septomyxa affinis* and like dehydrogenating microorganisms, to yield the corresponding 7α-methylestrones and 7α-methyl-estradiols.

The compounds of this invention can be prepared and administered to mammals, birds, humans, and animals, in a wide variety of oral or parenteral dosage forms singly, or in admixture with other coacting compounds. They can be administered with a pharmaceutical carrier which can be a solid material or a liquid in which the compound is dissolved, dispersed or suspended. The solid compositions can take the form of tablets, powders, capsules, pills, or the like, preferably in unit dosage forms for simple administration or precise dosages. The liquid compositions can take the form of solutions, emulsions, suspensions, syrups or elixirs. The oral forms are preferably used for the 17α-alkylated 17β-hydroxy compounds of this invention which possess particularly advantageous oral activity.

In carrying out the process of the present invention illustrated in Reaction Scheme A, the starting 6-dehydrotestosterone (I) is reacted with an excess of a methyl Grignard reagent, e.g., methyl magnesium iodide or methyl magnesium bromide, in the presence of cuprous chloride or equivalent catalyst. See "Grignard Reaction," Kharasch and Reinmuth, Prentice Hall, Inc. Publishers (1954), page 219, for a discussion of other catalysts. Cuprous chloride is preferred. Various inert solvents can be employed, e.g., benzene, toluene, the dimethyl ether of ethylene glycol, ether, tetrahydrofuran, or a mixture of these. The reaction temperature can vary between minus 40 degrees centigrade and the boiling point of the reaction mixture. A temperature between about sixty degrees centigrade and zero degrees centigrade is preferred. As the 17-oxygen function, and to a certain extent the 11-hydroxy group will also react with the Grignard reagent, more than one molar equivalent of the Grignard reagent should be employed to ensure complete reaction with the 3-keto-$\Delta^{4,6}$-diene system. A ratio of at least five moles of Grignard per mole of steroid is preferred. Methyl magnesium bromide produces the highest yield of desired product and is the preferred reagent.

The 7-methyltestosterones (II) so obtained can then, if desired, be converted to the corresponding 1-dehydro-7-methyltestosterones (IIa) by the procedures hereinbefore described. The 1-dehydro compounds (IIa) so obtained can be purified by procedures known in the art, for example, by recrystallization or by chromatography. Where the crude 1-dehydro compound (IIa) contains an appreciable amount of the unconverted starting material (II) the mixture can be separated by conversion of the latter to the corresponding 3-enamine. For example, refluxing the mixture of (II) and (IIa) in benzene in the presence of a secondary cyclic alkylene amine such as pyrrolidine for several hours converts the compound (II) to its 3-enamine whereas the compound (IIa) does not form an enamine under such conditions. The mixture of the compound (IIa) and the 3-enamine of (II) can then be separated by treatment with dilute mineral acid when the 3-enamine dissolves and the compound (IIa) can be recovered and purified further, if necessary, for example by recrystallization.

In the next step of the process of Reaction Scheme A, a 7-methyl-11-hydroxytestosterone or the corresponding 1-dehydro compound (II or IIa, R′=OH) is dehydrated by the process shown in the example, or by prior art procedure for dehydration of 11α- and 11β hydroxy steroids, e.g., [Fieser and Fieser, "Natural Products Related to Phenanthrene," Reinhold Publishing Corporation, New York, 1949, pages 408–409], to produce the corresponding 7-methyl-9(11)-dehydrotestosterone or 1-dehydro-7-methyl-9(11)-dehydrotestosterone (III). The compound (III) dissolved in a suitable solvent such as, for example, methylene chloride, tertiary butyl alcohol, dioxane, tertiary amyl alcohol, acetone, or the like, is reacted with a hypohalous acid, i.e., hypochlorous, hypobromous or hypoiodous acid to produce the corresponding 7-methyl-9α-halo-11β-hydroxytestosterone or 1-dehydro-7-methyl-9α-halo-11β-hydroxytestosterone (IV).

Instead of using the free acid it is usually more convenient to produce the hypohalous acid in situ by reacting an N-haloamide or an N-haloimide with a mineral acid. N-haloamides or an N-haloimides useful in this procedure include N-chloroacetamide, N-bromoacetamide, N-chlorosuccinimide, N-bromosuccinimide, N-iodosuccinimide, and the like. The mineral acid used to liberate the hypohalous acid is usually dilute perchloric or dilute sulfuric acid. The reaction is generally carried out at temperatures between zero and thirty degrees centigrade, however, lower or higher temperatures are operative for the process. The hypohalous acid releasing agent is generally used in equimolar proportion or in slight excess, e.g., a 25 percent excess. A large excess of the hypohalous acid-releasing agent, while operative, is undesirable since the excess of hypohalous acid has a tendency to react with other positions of the molecule. The reaction period is rather short and may vary between about four to five minutes to one hour. At the end of the reaction time excess hypohalous

acid is destroyed by the addition of sodium sulfite or other sulfites or hydrosulfites. The thus-produced product, a 7-methyl-9α-halo-11β-hydroxytestosterone or the 1-dehydro derivative thereof (IV), is isolated from the reaction mixture by adding an excess of water and extracting the reaction mixture with organic solvents such as methylene chloride, chloroform, benzene, toluene, ether, ethyl acetate, hexane hydrocarbons (Skellysolve B), or the like, or by filtration. The crude product thus obtained is purified by conventional procedures such as recrystallization or chromatography, as deemed necessary.

7-methyl-9β,11β-epoxytestosterones and the corresponding 1-dehydro compounds (V) are prepared by treating the appropriately substituted compound (IV) with a mild base. In this reaction the compound (IV) is dissolved in an organic solvent such as, for example, methanol, ethanol, isopropanol, dioxane, tertiary butyl alcohol, or tetrahydrofuran, and treated with a base, e.g., potassium acetate, sodium bicarbonate, or a sodium acylate e.g., sodium acetate. If the starting material is a 17-ester of a compound (IV) sodium or potassium acetate is preferred in order to avoid simultaneous hydrolysis of such ester. Heating of the reaction mixture is preferred and the reaction time is usually between three and twelve hours. Alternatively a methanolic solution of compound (IV) is stirred at room temperature with aqueous base such as sodium hydroxide, potassium hydroxide, barium hydroxide, or the like. The base is added slowly with continuous agitation and carried only to the point at which the reaction mixture remains basic to phenolphthalein for a period of about one-half minute. The thus-obtained 7-methyl-9β,11β-epoxytestosterone or 1-dehydro-7-methyl-9β,11β-epoxytestosterone (V) is separated from the reaction mixture by conventional means such as adding an excess of water to the reaction mixture and either filtering the thus-produced precipitate or extracting with water-immiscible solvent, e.g., ether, hexanes (Skellysolve B), pentanes, benzene, ether, ethyl acetate, chloroform, methylene chloride, carbon tetrachloride, or the like. Purification of the thus obtained compound (V) may be by conventional means such as recrystallization or chromatography.

7-methyl-9β,11β-epoxytestosterones and the corresponding 1-dehydro compounds (V) are converted to 7-methyl-9α-fluoro-11β-hydroxytestosterones and the corresponding 1-dehydro compounds (VI) by reaction with 48 percent aqueous hydrofluoric acid solution in a solvent. As solvents for this reaction, methylene chloride, ethylene dichloride, chloroform, carbon tetrachloride, or the like, are used with methylene chloride and chloroform preferred. The reaction in the preferred embodiment is carried out in the presence of acid catalysts such as perchloric acid, toluenesulfonic acid, sulfuric acid, or the like. The reaction temperature is preferably from twenty to thirty degrees centigrade. The period of reaction is from one to 24 hours. Instead of aqueous hydrofluoric acid, hydrogen fluoride gas, dissolved in a chilled solution of alcohol-free chloroform or methylene chloride, preferably containing tetrahydrofuran, can be used. In this case, a chilled solution of compound (V) in a convenient solvent such as chloroform, methylene chloride, carbon tetrachloride, or the like, contained in a polyethylene bottle, is admixed with a chilled solution of gaseous hydrogen fluoride in chloroform, methylene chloride, or carbon tetrachloride solution. The stoppered bottle is then allowed to stand for a period of between one hour and 24 hours at low temperatures, e.g., between minus forty and plus ten degrees centigrade, with temperatures between zero and minus 25 degrees centigrade preferred. After the reaction is terminated, the reaction mixture obtained by either of the two methods is neutralized with an aqueous base such as aqueous sodium bicarbonate, aqueous sodium carbonate, potassium carbonate or bicarbonate, or dilute sodium or potassium hydroxide, or the like, and the thus-obtained 7-methyl-9α-fluoro-11β-hydroxytestosterone, or ester thereof, or the corresponding 1-dehydro compound, is separated from the reaction mixture by conventional means such as extraction with water-immiscible organic solvents, for example, ether, ethyl acetate, hexanes (Skellysolve B), chloroform, carbon tetrachloride, methylene chloride, or the like. Evaporation of the extraction solvent gives the crude compound (VI) which can be purified by conventional means, e.g., recrystallization or chromatography.

In order to obtain 7-methyl-9α-halo-11-ketotestosterones or the corresponding 1-dehydro compounds (VII), any one of the before-mentioned 7-methyl-9α-halo-11β-hydroxytestosterone 17-esters or corresponding 1-dehydro compounds (IV, VI, R=acyloxy) or 7-17-dimethyl-9α-halo-11β-hydroxytestosterone or corresponding 1-dehydro compounds (IV, VI, R=β-hydroxy-α-methyl) is oxidized preferably by chromic acid in an acidic solvent, e.g., acetic acid, acetic acid plus benzene, dilute mineral acid plus methylene chloride, or the like.

Hydrolyzing a 7-methyltestosterone 17-acylate or corresponding 1-dehydro compound (II–VII, R=acyloxy) with an alkali metal base in aqueous alcoholic solution or dilute mineral acid produces the corresponding 7-methyltestosterone or 1-dehydro compound as the free 17-alcohol.

The pure 7-stereoisomers, each free from the other, can be obtained by fractional crystallization or carbon chromatography to obtain one of the isomers and then treatment of the residual mixture of isomers with chloranil which reacts with only the 7β-isomer leaving the 7α-isomer unchanged, and then separating that isomer from the resulting 6-dehydro compound as shown in Example 2. The 6-dehydro-7-methyl compound resulting from the chloranil reaction can be converted back to the 7β-methyl compound by selective hydrogenation using, for example, a palladium-on-charcoal catalyst as disclosed by Shepherd et al., J. Am. Chem. Soc. 77, 1212, 1955.

Any of the compounds III, V, VI, wherein the 1,2-bond is unsaturated can be prepared from the corresponding compound in which the 1,2-bond is saturated by 1-dehydrogenation using the procedures described above.

The 6-dehydrotestosterones employed as starting materials in Reaction Scheme A are prepared as described in U.S. 2,739,974 or by the reaction of testosterone with chloranil as shown in Example 2, or by reacting a 3β-hydroxy-5-androstene, having R' in the 11-position and R in the 17-position, R and R' being defined a hereinabove, with aluminum tertiary butoxide and para quinone in the manner described in Preparation 2. The starting 3β-hydroxy-5-androstenes can be prepared by the sodium borohydride reduction of a 3-enol ester of a testosterone in the manner described in Preparation 1.

In carrying out the process of the present invention as illustrated in Reaction Scheme B, the starting 6-dehydro-19-nortestosterone (VIII) is reacted with an excess of a methyl Grignard reagent, for example, methyl magnesium iodide, methyl magnesium bromide, and the like, in the presence of cuprous chloride or equivalent catalyst; see "Grignard Reaction," supra. Cuprous chloride is preferred. Various inert solvents can be employed, for example, benzene, toluene, ethylene glycol dimethyl ether, ether, tetrahydrofuran, and the like, or a mixture of any two of these solvents. The reaction temperature can vary between minus 40° C. and the boiling point of the reaction mixture. A temperature between about 0° C. and 60° C. is preferred. The Grignard reagent is preferably employed in the ratio of at least 5 moles of Grignard per mole of steroid. Methyl magnesium bromide produces the highest yield of desired product and is the preferred reagent.

Where the group Y is hydrogen in the compound (IX) so obtained said compound can be acylated to produce the corresponding 17-acyloxy compound (IX; Y=Ac). The acylation can be accomplished using methods known in the art, for example, by treatment with the appropriate acid anhydride or acid halide in the presence of a tertiary base such as pyridine.

The 7α-methyl-19-nortestosterone (IX) can be subjected to 11-hydroxylation as follows. The compound (IX) can be subjected to the action of the enzymes of an 11α-hydroxylating microorganism such as those of the genera Mucorales, Aspergillus, Penicillium, and Streptomyces using, for example, the procedures described in U.S. Patents 2,602,769, 2,649,400, 2,649,401, and 2,649,402. There is thus obtained the compound (XII) wherein Z=α-hydroxy and Y=hydrogen. Alternatively the compound (IX) can be subjected to the action of the enzymes of an 11β-hydroxylating microorganism such as Cunninghamella blakeslecana, Curvularia lunata, Trichothecium roseum, and the like using procedures well known in the art, for example, that described in Example 2 of U.S. Patent 2,602,769. There is thus obtained the compound XII wherein Z=β-hydroxy and Y=hydrogen.

Where the group Y is acyl in the compound (IX) said group will generally be removed during the microbiological hydroxylation procedures and in order to obtain the compound (XII) wherein Y is acyl it is necessary to acylate the free 17-hydroxy group using procedures such as those described above. Such acylation will also convert the 11α-hydroxy, when present, to the corresponding 11α-acyloxy group.

In order to obtain the compound (XII) wherein Z is keto, the corresponding 11α or β-hydroxy compound (XII; Z=α or β-OH and Y=Ac when R'' is hydrogen) is oxidized using procedures known in the art. For example, the oxidation can be effected using chromic acid, sodium dichromate, potassium dichromate and like oxidizing agents.

The compound (IX) wherein Y and R'' both represent hydrogen, i.e., 7α-methyl-19-nortestosterone, can be oxidized to the compound (X), i.e., 7α-methyl-19-nor-Δ4-androstene-3,17-dione, using procedures known in the art, for example, using chromic acid, sodium dichromate, potassium dichromate and like oxidizing agents.

The 7α-methyl-19-nor-Δ4-androstene-3,17-dione (X) so obtained can then be converted to the corresponding 11α-hydroxy, 11β-hydroxy, and 11-keto compound (XI) using the procedures described above for the 11-hydroxylation of compound (IX) and the oxidation of the 11-hydroxy compounds to 11-keto.

The compound (X) can also be converted to the compounds (XVII), (XIX) and (XX) of the invention using the following procedure. The 7α-methyl-19-nor-Δ4-androstene-3,17-dione (X) is first converted to the corresponding 3-enamine, for example, by reaction with a secondary cyclic alkylene amine

$$A \quad \text{XII}$$

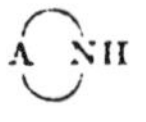

wherein A has the significance hereinbefore defined, if desired in the presence of an acid catalyst.

The secondary cyclic alkylene amines which can be used in the above reaction include pyrrolidine, piperidine, and C-alkyl substituted pyrrolidines, and piperidines such as 2,4-dimethylpyrrolidine, 3-propylpiperidine, 2-methylpyrrolidine, 3,4-dimethylpyrrolidine, 3-ethylpyrrolidine, 3-isopropylpyrrolidine, 3,3-dimethylpyrrolidine, and other lower alkyl C-substituted pyrrolidines, and piperidines. Pyrrolidine is the preferred amine for use in the above reaction. Advantageously, the amine is employed in excess of the required molar proportion. The reaction between the compound (X) and the amine is effected in a convenient manner by heating the reactants together in the presence of a suitable solvent, for example, a lower alkanol such as methanol, ethanol, and the like. The desired 3-enamine (XIII) generally separates from the reaction mixture after concentrating the latter and allowing to cool.

The 3-enamine (XIII) so obtained is then converted to the 3-enamine of the corresponding 17-alkylated compound (XV) by reaction with the appropriate alkylating agent. For example, the 3-enamine (XIII) can be reacted with the appropriate alkyl, alkenyl, or alkynyl magnesium halide in the presence of a solvent such as dimethyl ether, tetrahydrofuran, benzene and the like, to produce the corresponding compound (XV) wherein R''' is alkyl, alkenyl, or alkynyl as hereinbefore defined. Preferably, the Grignard reagent is employed in an excess of the order of 10 moles per mole of enamine (XIII). The resulting 17-alkylated 3-enamine (XV) is generally not isolated from the reaction mixture but is hydrolyzed in situ to the corresponding 7α-methyl-17-alkylated-19-nortestosterone (XVII) by treatment with an aqueous solution of a base such as sodium hydroxide, potassium hydroxide, and the like after first decomposing the reaction mixture with water, ammonium chloride, and the like.

Alternatively, the alkylating agent employed to convert the enamine (XIII) to the 17-alkylated compound (XV) in the case where R'' is alkyl or alkenyl, can be the appropriate alkyl or alkenyl lithium compound. The reaction is conducted advantageously in the presence of an inert solvent such as ether, benzene, toluene, and the like. The lithium compound is employed advantageously in excess of the stoichiometric proportion and is employed preferably in an amount of at least 1.5 moles per mole of compound (XIII). The reaction is ordinarily conducted at room temperature but may also be conducted at elevated temperatures up to the boiling point of the solvent employed. The 17-alkylated-3-enamine (XV) so formed is generally not isolated but is hydrolyzed in situ to the corresponding 3-keto compound (XVII) as hereinbefore described.

The compounds having the Formula XVII wherein R''' represents a 2 to 4 carbon atom alkynyl group can also be prepared by reacting the enamine (XIII) with an alkali metal derivative, for example, the sodium or potassium derivative of the corresponding alkyne. The reaction is carried out preferably in the presence of an inert solvent such as dimethylformamide or dimethylsulfoxide. The 17-alkynyl-3-enamine (XV) so obtained is not generally isolated from the reaction mixture but is hydrolyzed in situ as described above to obtain the desired compound (XVII).

The compound (XVII) where R''' represents alkynyl or alkenyl can be hydrogenated in the presence of a suitable hydrogenation catalyst such as palladium-on-charcoal to obtain the corresponding compounds in which R''' is a 2 to 4 carbon atom alkyl group.

The 7α-methyl-17-alkylated-19-nortestosterones (XVII; Y=H) so obtained can be acylated using the procedures hereinbefore described to obtain the corresponding 17-acyloxy compounds (XVII; Y=Ac).

The compounds (XVII) can be converted to the corresponding 11α-hydroxy and 11β-hydroxy compounds (XIX) using the microbiological oxidation procedures hereinbefore described, and the 11β-hydroxylated compounds (XIX) can be oxidized to the corresponding 11-keto compounds (XX) using the oxidation procedures hereinbefore described. The microbiological hydroxylations will generally result in the removal of the 17-acyl group if this is present in the starting compound (XVII). The free 17-hydroxy group in the resulting compound (XIX; Y=H) can be reacylated if desired using the procedures described above.

The compound (XIX) wherein R''' represents alkynyl or alkenyl can be hydrogenated in the presence of a suitable hydrogenation catalyst such as palladium-on-charcoal to obtain the corresponding compounds in which R''' is a 2 to 4 carbon atom alkyl group.

In an alternative method of preparation of the compounds XIX and XX, the compound XII, wherein R''=Y=H and Z=α- or β-OH, is subjected to an Oppenauer oxidation using procedures known in the art, for example, using aluminum tert-butoxide and acetone or cyclohexanone in the presence of an anhydrous organic solvent such as toluene, benzene, petroleum ether, dioxane, or other organic solvents or mixtures thereof. There is thus obtained 11-hydroxy-7α-methyl-19-nor-Δ4-andro-

stenedione (XIV; identical to XI wherein Z=α- or β-hydroxy).

The compound (XIV) so obtained is then converted to the corresponding 3-enamine (XVI) using the procedure described above for the preparation of the corresponding 11-desoxy 3-enamine (XII).

The 11-hydroxy-7α-methyl-19-nor-Δ4-androstenedione 3-enamine (XVI) so obtained is alkylated using any of the alkylating agents and alkylating procedures described above for the alkylation of the corresponding 11-desoxy 3-enamine (XIII). There is thus obtained the corresponding 17-alkylated-11-hydroxy-7α-methyl-19-nortestosterone 3-enamine (XVIII) which is generally not isolated as such from the reaction mixture after alkylation but is hydrolyzed in situ to the corresponding 11-hydroxy-7α-methyl-17-alkylated-19-nortestosterone (XIX), for example, by treatment with an aqueous solution of a base such as sodium hydroxide, potassium hydroxide, and the like.

The compounds having the Formula VIII, which are employed as starting materials in the processes of Reaction Scheme B, can be prepared as follows:

The preparation of 6-dehydro-19-nortestosterone acetate (VIII; R''=H, Y=CH₃CO) by reaction of 19-nortestosterone with acetic anhydride and acetyl chloride in pyridine solution, followed by bromination of the resulting 3,17β-diacetoxy-19-nor-Δ3,5-androstadiene and dehydrobromination of the 6-bromo-19-nortestosterone 17-acetate so formed, has been described in British Patent Specification 833,183. Replacing the acetic anhydride and acetyl chloride employed in the first step of the above process by the appropriate acid anhydride and acid chloride yields other 17-acylates having the formula (VIII; R''=H, Y=Ac). The corresponding 17-hydroxy compounds (VIII: R''=H, Y=H) can be prepared by deacylation of the 17-acylates using procedures well known in the art.

Replacing 19-nortestosterone by the appropriate 17-alkyl-19-nortestosterone and employing the appropriate acid anhydride and acid halide in the above-described process affords the requisite 17-alkyl-6-dehydro-19-nortestosorone 17-acylate (VIII: R''=alkyl, Y=acyl). The corresponding free 17-hydroxy compounds (VIII: R''=alkyl, Y=H) can be prepared by deacylation of the 17-acylates using procedures well known in the art, for example, using a base such as sodium hydroxide or potassium hydroxide in aqueous or aqueous alcoholic solution.

This invention also includes the compound 7α-methyl-17α-ethyltestosterone and the 17-acylates thereof. These compounds have androgenic and anabolic activity of improved therapeutic ratio and also possess antiestrogenic, gonadotropin-inhibiting activity, progestational, growth promoting, and central nervous system regulating activities which make them useful in the treatment of mammals in medical and veterinary practice.

The compound 7α-methyl-17α-ethyltestosterone can be prepared by reacting 6-dehydro-17α-ethyltestosterone (U.S. Patent 2,739,974) with a methyl Grignard reagent in the presence of a 1,6-addition-promoting agent, for example, cuprous chloride using the conditions hereinbefore described for the conversion of compound (I) to compound (II) in Reaction Scheme A.

Alternatively, 7α-methyl-17α-ethyltestosterone can be prepared from 7α-methyltestosterone by oxidizing the latter compound to 7α-methyl-Δ4-landrostene-3,17-dione using procedures known in the art, for example, using chromic acid, sodium dichromate, potassium dichromate and like oxidizing agents. The 7α-methyl-Δ4-landrostene-3,17-dione is then converted to the corresponding 3-enamine using pyrrolidine and like secondary cyclic alkylene amines, according to the procedures described above for the preparation of the 3-enamines (XIII) and (XVI). The 3-enamine of 7α-methyl-Δ4-landrostene-3,17-dione is then reacted with an ethyl Grignard reagent such as ethyl magnesium bromide, in the presence of a solvent such as dimethylether, tetrahydrofuran, benzene, and the like.

13

Preferably the ethyl Grignard reagent is employed in an excess of the order of 10 moles per mole of the 3-enamine. The resulting 3-enamine of 7α-methyl-17α-ethyltestosterone is generally not isolated from the reaction mixture but is hydrolyzed in situ to the corresponding 7α-methyl-17α-ethyltestosterone by treatment with an aqueous solution of a base such as sodium hydroxide, potassium hydroxide, and the like after first decomposing the reaction mixture with water, ammonium chloride, and the like.

In an alternative method of preparation the 3-enamine of 7α-methyl-Δ4-landrostene-3,17-dione is reacted with an alkali metal derivative, for example, the sodium or potassium derivative of acetylene. The reaction is carried out preferably in the presence of an inert solvent such as dimethylformamide or dimethylsulfoxide. The 3-enamine of 7α-methyl-17α-ethynyltestosterone so obtained is not generally isolated from the reaction mixture but is hydrolyzed in situ as described above to obtain 7α-methyl-17α-ethynyltestosterone. The latter compound is then hydrogenated in the presence of a suitable hydrogenation catalyst such as palladium-on-charcoal to obtain the desired 7α-methyl-17α-ethyltestosterone.

The 17-acylates of 7α-methyl-17α-ethyltestosterone can be prepared from the latter compound using procedures known in the art, for example, by treatment with the appropriate acid anhydride or acid halide in the presence of a tertiary base such as pyridine.

The compound 7α-methyl-17α-ethynyltestosterone (which is employed as described above as an intermediate in the preparation of 7α-methyl-17α-ethyltestosterone) and the corresponding 17-acylates are compounds having androgenic and anabolic activity of improved therapeutic ratio and also possess antiestrogenic, gonadotropin-inhibiting activity, progestational, growth-promoting, and central nervous system regulating activities which make them useful in the treatment of mammals in medical and veterinary practice.

The following preparations and examples are illustrative of the process and products of the present invention, but are not to be construed as limiting.

PREPARATION 1.—17α-METHYL-5-ANDROSTENE-3β,11β,17β-TRIOL

A solution of five grams of 11β-hydroxy-17α-methyltestosterone (U.S. Patent 2,735,854), 25 milliliters of acetic anhydride, 100 milligrams of para-toluenesulfonic acid, and 100 milliliters of toluene was heated in a nitrogen atmosphere at reflux for four and one-half hours. The solvent was removed by distillation under vacuum. The residue resisted crystallization. It was dissolved in 100 milliliters of 95 percent alcohol and three milliliters of ten percent sodium hydroxide and cooled to zero degrees centigrade.

A solution of five grams of sodium borohydride and 100 milliliters of seventy percent alcohol was added with stirring and cooling. After one hour, 2.5 grams of sodium borohydride in fifty milliliters of seventy percent alcohol was added. The solution was stored three days at five degrees centigrade, then fifteen milliliters of ten percent sodium hydroxide solution was added and the solution heated to nearly boiling. The alcohol was distilled off under vacuum. Ice and 3N hydrochloric acid were added to the concentrate with stirring. The product precipitated and was collected. It was washed with water, dilute hydrochloric acid then water and dried. The yield was 5.7 grams. This material was dissolved in fifty milliliters of tetrahydrofuran and 1.5 grams of lithium aluminum hydride was added slowly with stirring. After about three minutes the reaction mixture set to a hard gel. Fifteen milliliters of ether was added and the mixture stirred for one hour. Ethyl acetate and water were added. The aqueous phase was separated, extracted with ether and then with methylene chloride. The nonaqueous phase and the extracts were combined, dried over magnesium sulfate and filtered. The filtrate on standing overnight deposited 1.5 grams of crystals having a melting point of 223 to

14

230 degrees centigrade. The liquor was concentrated to dryness and triturated with methylene chloride to give an additional 1.3 grams with a melting point of 203 to 210 degrees centigrade. The two crops were combined and crystallized from fifteen milliliters of alcohol, containing 0.5 milliliters of water. The yield of 17α-methyl-5-androstene-3β,11β,17β-triol was 1.7 grams and the melting point 227 to 230 degrees centigrade. Recrystallization from ethyl acetate yielded 1.2 grams melting at 230 to 235 degrees centigrade and having a rotation of $[\alpha]_D$ minus 68 degrees (dioxane).

Analysis.—Calculated for $C_{20}H_{32}O_3$: C, 74.95; H, 10.07. Found: C, 74.53; H, 10.16.

Infrared spectra show OH bands at 3610 and 3280, isolated C=C at 1665 (weak) and alcohol C—O at 1146, 1085, 1054, and 1030 centimeters^{-1}.

In the same manner as described in Preparation 1, but employing 11α-hydroxy-17-methyltestosterone (U.S. 2,660,586), 17-methyltestosterone and 9(11)-dehydro-17-methyltestosterone as starting steroid, there is thus produced 17α-methyl-5-androstene-3β,11α,17β-triol, 17α-methyl-5-androstene-3β,17β-diol and 17α-methyl-5,9(11)-androstadiene-3β,17β-diol, respectively.

PREPARATION 2.—17α-METHYL-9(11)-DEHYDROTESTOSTERONE

A warm solution of one gram of 11α-hydroxy-17-methyltestosterone in dry pyridine was mixed with one gram of para-toluenesulfonyl chloride. The mixture was maintained at room temperature for eighteen hours and then poured into 25 milliliters of water. The mixture was stirred until the precipitated oil solidified. The solid was filtered, washed with water and dried to give 11α-(p-toluenesulfonyloxy)-17-methyltestosterone which, after crystallization from a mixture of methylene chloride and hexane hydrocarbons, was a light colored crystalline solid.

A mixture of one gram of the thus-produced 11α-(p-toluenesulfonyloxy)-17-methyltestosterone, 0.2 gram of sodium formate, 0.57 milliliter of water and fourteen milliliters of absolute ethanol was heated at its refluxing temperature for nineteen hours. The solution was cooled and then poured into fifty grams of a mixture of ice and water with stirring. The resulting precipitate was filtered and dried to give 9(11)-dehydro-17-methyltestosterone which, after crystallization from a mixture of methylene chloride and hexane hydrocarbons, was a light colored crystalline solid.

PREPARATION 3.—11β-HYDROXY-17α-METHYL-6-DEHYDROTESTOSTERONE

To a solution of two grams of 17α-methyl-5-androstene-3β,11β,17β-triol and twelve grams of para-quinone in 150 milliliters of toluene (dried by distilling off thirty milliliters) was added 2.0 grams of aluminum tertiary-butoxide. After refluxing for fifty minutes the solution was cooled and washed with dilute sodium hydroxide and water. The aqueous phases were extracted with methylene chloride. The nonaqueous solutions were combined and the methylene chloride removed by distillation. The toluene solution was poured into a 100 gram magnesium silicate (Florisil) column packed wet with hexanes (Skellysolve B) and eluted with increasing amounts of acetone in hexanes. The fraction eluted with 17 to 20 percent acetone yielded 0.6 gram of 11β-hydroxy-17α-methyl-6-dehydrotestosterone which on recrystallization from ethyl acetate-acetone gave 0.4 gram of purified product of melting point 246 to 254 degrees centigrade and having a rotation of $[\alpha]_D$ plus 150 degrees (chloroform) and ultraviolet absorption of

$$\lambda_{max}^{alc} 284.5\ m\mu, a_M 24,825$$

Analysis.—Calculated for: $C_{20}H_{28}O_3$: C, 75.91; H, 8.92. Found: C, 75.97; H, 9.13.

In the same manner as described in Preparation 3, but employing 17α-methyl-5-androstene-3β,11α,17β-triol, and 17α-methyl-5,9(11)-androstadiene-3β,17β-diol as starting steroid, there is thus-produced 6-dehydro-11α-hydroxy-17 - methyltestosterone and 6.9(11) - bisdehydrotestosterone, respectively.

PREPARATION 4.—6-DEHYDRO-17-METHYLTESTOSTERONE

A solution of forty grams of 17α-methyl-5-androstene-3β,17β-diol and 170 grams of para-quinone in 1.3 liters of toluene was distilled until 250 milliliters of distillate had been collected. To the remaining solution was added with stirring a solution of 32 grams of aluminum tertiary butoxide in 100 milliliters of dry toluene. The mixture was refluxed for fifty minutes and then about half the toluene evaporated under a stream of nitrogen. Ether was added and the solution washed with aqueous sodium hydroxide and then with water. The aqueous phases were extracted with ether which was combined with the ether phase and then dried and the solvent evaporated. The residue, dissolved in hexanes, was chromatographed through a column of 300 grams of magnesium silicate (Florisil) which was developed with 250 milliliter portions of solvent of the following composition and orde : two of hexanes, seven of hexane plus two percent acetone, four of hexanes plus four percent acetone, eight of hexanes plus six percent acetone, five of hexanes plus ten perecnt acetone, eleven of hexanes plus twelve percent acetone and four of hexanes plus twenty percent acetone. Fractions 22 to 26 were combined and recrystallized from a mixture of hexanes plus acetone to give 6.5 grams of 6-dehydro-17-methyltestosterone melting at 182 to 191 degrees centigrade, having an $[α]_D$ (chloroform) of +21 degrees,

$$a\ \lambda_{max}^{alc.}\ 284\ m\mu,\ a_M = 22,725$$

and the analysis below.

Analysis.—Calculated for $C_{20}H_{28}O_2$: C, 79.95; H, 9.39. Found: C, 79.60; H, 9.55.

PREPARATION 5.—11β-HYDROXY-6-DEHYDROTESTOSTERONE

0.5 gram of 11β-hydroxytestosterone was dissolved in fifty milliliters of tertiary butyl alcohol and then refluxed under nitrogen after the addition of 0.5 gram of recrystallized chloranil. After 2.5 hours the mixture was concentrated under a fast stream of nitrogen, diluted with methylene chloride and the solution washed with dilute sodium hydroxide, water and then dried. The dried solution was filtered and the solvent distilled. The residual 11β-hydroxy-6-dehydrotestosterone was dissolved in benzene and chromatographed over a 100 gram column of magnesium silicate. The column was eluted with hexane hydrocarbons (Skellysolve B) containing increasing proportions of acetone. The eluates were collected in 250 milliliter fractions and the solvent removed. The fraction containing the largest amount of residual solids contained substantially pure 11β-hydroxy-6-dehydrotestosterone.

Following the procedure of Preparation 5 but substituting as starting steroid testosterone, 11α-hydroxytestosterone, 11-ketotestosterone, 9(11) - dehydrotestosterone, 9(11) - dehydro - 17 - methyltestosterone and 11-keto-17-methyltestosterone, there is thus-produced 6-dehydrotestosterone, 6-dehydro-11α-hydroxytestosterone, 6-dehydro-11-ketotestosterone, 6,9(11)-bisdehydrotestosterone, 6,9(11)-bisdehydro-17-methyltestosterone and 6-dehydro-11-keto-17-methyltestosterone, respectively.

EXAMPLE 1

7,17-dimethyltestosterone

A mixture of 0.4 gram of cuprous chloride, twenty milliliters of 4M methylmagnesium bromide in ether and sixty milliliters of redistilled tetrahydrofuran was stirred and cooled in an ice bath during the addition of a mixture of 2.0 grams of 6-dehydro-17-methyltestosterone, sixty milliliters of redistilled tetrahydrofuran and 0.2 gram of cuprous chloride. The ice bath was removed and stirring was continued for four hours. Ice and water were than carefully added, the solution acidified with 3N hydro-

chloric acid and extracted several times with ether. The combined ether extracts were washed with a brine-sodium carbonate solution, brine and then dried over anhydrous magnesium sulfate, filtered and then poured over a 75 gram column of magnesium silicate (Florisil) packed wet with hexanes (Skellysolve B). The column was eluted with 250 milliliters of hexanes, 0.5 liter of two percent acetone, two liters of four percent acetone and 3.5 liters of six percent acetone in hexanes. Four 250 milliliter fractions were collected followed by 150 milliliter fractions. The residues from fractions eight to sixteen were combined and rechromatographed over a 125 gram column of magnesium silicate. The column was eluted with six percent acetone in hexanes which was collected in 150 milliliter portions. Fractions 18 to 29 were combined and dissolved in acetone, decolorized with charcoal, and recrystallized from acetone. One gram of a crystalline mixture of the 7-epimers of 7,17-dimethyltestosterone was obtained melting at 120 to 140 degrees centigrade.

$$\lambda_{max}^{alc.}\ 213\ m\mu\ a_M = 13,775,\ [α]_D + 55\ degrees\ (chloroform)$$

Analysis.—Calculated for $C_{21}H_{32}O_2$: C, 79.69; H, 10.19. Found: C, 79.18; H, 10.07.

The 7-isomers are separated one from the other according to the procedure described in Example 3. 7α,17-dimethyltestosterone melts at 163 to 165 degrees centigrade and 7β,17-dimethyltestosterone melts at 127 to 129 degrees centigrade.

EXAMPLE 2

1-dehydro-7α,17α-dimethyltestosterone

A mixture of 8.0 g. of 7α,17α-dimethyltestosterone, 8.0 g. of mercury, 6.5 ml. of acetic acid, 5.0 g. of selenium dioxide and 300 ml. of t-butyl alcohol was stirred and refluxed under nitrogen for 4 hours. An additional 2.0 grams of selenium dioxide was added and after refluxing for a total of 7 hours the reaction mixture was concentrated to about 200 milliliters under a fast stream of nitrogen. After diluting with a mixture of methylene chloride and ether, the solution was washed three times with freshly prepared ammonium sulfide, twice with diluted ammonium hydroxide and twice with water. The washed solution was dried, filtered and concentrated to dryness. The gummy product was dissolved in methylene chloride and poured on a 200 g. Florisil column packed wet with Skellysolve B. The column was washed with increasing amounts of acetone in Skellysolve B. Those fractions of eluted material which were identified as 1-dehydro-7α,17α-dimethyltestosterone by paper chromatogram analysis were combined and recrystallized from a mixture of acetone and Skellysolve B. There was thus obtained 1-dehydro-7α,17α-dimethyltestosterone in the form of a white crystalline solid having a melting point of 153 to 156 degrees centigrade; $[α]_D -6$ degrees (chloroform)

$$\lambda_{max}^{alc.}\ 243.5\ m\mu,\ a_M = 15,500$$

Analysis.—Calculated for $C_{21}H_{30}O_2$: C, 80.21; H, 9.62. Found: C, 80.29; H, 9.76.

EXAMPLE 3

7,17-dimethyl-11β-hydroxytestosterone

A solution was prepared by the addition of 100 milliliters of 3M methyl magnesium bromide in ether to a mixture of 1.6 grams of cuprous chloride in 240 milliliters of purified tetrahydrofuran. To this solution was added a solution of 8.0 grams of 6-dehydro-11β-hydroxy-17-methyltestosterone and 0.8 gram of partially dissolved cuprous chloride in 300 milliliters of tetrahydrofuran, under nitrogen and with stirring and cooling in an ice-salt bath. After fifteen minutes, the reaction mixture was poured into a mixture of ether and dilute hydrochloric acid and ice and saturated with sodium chloride. The ether phase was separated, washed with brine followed by dilute sodium hydroxide saturated with sodium chloride and then again with brine, and then dried over magnesium sulfate. The dried solution was filtered and concentrated to dryness. The residue was dissolved in methylene chloride which was then poured onto a 250 gram magnesium silicate (Florisil) chromatographic column. The column was developed with 250 milliliter portions of solvent of the following composition and order: three of methylene chloride, two of methylene chloride plus two percent acetone, two of methylene chloride plus three percent acetone, nine of methylene chloride plus four percent acetone, two of methylene chloride plus ten percent acetone, three of methylene chloride plus fifty percent acetone, and finally, one of acetone. Fractions ten to twenty, eluted with the four to ten percent acetone in methylene chloride, were combined, the solvent evaporated and the residue dissolved in hot methanol, filtered, the filtrate freed of solvent and the residue triturated with a mixture of acetone and hexane hydrocarbons. A 3.2 gram crystalline mixture of the 7-stereoisomers of 7,17-dimethyl-11β-hydroxytestosterone was obtained which melted at 218 to 224 degrees centigrade (presoftening), had a

$$\lambda_{max.}^{alc.} \ 243 \ m\mu, \ a_M = 15,175$$

and an [α]$_D$ +102 degrees in chloroform.

Analysis.—Calculated for $C_{21}H_{32}O_3$: C, 75.86; H, 9.70. Found: C, 75.56; H, 9.57.

The pure 7(β) isomer of 7,17-dimethyl-11β-hydroxytestosterone was obtained by six crystallizations of the crys...ine mixture of isomers described above from a mixture of acetone and methanol and melted at 242 to 246 degrees centigrade (dec.), had a

$$\lambda_{max.}^{alc.} \ 245.5 \ m\mu, \ a_M = 15,175$$

and an [α]$_D$ of +105 degrees in chloroform.

Analysis.—Calculated for $C_{21}H_{32}O_3$: C, 75.86; H, 9.70. Found: C, 75.59; H, 10.04.

To obtain the 7(α)-isomer 0.5 gram of the crystalline mixture of the 7 stereoisomers of 7,17-dimethyl-11β-hydroxytestosterone was refluxed in fifty milliliters of tertiary butyl alcohol with 0.5 gram of recrystallized chloranil under nitrogen for 2.5 hours. The reaction mixture was concentrated under a fast stream of nitrogen, diluted with methylene chloride and the solution washed with dilute sodium hydroxide, water and then dried, filtered and the solvent removed. The residue, showing

$$\lambda_{max.}^{alc.} \ at \ 245 \ and \ 291 \ m\mu$$

was combined with the product from an identical run and chromatographed through a 100 gram magnesium silicate column developed with 250 milliliter portions of solvent of the following composition and order: two each of hexane hydrocarbons (Skellysolve B), hexanes plus four percent acetone, hexanes plus eight percent acetone, hexanes plus twelve percent acetone, hexanes plus fourteen percent acetone, hexanes plus sixteen percent acetone, hexanes plus eighteen percent acetone, hexanes plus twenty percent acetone, hexanes plus twenty-four percent acetone, hexanes plus tweny-eight percent acetone, and two of acetone. The residues from fractions fifteen to eighteen, eluted with eighteen percent acetone, were combined and crystallized from acetone to give 100 milligrams of 7,17-dimethyl-11β-hydroxy-6-dehydro-testosterone, melting point 242 to 2.. degrees centigrade (dec.),

$$\lambda_{max.}^{alc.} \ 295.5 \ m\mu, \ a_M = 23,250, \ [\alpha]_D +310 \ degrees \ (chloroform)$$

Analysis.—Calculated for $C_{21}H_{30}O_3$: C, 76.32; H, 9.15. Found: C, 76.49; H. 9.53.

The residues from fractions eleven to fourteen, eluted with sixteen to eighteen percent acetone, were combined and chromatographed through a fifty gram 1:1 charcoal (Darco)-diatomaceous earth (Celite) column. The column was developed with solvent of the following composition and order: nine-100 milliliter portions of methanol, five-100 milliliter portions of a 1:1 mixture of methanol and acetone, seven-fifty milliliter portions of a 1:1 mixture of methanol and acetone, seven-fifty milliliter

portions of a 1:2 mixture of methanol and acetone, three-fifty milliliter portions of acetone and four-fifty milliliter portions of a 1:4 mixture of acetone and methylene chloride. Fractions twelve to twenty were combined, the solvent evaporated and the residue crystallized from acetone to give sixty milligrams of the 7(α)-epimer of 7,17-dimethyl-11β-hydroxytestosterone, melting point 225 to 230 degrees centigrade (presoftening).

$$\lambda_{max.}^{alc.} \ 243 \ m\mu, \ a_M = 15,825$$

Analysis.—Calculated for $C_{21}H_{32}O_3$: C, 75.86; H, 9.70. Found: C, 75.65; H, 9.96.

EXAMPLE 4

1-dehydro-7α,17-dimethyl-11β-hydroxytestosterone

Following the procedure of Example 2, but substituting 7α,17-dimethyl-11β-hydroxytestosterone for 7α,17α-dimethyltestosterone, there is obtained 1-dehydro-7α,17-dimethyl-11β-hydroxytestosterone.

EXAMPLE 5

7,17-dimethyl-9(11)-dehydrotestosterone

Following the procedure of Examples 1 and 3, but substituting 17-methyl-6,9(11)-bisdehydrotestosterone as the starting steroid, there are produced the 7α and 7β-epimers of 7,17-dimethyl-9(11)-dehydrotestosterone. 7α,17-dimethyl-9(11)-dehydrotestosterone is a white crystalline solid having a metling point of 172 to 176° C;

$$\lambda_{max.}^{alc.} \ 240 \ m\mu, \ a_M = 16,800$$

The foregoing compound is also obtained from 7α,17α-dimethyl-11α-hydroxytestosterone [M.P. 230 to 234.5 degrees centigrade, [α]$_D$ +81 degrees (chloroform)

$$\lambda_{max.}^{alc.} \ 243 \ m\mu$$

obtained by 11α-hydroxylation of 7α,17α-dimethyltestosterone using the procedure described in U.S. Patent 2,602,769] by 11α-tosylation and reaction of the 11α-tosylate with sodium formate in aqueous alcohol solution according to the procedure described in U.S. Patent 2,793,218, Example 3.

EXAMPLE 6

7,17-dimethyl-1,9(11)-bisdehydrotestosterone

Following the procedure of Example 2, but substituting 7,17-dimethyl-9(11)-dehydrotestosterone for 7α,17α-dimethyltestosterone, there is obtained 7,17-dimethyl-1,9(11)-bis-dehydrotestosterone.

EXAMPLE 7

7-methyl-11β-hydroxytestosterone

Following the procedure of Examples 1 and 3, but substituting 11β-hydroxy-6-dehydrotestosterone as the starting steroid, there is produced 7-methyl-11β-hydroxytestosterone.

Similarly, 6-dehydrotestosterone and 6-dehydrotestosterone acetate are converted to 7-methyltestosterone, 6-dehydro-11β-hydroxytestosterone 17-acetate and 6-dehydro-11β-hydroxytestosterone to 7-methyl-11α-hydroxytestosterone, 6-dehydro-11α-hydroxy-17-methyltestosterone to 7,17-dimethyl-11α-hydroxytestosterone, 6-dehydro-11-ketotestosterone acetate and 6-dehydro-11-ketotestosterone to 7-methyl-11-ketotestosterone, 6,9(11)-bisdehydrotestosterone acetate and 6,9(11)-bisdehydrotestosterone to 7-methyl-9(11)-dehydrotestosterone and 6-dehydro-11-keto-17-methyltestosterone to 7,17-dimethyl-11-ketotestosterone.

The 7-isomers of each of the above 7-methyltestosterones described in Examples 1, 3, 5, and 7 can be separated by fractional crystallization to remove the more insoluble isomer and reaction of the resulting mixture from the mother liquors with chloranil in the manner described in Example 3 to produce the corresponding 7-methyl-6-dehydrotestosterone, which compounds also

19

possess androgenic and anabolic activity, and then separating the residual 7-epimer of 7-methyltestosterone therefrom.

EXAMPLE 8

1-dehydro-7-methyl-11β-hydroxytestosterone

Following the procedure of Example 2, but substituting 7-methyl-11β-hydroxytestosterone for 7α,17α-dimethyltestosterone, there is obtained 1-dehydro-7-methyl-11β-hydroxytestosterone.

Similarly, 7-methyltestosterone, 7-methyl-11α-hydroxytestosterone, 7,17-dimethyl-11α-hydroxytestosterone, 7-methyl-11-ketotestosterone, 7 - methyl-9(11)-dehydrotestosterone and 7,17-dimethyl-11-ketotestosterone are converted to 1-dehydro-7-methyltestosterone, 1-dehydro-11α-hydroxy-7-methyltestosterone, 1 - dehydro-7,17-dimethyl-11α-hydroxytestosterone, 1-dehydro-7-methyl-11-ketotestosterone, 7-methyl-1,9(11)-bisdehydrotestosterone, and 1 - dehydro - 7,17 - dimethyl - 11 - ketotestosterone, respectively.

EXAMPLE 9

7-methyl-11β-hydroxytestosterone 17-acetate

A solution of 1.0 gram of 7-methyl-11β-hydroxytestosterone, dissolved in six milliliters of dried and redistilled pyridine, was treated with six milliliters of acetic anhydride. After standing at room temperature for seventeen hours, it was poured into ice water. The mixture was filtered after two hours of standing and the precipitate was washed with water and dried in vacuo. Upon recrystallization from an acetone-hexane mixture substantially pure 7-methyl-11β-hydroxytestosterone 17-acetate was obtained.

In the same manner as given in Example 9, by the reaction of 7-methyl-11β-hydroxytestosterone with propionic anhydride, 7-methyl-11β-hydroxytestosterone 17-propionate was obtained.

In the same manner as given in Example 9, by reaction of 1-dehydro-7-methyl-11β-hydroxytestosterone with acetic anhydride or propionic anhydride there are obtained the 17-acetate and 17-propionate, respectively, of 1-dehydro-7-methyl-11β-hydroxytestosterone.

EXAMPLE 10

7-methyl-11β-hydroxytestosterone 17-benzoate

Three-tenths gram (0.3 gram) of 7-methyl-11β-hydroxytestosterone, suspended in twelve milliliters of dry benzene, was treated with 0.3 milliliter of distilled benzoyl chloride and 0.3 milliliter of dry pyridine. The mixture was stirred for seventeen hours at room temperature. After refrigeration, the product was collected on a filter, washed with benzene and ether, and dried. Recrystallization from ethyl acetate gave substantially pure 7-methyl-11β-hydroxytestosterone 17-benzoate.

In the same manner as given in Examples 5 and 6, the 17β-cyclopentylpropionate, butyrate, isobutyrate, valerate, isovalerate, hexanoate, heptanoate, octanoate, phenylacetate, p-hexyloxyphenylpropionate, and other like 17-esters of 7-methyl-11β-hydroxytestosterone and 1-dehydro-7-methyl-11β-hydroxytestosterone are prepared by the reaction of 7-methyl-11β-hydroxytestosterone and 1-dehydro-7-methyl-11β-hydroxytestosterone with the selected acid anhydride or halide. Treatment of 7-methyl-11β-hydroxytestosterone with formic acid produces 7-methyl-11β-hydroxytestosterone 17-formate.

Similarly, following the procedure of Examples 9 and 10 and the paragraphs following, 7-methyltestosterone, 1-dehydro-7-methyltestosterone, 7 - methyl-11-ketotestosterone and 1-dehydro-7-methyl-11-ketotestosterone are converted to their 17-acetate, 17-propionate, 17-benzoate and the other esters named therein.

Substituting 7-methyl-11α-hydroxytestosterone as the starting steroid in the reactions described in Examples 5 and 6 and the paragraph following is productive of the

20

corresponding 11α,17-diesters of 7-methyl-11α-hydroxytestosterone.

EXAMPLE 11

7-methyl-11-ketotestosterone 17-benzoate

A solution of 1.5 grams of 7-methyl-11β-hydroxytestosterone 17-benzoate in eighty milliliters of acetic acid was treated with a solution of 0.74 gram of chromic acid anhydride in four milliliters of water and eighty milliliters of acetic acid and allowed to stand at room temperature for five hours. The excess chromic acid was destroyed by the addition of ten milliliters of methanol and the solution was concentrated in vacuo on a water bath. The residue, after trituration with water, was extracted with ether and the ether solution washed with dilute sodium hydroxide solution and water, and then dried over anhydrous sodium sulfate. Upon evaporation of the ether there was obtained 7-methyl-11-ketotestosterone 17-benzoate.

EXAMPLE 12

7-methyl-11-ketotestosterone 17-acetate

A solution of 7-methyl-11β-hydroxytestosterone 17-acetate in acetic acid was agitated for twelve hours with an aqueous solution of chromic acid anhydride. The steroid product was extracted thoroughly with benzene which was washed with a sodium bicarbonate solution and then water, dried over anhydrous sodium sulfate, and evaporated to give 7-methyl-11-ketotestosterone 17-acetate.

In the same manner as given in Examples 11 and 12, 7-methyl-11-ketotestosterone 17-formate, 17-butyrate, 17-isobutyrate, 17-valerate, 17-isovalerate, 17-hexanoate, 17-heptanoate, 17-octanoate, 17-benzoate, 17-phenylacetate, 17 - (β-cyclopentyl)-propionate, 17-p-butyloxyphenylpropionate, and like 17-esters of 7-methyl-11-ketotestosterone are prepared by reaction of the corresponding 7-methyl-11β-hydroxytestosterone 17-ester with chromic anhydride in acetic acid or with an acidified dichromate solution.

Following the procedure of Example 11, 7,17-dimethyl-11β-hydroxytestosterone is converted to 7,17-dimethyl-11-ketotestosterone.

EXAMPLE 13

7-methyl-11-ketotestosterone

A solution of 1.0 gram of 7-methyl-11-ketotestosterone 17-propionate in fifty milliliters of 1 normal methanolic potassium hydroxide solution containing three milliliters of water was refluxed for a period of thirty minutes. The solution was poured onto ice and the mixture neutralized with dilute sulfuric acid. After standing, the resulting precipitate was recovered, washed with water and dried. The aqueous filtrate was extracted with methylene chloride to recover an additional amount of material. Substantially pure 7-methyl-11-ketotestosterone is obtained when this residue is recrystallized from methylene chloride.

EXAMPLE 14

7-methyl-9(11)-dehydrotestosterone

A two-phase mixture of 2.5 grams of 7-methyl-11β-hydroxytestosterone, 250 milliliters of benzene, 200 milliliters of ether, 100 milliliters of concentrated hydrochloric acid, and 100 milliliters of water was heated under reflux for eighteen hours with vigorous stirring. After cooling, the two layers were separated and the aqueous layer extracted three times with 75-milliliter portions of ether. The ether extracts were combined with the benzene-ether layer, and then washed with dilute aqueous potassium carbonate solution and with water. The washed solution was dried over anhydrous sodium sulfate and, after removal of the drying agent, the solvent was evaporated. The residue was recrystallized from a mixture of methylene chloride and hexane hydrocarbons (Skellysolve B) to provide 7-methyl-9(11)-dehydrotestosterone.

21

Following the procedure of Example 14, 1-dehydro-7-methyl-11β-hydroxytestosterone is converted to 7-methyl-1,9(11)-bisdehydrotestosterone.

EXAMPLE 15

7-methyl-9(11)-dehydrotestosterone 17-propionate

A solution of 250 milligrams of 7-methyl-9(11)-dehydrotestosterone in thirty milliliters of benzene was prepared, and eighteen milliliters of benzene was distilled to dry the solution. After cooling, the dried solution was treated with two milliliters of dry pyridine and two milliliters of propionic anhydride and maintained at a temperature of about 26 degrees centigrade for 22 hours. The mixture was then treated with 25 milliliters of water and extracted with ether. The ether extract was washed with dilute aqueous hydrochloric acid and then with dilute aqueous sodium hydroxide solution, followed by water. The solution was dried over anhydrous sodium sulfate, and, after removing the drying agent, the solvent was evaporated in vacuo. The residue was crystallized from absolute methanol to yield substantially pure 7-methyl-9(11)-dehydrotestosterone 17-propionate.

In the same manner, but employing benzoyl chloride, 7-methyl-9(11)-dehydrotestosterone 17-benzoate is prepared.

Following the procedure of Example 15, 7-methyl-1,9(11)-bisdehydrotestosterone is converted to its 17-propionate.

EXAMPLE 16

7-methyl-9(11)-dehydrotestosterone 17-(β-cyclopentylpropionate)

A solution of 250 milligrams of 7-methyl-9(11)-dehydrotestosterone in 25 milliliters of benzene was prepared and dried by distilling twelve milliliters of benzene from the solution. After cooling, the solution was treated with 0.25 milliliter of dry pyridine and 0.25 milliliter of β-cyclopentylpropionyl chloride and was maintained at about 26 degrees centigrade for five hours, during which time pyridine hydrochloride separated. The resulting mixture was treated with twenty milliliters of water and then extracted with ether. After washing the ether extract with dilute aqueous hydrochloric acid, dilute aqueous sodium hydroxide, and water, it was dried over anhydrous sodium sulfate. After removal of the drying agent, the solvent was evaporated to give a residue of 7-methyl-9(11)-dehydrotestosterone 17-(β-cyclopentylpropionate).

In the same manner, but replacing 7-methyl-9(11)-dehydrotestosterone by 7-methyl-1,9(11)-bisdehydrotestosterone, there is obtained 7-methyl-1,9(11)-bisdehydrotestosterone 17-(β-cyclopentylpropionate).

In the same manner reacting 7-methyl-9(11)-dehydrotestosterone or 7-methyl-1,9(11)-dehydrotestosterone with the appropriate acylating agent provides other representative 17-cycloalkylalkanoates of 7-methyl-9(11)-dehydrotestosterone or 7-methyl-1,9(11)-dehydrotestosterone, including the 17-cyclopentylformate, cyclohexylformate, cyclopentylacetate, cyclobutylformate, α-cyclopentylpropionate, cyclohexylacetate, cyclopropylformate, cycloheptylformate, β-(methylcyclopentyl)-acetate, β-cyclobutylpropionate, and other 17-cycloalkylalkanoates.

In the same manner as shown in Examples 15 and 16, other acylates of 7-methyl-9(11)-dehydrotestosterone or 7-methyl-1,9(11)-bisdehydrotestosterone are prepared by reacting 7-methyl-9(11)-dehydrotestosterone or 7-methyl-1,9(11)-bisdehydrotestosterone, preferably in pyridine solution, with the acyl halide or the anhydride of a hydrocarbon carboxylic acid preferably containing from one to twelve carbon atoms, inclusive. Other representative esters of 7-methyl-9(11)-dehydrotestosterone or 7-methyl-1,9(11)-bisdehydrotestosterone thus prepared include the acetate, butyrate, isobutyrate, valerate, isovalerate, hexanoate, heptanoate, octanoate, phenylacetate, phenylpropionate, p-hexyloxyphenylpropionate, and trimethylacetate.

22

EXAMPLE 17

7-methyl-9α-bromo-11β-hydroxytestosterone 17-propionate

Two grams of 7-methyl-9(11)-dehydrotestosterone 17-propionate, dissolved in 100 milliliters of acetone, were cooled to fifteen degrees centigrade and the solution was thereupon treated with two grams of N-bromoacetamide, dissolved in fifty milliliters of water. Maintaining the bath temperature at twelve degrees centigrade, a solution of ten milliliters of 0.8 N perchloric acid was added. Five minutes later another ten milliliters of perchloric acid was added and after ten more minutes a final twenty milliliters of the same 0.8 N perchloric acid was added. At the end of twenty minutes total reaction time, a saturated solution of sodium sulfite was added slowly with mixing. The mixture was thereupon diluted with 200 milliliters of water and the product, thus separated, was recovered by filtration, washed well with water and dried over anhydrous sodium sulfate, and the solvent separated by distillation, leaving a residue of 7-methyl-9α-bromo-11β-hydroxytestosterone 17-propionate.

In the same manner as given in Example 17, 7-methyl-9(11)-dehydrotestosterone 17-benzoate, 7-methyl-9(11)-dehydrotestosterone 17-acetate, 7-methyl-9(11)-dehydrotestosterone 17-butyrate, 7-methyl-9(11)-dehydrotestosterone 17-isobutyrate, 7-methyl-9(11)-dehydrotestosterone 17-valerate, 7-methyl-9(11)-dehydrotestosterone 17-hexanoate, 7-methyl-9(11)-dehydrotestosterone 17-(β-cyclophenylpropionate) and 7-methyl-9(11)-dehydrotestosterone 17-phenylacetate gave the corresponding 7-methyl-9α-bromo-11β-hydroxytestosterone 17-acylates by reaction with N-bromoacetamide in acetone solution in the presence of aqueous perchloric acid.

Using the procedure described in Example 17, but replacing 7-methyl-9(11)-dehydrotestosterone 17-propionate by 7-methyl-1,9(11)-bisdehydrotestosterone 17-propionate, there is obtained 1-dehydro-7-methyl-9α-bromo-11β-hydroxytestosterone 17-propionate. By employing other 17-acylates of 7-methyl-1,9(11)-bisdehydrotestosterone in place of the 17-propionate there are obtained the corresponding 17-acylates of 1-dehydro-7-methyl-9α-bromo-11β-hydroxytestosterone.

EXAMPLE 18

7-methyl-9α-chloro-11β-hydroxytestosterone 17-propionate

One gram of 7-methyl-9(11)-dehydrotestosterone 17-propionate, dissolved in fifty milliliters of tertiary butyl alcohol, was treated at room temperature, about twenty to 25 degrees centigrade, with one gram of N-chlorosuccinimide, dissolved in tertiary butyl alcohol. To this solution was added fifty milliliters of 0.1 N sulfuric acid. The mixture was stirred for a period of thirty minutes at room temperature and thereupon diluted with 300 milliliters of water and extracted with three fifty-milliliter portions of methylene chloride. The methylene chloride extracts were dried over anhydrous sodium sulfate and evaporated to give a residue which was recrystallized twice from methanol to give 7-methyl-9α-chloro-11β-hydroxytestosterone 17-propionate.

EXAMPLE 19

7,17-dimethyl-9α-bromo-11β-hydroxytestosterone

One gram of 7,17-dimethyl-9(11)-dehydrotestosterone, dissolved in dioxane (fifty milliliters), was reacted at about 24 degrees centigrade with one gram of N-bromosuccinimide, dissolved in fifty milliliters of dioxane. To this solution was added fifty milliliters of 0.1 N sulfuric acid and the mixture was agitated at room temperature for a period of one hour. Thereafter, 300 milliliters of water was added and the reaction mixture was extracted with three fifty-milliliter portions of methylene chloride. The methylene chloride solution was washed with sodium thiosulfate solution and then with water and then dried over anhydrous sodium sulfate. Evaporation of the dried methylene chloride solution gave a residue which, after recrystallization from methanol, gave 7,17-dimethyl-9α-bromo-11β-hydroxytestosterone.

Using the procedure shown in Example 19, but substituting 7,17-dimethyl-1,9(11)-bisdehydrotestosterone for 7,17-dimethyl-9(11)-dehydrotestosterone, there is obtained 1-dehydro-7,17-dimethyl-9α-bromo-11β - hydroxytestosterone.

In the same manner as shown in Examples 17 to 19, inclusive, reacting 7-methyl-9(11)-dehydrotestosterone 17-acylate or 7-methyl-1,9(11)-bisdehydrotestosterone 17-acylate in tertiary butyl alcohol, dioxane, acetone, or the like, with a hypohalous acid, preferably produced by reaction of a strong acid such as perchloric, sulfuric, trichloroacetic acid and an N-haloamide or an N-haloimide especially N-haloacetamide or N-halosuccinimide produces the corresponding 7-methyl-9α-halo-11β - hydroxytestosterone 17-acylate or 1-dehydro-7-methyl-9α-halo-11β-hydroxytestosterone 17-acylate. Other such 7-methyl-9α-halo-11β-hydroxytestosterone acylates and 1-dehydro-7-methyl-9α-halo-11β-hydroxytestosterone 17-acylates thus produced include the 17-acetate, propionate, butyrate, valerate, isovalerate, β-cyclopentylpropionate, benzoate, phenylacetate, toluate, β-cyclopentylpropionate of 7-methyl-9α-iodo-11β-hydroxytestosterone, 1-dehydro-7methyl-9α-iodo-11β-hydroxytestosterone, 7-methyl-9α-chloro-11β-hydroxytestosterone, and 1-dehydro - 7 - methyl-9α-chloro-11β-hydroxytestosterone.

If 7-methyl-9α-halo-11β-hydroxytestosterone 17 - acylates are desired wherein the acyl radical is of an unsaturated acid such as acrylic, crotonic, cinnamic, fumaric, or maleic acid or the like, the selected 7-methyl-9α-halo-11β-hydroxytestosterone is reacted with the acid halide of such unsaturated acid to give the corresponding 7-methyl-9α-halo-11β-hydroxytestosterone 17-acylate.

EXAMPLE 20

7-methyl-9β,11β-epoxytestosterone 17-propionate

A solution of 1.36 grams of 7-methyl-9α-bromo-11β-hydroxytestosterone propionate, dissolved in fifty milliliters of methanol was titrated with 0.1 N aqueous sodium hydroxide until the solution remained basic to phenolphthalein upon standing for a period of thirty seconds. About 32 milliliters of base, equal to one equivalent, was required. Thereafter 300 milliliters of water was slowly added with stirring. The mixture was cooled and thereafter filtered and the precipitate thus obtained washed with water and dried over anhydrous sodium sulfate to give crude 7-methyl-9β,11β - epoxytestosterone 17 - propionate which was recrystallized from dilute methanol to give a substantially pure sample.

Using the procedure described in Example 20, but replacing 7-methyl-9α-bromo-11β-hydroxytestosterone propionate by 1 - dehydro - 7-methyl-9α-bromo-11β-hydroxytestosterone propionate, there is obtained 1-dehydro-7-methyl-9β,11β-epoxytestosterone 17-propionate.

In the same manner given in Example 20, 7-methyl-9α-bromo-11β-hydroxytestosterone was titrated with aqueous sodium hydroxide solution until the reaction mixture became basic to phenolphthalein for about one-half minute. The solution was then diluted with water and filtered to give a precipitate of 7-methyl-9β,11β- epoxytestosterone.

EXAMPLE 21

7,17-dimethyl-9β,11β-epoxytestosterone

A mixture of 7,17-dimethyl-9α-bromo-11β-hydroxytestosterone, potassium acetate and tertiary butyl alcohol was heated on a water bath for a period of one hour. The mixture was thereupon poured into ice water and the resulting precipitate collected on filter and recrystallized to give substantially pure 7,17-dimethyl-9β,11β-epoxytestosterone.

Using the procedure of Example 21, but replacing 7,17-dimethyl - 9α-bromo-11β-hydroxytestosterone by 1-dehydro - 7,17 - dimethyl-9α-bromo-11β-hydroxytestosterone, there is obtained 1-dehydro-7,17-dimethyl-9β,11β-epoxytestosterone.

In the same manner as shown in Example 21, other 7-methyl-9β,11β-epoxytestosterone 17-acylates are produced by reacting the 7-methyl-9α-halo-11β-hydroxytestosterone 17-acylates and the 1-dehydro-7-methyl-9α-halo-11β-hydroxytestosterone 17 - acylates described in Example 19 with a mild base. Representative 17-acylates thus produced include the 17-acetate, butyrate, isobutyrate, valerate, isovalerate, hexanoate, heptanoate, octanoate, toluate, trimethylacetate, acrylate, crotonate, and β-cyclopentylpropionate of 7-methyl-9β,11β-epoxytestosterone and 1-dehydro-7-methyl-9β,11β-epoxytestosterone.

EXAMPLE 22

7-methyl-9α-fluoro-11β-hydroxytestosterone 17-propionate

A chilled solution of 1.13 grams of 7-methyl-9β-11β-epoxytestosterone 17-propionate in twenty milliliters of alcohol-free chloroform was added to a chilled solution of alcohol-free chloroform into which hydrogen fluoride gas had been introduced for a period of three minutes. The mixture, contained in a polyethylene bottle, was maintained at minus fifteen degrees centigrade for a period of four hours and thereafter was poured into an excess of a saturated sodium bicarbonate solution. The aqueous layer was separated from the chloroform layer and extracted three times with chloroform. The combined chloroform layer and extracts were washed with water, dried over anhydrous sodium sulfate and the solvent evaporated to give a residue of 7-methyl-9α-fluoro-11β-hydroxytestosterone 17-propionate which was purified by chromatography over 100 grams of anhydrous magnesium silicate (Florisil) developed with from 20 to 1 to 9 to 1 mixture of hexane hydrocarbons (Skellysolve B) and acetone. The solvent was evaporated from the eluate fractions leaving 7-methyl-9α-fluoro-11β-hydroxytestosterone 17-propionate as the main solid fraction.

Using the procedure shown in Example 22, but replacing 7 - methyl - 9β,11β - epoxytestosterone 17-propionate by 1-dehydro-7-methyl-9β,11β-epoxy-testosterone 17-propionate, there is obtained 1-dehydro-7-methyl-9α-fluoro-11β-hydroxytestosterone 17-propionate.

EXAMPLE 23

7,17-dimethyl-9α-fluoro-11β-hydroxytestosterone

In the same manner as shown in Example 22, 7,17-dimethyl - 9β,11β-epoxytestosterone and 1-dehydro-7,17-dimethyl-9β,11β-epoxytestosterone were treated with hydrogen fluoride gas dissolved in alcohol-free chloroform to give 7,17-dimethyl-9α-fluoro-11β-hydroxytestosterone and 1 - dehydro-7,17-dimethyl-9α-fluoro-11β-hydroxytestosterone, respectively.

In the same manner as given in Example 22, reacting any of the 9β,11β-epoxides described in Example 21 and the paragraphs following, in methylene chloride with hydrogen fluoride or with aqueous hydrofluoric acid in the presence of perchloric acid is productive of the corresponding 7-methyl-9α-fluoro-11β-hydroxytestosterone acylate and 1-dehydro-7-methyl-9α-fluoro-11β-hydroxytestosterone acylate, e.g., 7 -methyl - 9α-fluoro-11β-hydroxytestosterone 17-benzoate and 17-phenylacetate, 7-methyl-9α - fluoro-11β-hydroxytestosterone 17-acetate, 7-methyl-9α - fluoro-11β-hydroxytestosterone 17-(β-cyclopentylpropionate), 1 - dehydro-7-methyl-9α-fluoro-11β-hydroxytestosterone 17 - acetate and 17 - propionate, and other 7-methyl - 9α-fluoro-11β-hydroxytestosterone 17-acylates including the 17-butyrate, isobutyrate, valerate, isovalerate, hexanoate, heptanoate, octanoate, phenylpropionate, toluate, cinnamate, p-isobutyloxyphenylpropionate, and trimethylacetate.

EXAMPLE 24

7-methyl-9α-fluoro-11-ketotestosterone 17-propionate

A solution of 0.779 gram of 7-methyl-9α-fluoro-11β-hydroxytestosterone 17-propionate in forty milliliters of glacial acetic acid was treated with a solution of 0.37 gram of chromium trioxide, dissolved in two milliliters of water and forty milliliters of glacial acetic acid. The reaction mixture was allowed to stand at room temperature for a period of five hours. Thereafter, ten milliliters of methanol was added, then 200 milliliters of water, and the mixture was extracted with ether, the ether fraction washed with sodium bicarbonate solution and water, evaporated, the residue recrystallized from methylene chloride-hexane hydrocarbons solution and finally from dilute acetone to give 7 - methyl-9α-fluoro-11-ketotestosterone 17-propionate.

Following the procedure of Example 20, 7,17-dimethyl-9α-fluoro-11β-hydroxytestosterone was converted to 7,17-dimethyl-9α-fluoro-11-ketotestosterone, 1-dehydro-7-methyl - 9α - fluoro-11β-hydroxytestosterone 17-propionate was converted to 1-denydro-7-methyl-9α-fluoro-11-ketotestosterone 17 - propionate, and 1 - dehydro-7,17-dimethyl-9α-fluoro-11β-hydroxytestosterone was converted to 1-dehydro-7-17-dimethyl-9α-fluoro-11β-hydroxytestosterone.

In the same manner as shown in Example 20, 7-methyl-9α-chloro-11β-hydroxytestosterone 17-propionate was oxidized with chromium trioxide in glacial acetic acid to give 7-methyl-9α-chloro-11-ketotestosterone 17-propionate. 7-methyl - 9α - iodo-11β-hydroxytestosterone 17-propionate gave 7-methyl-9α-iodo-11-ketotestosterone 17-propionate, 7 - methyl-9α-fluoro-11β-hydroxytestosterone 17-benzoate gave 7 - methyl-9α-fluoro-11-ketotestosterone 17-benzoate and 7-methyl-9α-fluoro-11β-hydroxytestosterone 17-phenylacetate gave 7-methyl-9α-fluoro-11-ketotestosterone 17-phenylacetate.

In the same manner given in Example 20, oxidizing the corresponding 9α-halo-11β-hydroxy compound in glacial acetic acid solution with chromic trioxide produced the following compounds: 7-methyl - 9α-fluoro-11-ketotestosterone 17-acetate; 7 - methyl - 9α-fluoro-11-ketotestosterone 17 - (β - cyclopentylpropionate); 7-methyl-9α-fluoro-11-ketotestosterone 17-butyrate, isobutyrate, valerate, isovalerate, hexanoate, heptanoate, octanoate, phenylpropionate, toluate, and trimethyl- acetate- 1-dehydro-7-methyl-9α-fluoro-11-ketotestosterone 17-acetate and 17-(β-cyclopentylpropionate).

7-methyl-9α-fluoro-11-ketotestosterone 17-acylates and 1 - dehydro - 7-methyl-9α-fluoro-11-ketotestosterone 17-acylates may also be obtained by acylation of the free 7-methyl-9α-fluoro-11-ketotestosterone or free 1-dehydro-7-methyl-9α-fluoro-11-ketotestosterone with acyl halides or acid anhydride, preferably of hydrocarbon carboxylic acids containing from one to twelve carbon atoms, inclusive, and in the preferred embodiment in pyridine solution. This method is preferred for obtaining 7-methyl-9α-fluoro-11-ketotestosterone 17-acylates and 1-dehydro-7-methyl-9α-fluoro-11-ketotestosterone 1'-acylates wherein the 17-acyloxy group is easily attacked by chromic acid such as in cases wherein an unsaturated acid, e.g., acrylic, crotonic, or similar acids are desired.

In the same manner as shown for the production of 7 - methyl - 9α - fluoro-11-ketotestosterone 17-acylates other 7 - methyl - 9α-halo-11-ketotestosterone 17-acylates and the corresponding 1-dehydro compounds are produced by either oxidizing the corresponding 7-methyl-9α-halo-11β-hydroxy-testosterone 17-acylate or corresponding 1-dehydro compound or by esterifying the 7-methyl-9α-halo - 11 - ketotestosterone or correspon ling 1-dehydro compound wherein the halogen atom is chlorine, bromine, or iodine. In this manner, the acetates, butyrates, isobutyrates, valerates, isovalerates, hexanoates, heptanoates, octanoates, benzoates, phenylacetates, toluates, cinnamates, and other esters of 7-methyl-9α-chloro, 7-methyl-

26

9α-bromo and 7-methyl-9α-iodo-11-ketotestosterone, and the corresponding 1-dehydro compounds, are produced.

EXAMPLE 25

7-methyl-9α-fluoro-11-ketotestosterone

A solution of 0.5 gram of 7-methyl-9α-fluoro-11-ketotestosterone 17-propionate, eighty milligrams of potassium hydroxide in ten milliliters of ethanol and one milliliter of water was heated on the water bath for a period of one hour. Thereafter the mixture was poured in fifty milliliters of water and neutralized with dilute hydrochloric acid. The aqueous reaction mixture was thereupon extracted with three fifty-milliliter portions of methylene chloride, the methylene chloride solution was washed repeatedly with water, dried over anhydrous sodium sulfate and evaporated and the residues thus obtained recrystallized from acetone-Skellysolve B hexanes to give 7-methyl-9α-fluoro-11-ketotestosterone.

Using the procedure described in Example 25, but substituting 1-dehydro-7-methyl-9α-fluoro-11-ketotestosterone 17-propionate for 7-methyl-9α-fluoro-11-ketotestosterone 17-propionate, there is obtained 1-dehydro-7-methyl-9α-fluoro-11-ketotestosterone.

EXAMPLE 26

7-methyl-9α-fluoro-11β-hydroxytestosterone

A solution of one gram of 7-methyl-9α-fluoro-11β-hydroxytestosterone 17-acetate in methanol was freed of oxygen gas by bubbling nitrogen therethrough. A solution of one gram of potassium bicarbonate in ten milliliters of water was similarly freed of oxygen. The two solutions were mixed at a temperature of between eighteen and twenty degrees centigrade and in a nitrogen atmosphere. The mixture was stirred at room temperature for twenty hours while protecting it from atmospheric oxygen with nitrogen. At the end of twenty hours the solution was neutralized by the addition of ice water containing acetic acid. The neutralized solution was concentrated to about sixty milliliters by distillation at room temperature at reduced pressure and then chilled in a refrigerator for about sixteen hours. The thus-precipitated 7-methyl-9α-fluoro-11β-hydroxytestosterone was filtered, washed with water, dried and recrystallized to give 7-methyl-9α-fluoro-11β-hydroxytestosterone.

Using the procedure described in Example 26, but substituting 1-dehydro - 7 - methyl-9α-fluoro-11β-hydroxytestosterone 17-acetate for 7-methyl-9α-fluoro-11β-hydroxytestosterone 17-acetate, there is obtained 1-dehydro-7-methyl-9α-fluoro-11β-hydroxytestosterone.

EXAMPLE 27

7α-methyl-19-nortestosterone acetate

To 30 ml. of tetrahydrofuran (prepared by percolating commercial grade tetrahydrofuran through a column of neutral alumina and discarding the first 15 ml. of percolate) cooled in an ice-bath was added, with stirring under an atmosphere of nitrogen, 25 ml. of a 3 M solution of methylmagnesium bromide in ether followed of 0.4 g. of cuprous bromide. To the stirred mixture so obtained was added a slurry of a small amount of cuprous bromide in a solution of 3 g. of 6-dehydro-19-nortestosterone 17-acetate in 50 ml. of tetrahydrofuran (previously treated as described above). The resulting mixture was stirred with cooling for a further ten minutes and was then poured into a mixture of ice-diluted hydrochloric acid saturated with sodium chloride-ether which was purged with nitrogen. The ether phrase was separated and washed successively with brine, diluted sodium hydroxide-brine, and finally with brine. The ether extracts were combined and dried over anhydrous magnesium sulfate. The dried solution was filtered and the filtrate was evaporated to dryness. The residue was dissolved in 5 ml. of pyridine and 5 ml. of acetic anhydride. After standing at room temperature for 18 hrs., ice and water were added and the product was extracted with ether. The extract was washed with dilute acid, dilute sodium hydroxide and water, dried and the solvent removed. The residue was dissolved in methylene chloride and chromatographed on a column of magnesium silicate (Florisil). The column was eluted with Skellysolve B hexanes containing increasing proportions of acetone and those fractions, which were found by infrared analysis to contain the desired 7α-methyl-19-nortestosterone 17-acetate, were combined and evaporated to dryness. The oily residue was dissolved in acetone and chromatographed on a 30 g. 2:1 Celite: Darco column packed wet with acetone. The column was eluted with acetone and the first 750 ml. of eluate was evaporated to dryness. The residue was recrystallized from aqueous methanol. There was thus obtained 1 g. of 7α-methyl-19-nortestosterone 17-acetate in the form of a crystalline solid having a melting point of 111 to 114° C.; [α]$_D$ +48° (chloroform). The ultraviolet absorption spectrum of this compound (in solution in ethanol) exhibited a maximum at 240 millimicrons (ε=17,350).

Analysis.—Calcd. for $C_{21}H_{30}O_2$: C, 76.32; H, 9.15. Found: C, 76.28; H, 9.44.

EXAMPLE 28

7α-methyl-19-nortestosterone

A solution of 3 g. of 7α-methyl-19-nortestosterone-17-acetate in 40 ml. of a 5 percent solution of potassium carbonate in 80 percent aqueous methanol was heated under reflux in an atmosphere of nitrogen for 2 hours. The reaction mixture was extracted with ether and the ethereal extract was washed with water and dried over anhydrous magnesium sulfate. The dried ether solution was filtered and the filtrate was evaporated to dryness. The residue was triturated with ether and the solid which separated was isolated by filtration. There was thus obtained 7α-methyl-19-nortestosterone in the form of a crystalline solid having a melting point of 140 to 145.5° C. An analytical sample having a melting point of 145 to 146° C. and [α]$_D$ +55° (chloroform) was obtained by recrystallization from a mixture of acetone and Skellysolve B (a mixture of hexanes). The ultraviolet absorption spectrum of this compound (in solution in ethanol) exhibited a maximum at 241 millimicrons (ε=17,150).

Analysis.—Calcd. for $C_{19}H_{28}O_2$: C, 79.17; H, 9.78. Found: C, 79.13; H, 10.19.

EXAMPLE 29

7α-methyl-19-nor-Δ^4-androstene-3,17-dione

To a slurry of 1.4 g. of chromium trioxide in 15 ml. of pyridine was added with stirring and cooling, a solution of 1.4 g. of 7α-methyl-19-nortestosterone in 15 ml. of pyridine. After the addition was complete, the reaction mixture was stirred at room temperature (approximately 20° C.) for 20 hours and was then diluted with a mixture of equal parts of benzene and ether. The resulting mixture was filtered through a bed of diatomaceous earth (Celite). The filter bed was washed well with a mixture of equal parts of ether and benzene, then with water and finally with the mixed solvent. The filtrate and the organic layer of the washings were combined and washed several times with water. Each aqueous washing was back-extracted with a mixture of equal parts of ether and benzene. The combined organic layers were then dried and evaporated to dryness. The residue was triturated with ether and the solid material was isolated by filtration. There was thus obtained 1.4 g. of 7α-methyl-19-nor-Δ^4-androstene-3,17-dione in the form of a crystalline solid having a melting point of 195 to 198° C. An analytical sample having a melting point of 201 to 204° C. was obtained by recrystallization from acetone. The ultraviolet absorption spectrum of this compound (in solution in ethanol) exhibited a maximum of 239.5 millimicrons (ε=17,000).

Analysis.—Calcd. for $C_{19}H_{26}O_2$: C, 79.69; H, 9.15. Found: C, 79.66; H, 8.87.

EXAMPLE 30

7α-methyl-19-nor-Δ^4-androstene-3,17-dione 3-pyrrolidinyl enamine

To a solution of 10 mg. of 7α-methyl-19-nor-Δ^4-androstene-3,17-dione in a little boiling methanol was added 1 drop of pyrrolidine. The resulting solution was concentrated by evaporation and allowed to cool. The crystalline solid which separated was isolated by filtration, washed with a small quantity of methanol and dried. There was thus obtained 7α-methyl-19-nor-Δ^4-androstene-3,17-dione 3-pyrrolidinyl enamine in the form of a crystalline solid having a melting point of 151 to 160° C. The ultraviolet absorption spectrum of the compound (in solution in ether) exhibited a maximum at 282 millimicrons

(ε=23,450)

The infrared absorption spectrum of the compound (mineral oil mull) exhibited maxima at 1735, 1635, 1600, 1200, 1180, 1155 and 1035 reciprocal centimeters.

EXAMPLE 31

7α-methyl-17α-ethinyl-19-nortestosterone

A volume of 1 ml. of a 20 percent by weight suspension of sodium acetylide in xylene was centrifuged and the solid which separated was taken up in 6 ml. of redistilled dimethylsulfoxide. To the resulting mixture was added the 3-pyrrolidyl enamine from 0.5 g. of 7α-methyl-19-nor-Δ^4-androstene-3,17-dione prepared as described in Example 30. The mixture so obtained was maintained under an atmosphere of nitrogen for five hours at the end of which time the excess sodium acetylide was destroyed by dropwise addition of water. About 2 ml. of water and 5 ml. of methanol was added to obtain a clear solution which was then heated on a steam bath for 1 hour. The mixture so obtained was extracted with ether and ethereal extract was washed successively with dilute hydrochloric acid, dilute sodium carbonate and water before being dried over anhydrous magnesium sulfate. The dried solution was filtered and the filtrate was evaporated to dryness. The residue was triturated with a mixture of ether and Skellysolve B and recrystallized twice from a mixture of acetone and Skellysolve B. There was thus obtained 0.161 g. of 7α-methyl-17α-ethinyl-19-nortestosterone in the form of a crystalline solid having a melting point of 197 to 199.5° C. The ultraviolet spectrum of the compound (in solution in ethanol) exhibited a maximum at 240.5 millimicrons. The infrared absorption spectrum of the compound (mineral oil mull) exhibited maxima at 3390, 3240, 2100, 1663 and 1623 reciprocal centimeters.

Analysis.—Calcd. for $C_{21}H_{28}O_2$: C, 80.72; H, 9.03. Found: C, 80.44; H, 9.05.

EXAMPLE 32

17α-ethyl-7α-methyl-19-nortestosterone

A suspension of 30 mg. of 1 percent palladium-on-charcoal catalyst in 20 milliliters of dioxane (purified as described by Fieser, Methods of Organic Chemistry, 2d Edition, p. 368) was saturated with hydrogen at atmospheric pressure. To the suspension was added 100 mg. of 7α-methyl-17α-ethinyl-19-nortestosterone and the mixture was hydrogenated at atmospheric pressure until 2 equivalents of hydrogen had been consumed. The reaction mixture was filtered through a bed of diatomaceous earth (Celite) and the filtrate was evaporated to dryness. The residue was combined with that obtained from a similar run employing 50 mg. of starting material. The combined residues were dissolved in methylene chloride and chromatographed on a column of 50 grams of magnesium silicate (Florisil) which had been packed wet with Skellysolve B. The column was eluted with Skellysolve B containing increasing proportions of acetone and those fractions, which, on the basis of infrared analysis, contained the desired 17α-ethyl-7α-methyl-19-nortestosterone, were combined and evaporated to dryness. The residue was recrystallized twice from a mixture of Skellysolve B and ether. There was thus obtained 17α-ethyl-7α-methyl-19-nortestosterone in the form of a crystalline solid having a melting point of 138 to 139° C. The ultraviolet spectrum of the compound (in solution in ethanol) exhibited a maximum of 241 millimicrons (ϵ=17,000).

Analysis.—Calcd. for $C_{21}H_{32}O_2$: C, 79.69; H, 10.19. Found: C, 79.43; H, 10.23.

EXAMPLE 33

7α,17α-dimethyl-19-nortestosterone

A solution of 2.75 g. of 7α-methyl-19-nor-Δ⁴-androstene-3,17-dione 3-pyrrolidyl enamine in 70 ml. of tetrahydrofuran is added over a short period with stirring under an atmosphere of nitrogen to 25 ml. of a 3 M solution of methylmagnesium bromide in diethyl ether. The resulting mixture is distilled until the vapor temperature reaches 55° C. and the residue is then heated under reflux for approximately 4 hours. To the mixture so obtained is added carefully with stirring an iced ammonium chloride solution followed by 130 ml. of methanol and 25 ml. of 5% aqueous sodium hydroxide. The mixture is stirred at 40° C. under nitrogen for several hours and is concentrated to about one third volume under reduced pressure. The resulting mixture is diluted with water and extracted with ether. The ether extract is washed successively with water, dilute hydrochloric acid, dilute aqueous sodium carbonate, and water before being dried over anhydrous sodium sulfate and filtered. The filtrate is evaporated to dryness and the residue is dissolved in methylene chloride and chromatographed over 100 grams of magnesium silicate (Florisil). The column is eluted with Skellysolve B containing increasing proportions of acetone and those fractions of the eluate which on infrared absorption analysis show no C-17 carbonyl absorption are combined and evaporated to dryness. The residue is recrystallized from a mixture of acetone and Skellysolve B. There is thus obtained 7α,17α-dimethyl-19-nortestosterone in the form of a crystalline solid.

Using the above procedure but replacing methylmagnesium bromide by propylmagnesium bromide, isopropylmagnesium bromide, butylmagnesium bromide, allylmagnesium bromide, and 2-butenylmagnesium bromide, there are obtained 7α-methyl-17α-propyl-19-nortestosterone, 7α-methyl-17α-isopropyl-19-nortestosterone, 7α-methyl-17α-butyl-19-nortestosterone, 7α-methyl-17α-allyl-19-nortestosterone and 7α-methyl-17α-(α-methallyl)-19-nortestosterone, respectively.

EXAMPLE 34

7α,17α-dimethyl-11α-hydroxy-19-nortestosterone

A medium is prepared of 20 g. of cornsteep liquor (60% solids) and 10 g. of commercial dextrose, diluted to 1 liter and adjusted to a pH of 4.8 to 5.0. A volume of 10 l. of this sterilized medium is inoculated with a 24 hr. vegetative growth of culture *Rhizopus nigricans* (strain; ATCC 6227b) and incubated for 24 hrs. at a temperature of about 28° C. using a rate of aeration of 0.3 l. per minute and stirring at 300 r.p.m. After 24 hr. of agitation, a solution of 2 g. of 7α,17α-dimethyl-19-nortestosterone in 20 ml. of dimethylformamide is added to the inoculated medium. After an additional 72 hr. period of incubation, the fermentation liquor and mycelium are extracted with three 1 l. portions of methylene chloride. The extracts are combined and washed with aqueous sodium bicarbonate solution and then with water before being dried and evaporated to dryness. The residue is dissolved in methylene chloride and chromatographed over a column of synthetic magnesium silicate (Florisil). The column is eluted with Skellysolve B containing increasing proportions of acetone. Those fractions of the eluate which are found by weight profile and paper chromatogram analysis to contain

the desired 7α,17α-dimethyl-11α-hydroxy-19-nortestosterone are combined and recrystallized from a mixture of acetone and Skellysolve B. There is thus obtained 7α,17α-dimethyl-11α-hydroxy-19-nortestosterone in the form of a crystalline solid.

Similarly, using the procedure described above, but replacing 7α,17α-dimethyl-19-nortestosterone by 17α-ethyl-7α-methyl-19-nortestosterone, 17α-ethinyl-7α-methyl-19-nortestosterone, 7α-methyl-17α-propyl-19-nortestosterone, 7α-methyl-17α-butyl-19-nortestosterone or 7α-methyl-17α-allyl-19-nortestosterone, there are obtained 17α-ethyl-7α-methyl-11α-hydroxy-19-nortestosterone, 17α-ethinyl-17α-methyl-11α-hydroxy-19-nortestosterone, 7α-methyl-17α-propyl-11α-hydroxy-19-nortestosterone, 7α-methyl-17α-butyl-11α-hydroxy-19-nortestosterone and 7α-methyl-17α-allyl-11α-hydroxy-19-nortestosterone, respectively.

EXAMPLE 35

7α,17α-dimethyl-11β-hydroxy-19-nortestosterone

A seed culture of *Cunninghamella blakesleeana* (ATCC 86885), obtained from spores grown on a 2% agar, 5% malt extract solids at a pH of 6.0, is prepared by growth in a medium containing, per liter of tap water, 10 g. of dextrose (Cerelose) and 20 g. of liquid corn steep liquor (60% solids), adjusted to a pH of about 5 with 25% aqueous sodium hydroxide.

Five 1 l. portions of the above medium are inoculated with the seed culture and growth is continued with aeration and shaking for 48 hours. Then 0.2 g. of 7α,17α-dimethyl-19-nortestosterone in 30 ml. of alcohol is added to each flask and fermentation is conducted for another 48 hours. The mycelium is filtered from the beer and the beer is extracted four times with one-fourth by volume amounts of methylene chloride containing 25% by volume of ethyl acetate. The extracts are evaporated to dryness. The residue is redissolved in 150 ml. of methylene chloride and chromatographed on a column of magnesium silicate (Florisil) which is developed with hexanes containing increasing proportions of acetone. Those fractions of the eluate which are found by weight profile and paper chromatogram analysis to contain the desired 7α,17α-dimethyl-11β-hydroxy-19-nortestosterone are combined and recrystallized from a mixture of acetone and Skellysolve B. There is thus obtained 7α,17α-dimethyl-11β-hydroxy-19-nortestosterone in the form of a crystalline solid.

Similarly, using the procedure described above, but replacing 7α,17α-dimethyl-19-nortestosterone by 17α-ethyl-7α-methyl-19-nortestosterone, 17α-ethinyl-7α-methyl-19-nortestosterone, 7α-methyl-17α-propyl-19-nortestosterone, 7α-methyl-17α-butyl-19-nortestosterone, or 7α-methyl-17α-allyl-19-nortestosterone, there are obtained 17α-ethyl-7α-methyl-11β-hydroxy-19-nortestosterone, 17α-ethinyl-7α-methyl-11β-hydroxy-19-nortestosterone, 7α-methyl-17α-propyl-11β-hydroxy-19-nortestosterone, 7α-methyl-17α-butyl-11β-hydroxy-19-nortestosterone and 7α-methyl-17α-allyl-11β-hydroxy-19-nortestosterone, respectively.

EXAMPLE 36

7α,17α-dimethyl-11-keto-19-nortestosterone

A solution of 1.5 g. of 7α,17α-dimethyl-11α-hydroxy-19-nortestosterone in 80 ml. of acetic acid is treated with a solution of 0.74 g. of chromic acid anhydride in 4 ml. of water and 80 ml. of acetic acid and the mixture is allowed to stand at room temperature for 5 hr. The excess chromic acid is destroyed by the addition of 10 ml. of methanol and the resulting solution is concentrated in vacuo with heating on a water-bath. The residue is triturated with water and then extracted with ether. The ether solution is washed with dilute sodium hydroxide solution and water before being dried over anhydrous sodium sulfate. The dried ether solution is evaporated to dryness and the residue is recrystallized from aqueous acetone. There is thus obtained 7α,17α-dimethyl-11-keto-19-nortestosterone in the form of a crystalline solid.

The above compound is also obtained by employing 7α,17α-dimethyl-11β-hydroxy-19-nortestosterone as starting material in the above procedure.

Similarly, using the above procedure, but replacing 7α,17α-dimethyl-11α-hydroxy-19-nortestosterone by 17α-ethyl-7α-methyl-11α-hydroxy-19-nortestosterone, 17α-ethinyl-7α-methyl-11α-hydroxy-19-nortestosterone, 7α-methyl-17α-propyl-11-hydroxy-19-nortestosterone, 7-methyl-17α-butyl-11α-hydroxy-19-nortestosterone, 7α-methyl-17α-allyl-11α-hydroxy-19-nortestosterone, or the corresponding 11β-epimers, there are obtained 7α-methyl-17α-allyl-11α-hydroxy-19-nortestosterone, 17α-ethinyl-7α-methyl-11-keto-19-nortestosterone, 7α-methyl-17α-propyl-11-keto-19-nortestosterone, 7α-methyl-17α-butyl-11-keto-19-nortestosterone, and 7α-methyl-17α-allyl-11-keto - 19 - nortestosterone, respectively.

EXAMPLE 37

7α-methyl-11α-hydroxy-19-nor-Δ4-androstene-3,17-dione

Using the procedure described in Example 34, but replacing 7α,17α-dimethyl-19-nortestosterone by 7α-methyl-19-nor-Δ4-androstene - 3,17 - done, there is obtained 7α-methyl-11α-hydroxy-19-nor-Δ4-androstene-3,17-dione.

EXAMPLE 38

7α-methyl-11β-hydroxy-19-nor-Δ4-androstene-3,17-dione

Using the procedure described in Example 35, but replacing 7α,17α-dimethyl-19-nortestosterone by 7α-methyl-19-nor-Δ4-androstene-3,17-dione, there is obtained 7α-methyl-11β-hydroxy-19-nor-Δ4-androstene-3,17-dione.

EXAMPLE 39

7α-methyl-11β-hydroxy-19-nortestosterone

Using the procedure described in Example 35, but replacing 7α,17α-dimethyl-19-nortestosterone by 7α-methyl-19-nortestosterone, there is obtained 7α-methyl-11β-hydroxy-19-nortestosterone.

EXAMPLE 40

7α-methyl-11α-hydroxy-19-nortestosterone

Using the procedure described in Example 34, but replacing 7α,17α-dimethyl-19-nortestosterone by 7α-methyl-19-nortestosterone, there is obtained 7α-methyl-11α-hydroxy-19-nortestosterone.

EXAMPLE 41

7α-methyl-11β-hydroxy-19-nor-Δ4-androstene-3,17-dione

A solution of 1.6 g. of 7α-methyl-11β-hydroxy-19-nortestosterone in a mixture of 35 ml. of toluene and 15 ml. of cyclohexanone is heated until about 10 ml. are distilled to dry the solution. To the dry solution so obtained is added 1.5 g. of aluminum tertiary butoxide and the resulting solution is refluxed until the reaction is complete. An excess of a saturated aqueous solution of sodium potassium tartrate is added and the solvents are then removed by steam distillation. The residue is extracted with methylene chloride and the methylene chloride extract is dried and chromatographed on a magnesium silicate (Florisil) column. The column is developed with Skellysolve B hexanes containing increasing proportions of acetone and those fractions which, by paper chromatogram analysis, are shown to contain the desired 7α-methyl-11β-hydroxy-19-nor-Δ4-androstene-3,17-dione, are combined and evaporated to dryness. The residue is recrystallized from aqueous acetone. There is thus obtained 7α-methyl-11β-hydroxy-19-nor-Δ4-androstene-3,17 - dione in the form of a crystalline solid.

Using the above procedure, but replacing 7α-methyl-11β-hydroxy-19-nortestosterone by 7α - methyl - 11α - hydroxy-19-nortestosterone, there is obtained 7α-methyl-11α-hydroxy-19-nor-Δ4-androstene-3,17-dione.

EXAMPLE 42

7α-methyl-11β-hydroxy-19-nor-Δ4-androstene-3,17-dione 3-pyrrolidinyl enamine

Using the procedure described in Example 30, but replacing 7α-methyl-19-nor-Δ4-androstene-3,17-dione by 7α-methyl-11β-hydroxy-19-nor-Δ4 - androstene - 3,17 - dione, there is obtained the 3-pyrrolidinyl enamine of 7α-methyl-11β-hydroxy-19-nor-Δ4-androstene-3,17-dione.

Similarly, using the procedure of Example 30, but replacing 7α-methyl-19-nor-Δ4-androstene-3,17-dione by 7α-methyl-11α-hydroxy-19-nor-Δ4 - androstene - 3,17 - dione, there is obtained the 3-pyrrolidinyl enamine of 7α-methyl-11α-hydroxy-19-nor-Δ4-androstene-3,17-dione.

EXAMPLE 43

7α-methyl-17α-ethinyl-11β-hydroxy-19-nortestosterone

Using the procedure described in Example 31, but replacing the 3-pyrrolidyl enamine of 7α-methyl-19-nor-Δ4-androstene-3,17-dione by the 3-pyrrolidyl enamine of 7α-methyl-11β-hydroxy-19-nor-Δ4 - androstene - 3,17 - dione, there is obtained 7α-methyl-17α-ethinyl-11β-hydroxy-19-nortestosterone in the form of a crystalline solid.

Similarly, using the procedure of Example 31, but replacing the 3-pyrrolidyl enamine of 7α-methyl-19-nor-Δ4-androstene-3,17-dione by the 3-pyrrolidyl enamine of 7α-methyl-11α-hydroxy-19-nor-Δ4 - androstene - 3,17 - dione, there is obtained 7α-methyl-17α-ethinyl-11α-hydroxy-19-nortestosterone.

EXAMPLE 44

7α,17α-dimethyl-11β-hydroxy-19-nortestoterone

Using the procedure described in Example 33, but replacing the 3-pyrrolidyl enamine of 7α-methyl-19-nor-Δ4-androstene-3,17-dione by the 3-pyrrolidyl enamine of 7α-methyl-11β-hydroxy-19-nor - Δ4 - androstene - 3,17-dione, there is obtained 7α,17α-dimethyl-11β-hydroxy - 19 - nortestosterone in the form of a crystalline solid.

Similarly, using the procedure described in Example 33, but replacing the 3-pyrrolidyl enamine of 7α-methyl-19-nor-Δ4-androstene-3,17-dione by the 3-pyrrolidyl enamine of 7α-methyl-11α-hydroxy-19-nor-Δ4-androstene-3,17-dione, there is obtained 7α,17α-dimethyl-11α-hydroxy-19-nortestosterone in the form of a crystalline solid.

EXAMPLE 45

7α-methyl-17α-ethinyl-19-nortestosterone 17-acetate

A mixture of 1 g. of 7α - methyl - 17α-ethinyl-19-nortestosterone, 20 ml. of acetic anhydride and 1 ml. of pyridine is stirred and heated at 140° C. for 1 hour under a nitrogen atmosphere. The reaction mixture is then cooled to room temperature and stirred with 100 ml. of water for 2 hours. The product which separates is isolated by filtration. This product is a mixture of the desired 7α-methyl-17α-ethinyl-19-nortestosterone 17-acetate and the corresponding 3-enol 3,17-diacetate and the latter compound is hydrolyzed to the desired compound by heating the above product under reflux for 1 hr. with 100 ml. of methanol containing 2 ml. of concentrated hydrochloric acid. The reaction product so obtained is diluted with water and extracted with ether. The ether extract is dried over anhydrous magnesium sulfate and evaporated to dryness. The residue is dissolved in methylene chloride and chromatographed on a column of magnesium silicate (Florisil). The column is eluted with Skellysolve B containing increasing proportions of acetone and the fraction of the eluate, which is shown by paper chromatogram analysis to contain the desired product, is evaporated to dryness. The solid so obtained is recrystallized from aqueous methanol. There is thus obtained 7α-methyl-17α-ethinyl-19-nortestosterone 17-acetate in the form of a crystalline solid.

Similarly, by reacting 7α - methyl - 17α-ethinyl-19-nortestosterone with the appropriate hydrocarbon car-

33

boxylic acid anhydride, for example, at temperatures between about 80° C. and 150° C. using the above procedure there are produced other 17-acylates thereof such as the 17-propionate, 17-butyrate, 17-valerate, 17-hexanoate, 17-trimethylacetate, 17-isobutyrate, 17-isovalerate, 17-cyclohexanecarboxylate, 17-cyclopentylpropionate, 17-p-hexyloxypropionate, 17-benzoate, 17-hemisuccinate, 17-henylacetate, 17-acrylate, 17-crotonate, 17-undecylenate, 17-propiolate, 17-cinnamate, 17-maleate, and 17-citraconate.

Similarly, by reacting other 7α-methyl-19-nortestosterones and 7α-methyl-17α-(lower aliphatic hydrocarbon substituted)-19-nortestosterones with the appropriate hydrocarbon carboxylic acid anhydride using the above procedure there are obtained the corresponding 17-acylates such as

7α-methyl-19-nortestosterone 17-propionate,
11-keto-7α-methyl-19-nortestosterone 17-cyclopentylpropionate,
11α-butyroxy-7α-methyl-19-nortestosterone 17-butyrate,
7α,17α-dimethyl-19-nortestosterone 17-acetate,
7α-methyl-17α-ethyl-19-nortestosterone 17-propionate,
11-keto-7α-methyl-17α-ethinyl-19-nortestosterone 17-acetate,
7α-methyl-17α-propyl-19-nortestosterone 17-acetate,
7α-methyl-17α-isopropyl-19-nortestosterone 17-propionate,
7α-methyl-17α-butyl-19-nortestosterone 17-valerate,
7α-methyl-17α-(α-methallyl)-19-nortestosterone 17-acetate,
11α-acetoxy-7α-methyl-17α-isopropyl-19-nortestosterone 17-acetate,
11α-propionyloxy-7α-methyl-17α-ethyl-19-nortestosterone 17-propionate,
11α-acetoxy-7α-methyl-17α-allyl-19-nortestosterone 17-acetate,
11β-hydroxy-7α-methyl-17α-isopropyl-19-nortestosterone 17-propionate,
11β-hydroxy-7α-methyl-17α-isobutyl-19-nortestosterone 17-acetate, and
11β-hydroxy-7α-methyl-17α-allyl-19-nortestosterone 17-isobutyrate.

EXAMPLE 46
7α-methyl-17α-ethyltestosterone

A. 7α-methyl-Δ4-androstene-3,17-dione
To a solution of 20 g. of sodium dichromate dihydrate in 200 ml. of acetic acid was added 20 g. of 7α-methyltestosterone with stirring and cooling in a cold water bath. The reaction mixture was allowed to stand for several hours and was then poured into ca. 1 litre of water. The precipitate so formed was isolated by filtration, washed with water and dried. The material (18.7 g.; M.P. 186 to 191° C.) so obtained was recrystallized from a mixture of acetone and Skellysolve B. There was thus obtained 15.6 g. of 7α-methyl-Δ4-androstene-3,17-dione in the form of a crystalline solid having a melting point of 194 to 196° C.; [α]D+196° (chloroform). The ultraviolet spectrum of the compound (in solution in ethanol) exhibited a maximum at 241 millimicrons (ε=17,250).
Analysis.—Calcd. for $C_{20}H_{28}O_2$: C, 79.95; H, 9.39. Found: C, 79.81; H, 9.33.

B. 7α-methyl-17α-ethynyltestosterone
The 7α-methyl-Δ4-androstene-3,17-dione (15.6 g.) obtained as described above, was dissolved in the minimum amount of boiling methanol with nitrogen bubbling through and 10 ml. of pyrrolidine was added. The mixture was cooled and the solid which had separated was isolated by filtration, washed with fresh methanol and ether and dried for about 15 minutes at 60° C. There was thus obtained the 3-pyrrolidyl enamine of 7α-methyl-Δ4-androstene-3,17-dione in the form of a crystalline solid having a melting point of 199 to 205° C. with decomposition; [α]D−190° (pyridine). The ultraviolet spectrum of the

34

compound (in solution in ether) exhibited a maximum at 282 millimicrons (ε=29,900).
Analysis.—Calcd. for $C_{24}H_{35}NO$: C, 81.53; H, 9.98; N, 3.95. Found: C, 81.57; H, 9.76; N, 3.77.

While the above enamine was being dried, 25 ml. of a suspension (0.2 g./ml.) of sodium acetylide in xylene was centrifuged. The solid so isolated was suspended in 160 ml. of redistilled dimethylsulfoxide. To this suspension was added a slurry of the whole of the above enamine in 100 ml. of dimethylsulfoxide. The reaction mixture was stirred under an atmosphere of nitrogen for 3 hrs. after which time 30 ml. of water and 50 ml. of methanol were added. The resulting mixture was heated to 50 to 60° C. for 1 hr. and was then stirred overnight at room temperature. The reaction mixture was then diluted with water and extracted with three 100 ml. portions of methylene chloride. The methylene chloride extracts were combined, washed with dilute hydrochloric acid and with water and then evaporated to dryness to give 2 g. of material. The aqueous washings from the above extraction were combined and made basic by the addition of sodium hydroxide solution. The solution so obtained was extracted several times with methylene chloride and the combined methylene chloride extracts were washed successively with dilute hydrochloric acid, dilute sodium carbonate and water before being dried over anhydrous sodium sulfate. The dried solution was filtered and the filtrate was evaporated to dryness. The residue (3.9 g.) was combined with the 2 g. of material obtained as described above and an acetone solution of the combined material was treated with a mixture of decolorizing charcoal (Darco), diatomaceous earth (Celite) and magnesium silicate (Florisil). The mixture was filtered and the filtrate was evaporated to dryness. The residue was recrystallized from a mixture of acetone and hexanes (Skellysolve B). There was thus obtained 3.9 g. of 7α-methyl-17a-ethynyltestosterone in the form of a crystalline solid having a melting point of 190 to 192.5° C. An analytical sample having a melting point of 191 to 193° C. and [α]D+41° (chloroform) was prepared by recrystallization from ethyl acetate. The ultraviolet spectrum of the compound (in solution in ethanol) exhibited a maximum at 242 millimicrons (ε=16,550).
Analysis.—Calcd. for $C_{22}H_{30}O_2$: C, 80.93; H, 9.26. Found: C, 80.86; H, 9.33.

C. 7α-methyl-17α-ethyltestosterone
A suspension of 0.2 g. of 1% palladium-on-charcoal catalyst in 40 ml. of dioxane was saturated with hydrogen at atmospheric pressure. To the suspension was added 1 g. of 7α-methyl-17α-ethynyltestosterone and the mixture was shaken in the presence of hydrogen until the theoretical quantity of hydrogen had been absorbed. The mixture was then filtered and the filtrate was evaporated to dryness under reduced pressure. The residue was recrystallized from a mixture of ether, methylene chloride, and Skellysolve B. There was thus obtained 0.8 g. of 7α-methyl-17α-ethyl-testosterone in the form of a crystalline solid having a melting point of 140.5 to 143° C. The ultraviolet spectrum of the compound (in solution in ethanol) exhibited a maximum at 242 millimicrons (ε=16,350).
Analysis.—Calcd. for $C_{22}H_{34}O_2$: C, 79.95; H, 10.37. Found: C, 80.15; H, 10.39.

EXAMPLE 47
7α-methyl-17α-ethyltestosterone 17-propionate

To a solution of 5 g. of 7α-methyl-17α-ethyltestosterone in 20 ml. of pyridine is added 5 ml. of propionic anhydride. The resulting solution is refluxed under nitrogen until the hydroxyl absorption in the infrared region is gone before being diluted with crushed ice and water. The solid which separates is isolated by filtration and recrystallized from aqueous acetone. There is thus obtained 7α-methyl-17α-ethyltestosterone 17-propionate in the form of a crystalline solid.

35

Using the above procedure, but replacing propionic anhydride by the appropriate hydrocarbon carboxylic acid anhydride, there are obtained other 17-acylates of 7α-methyl-17α-ethyltestosterone such as the 17-acetate, 17-butyrate, 17-valerate, 17-hexanoate, 17-trimethylacetate-17-isobutyrate, 17-isovalerate, 17-cyclohexanecarboxylate, 17β - cyclopentylpropionate, 17 - p-hexyloxyphenylpropionate, 17-benzoate, 17-hemisuccinate, 17-phenylacetate, 17-acrylate, 17-crotonate, 17-undecylenate, 17-propiolate, 17-cinnamate, 17-maleate, and 17-citraconate.

We claim:

1. A 7α-methyl-19-nortestosterone having the formula:

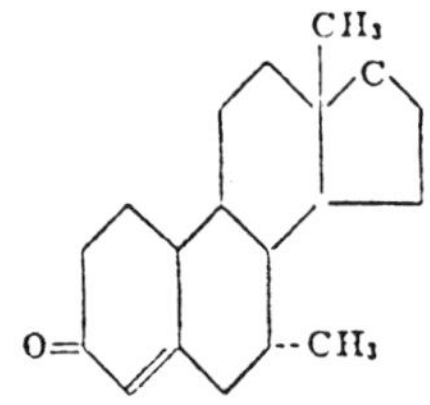

wherein C represents a group selected from the class consisting of

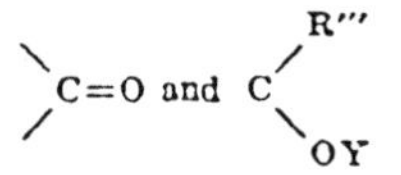

wherein R''' is selected from the class consisting of hydrogen and a lower aliphatic hydrocarbon radical containing

36

from 1 to 4 carbon atoms, inclusive, and Y is selected from the class consisting of hydrogen and the acyl radical of a hydrocarbon carboxylic acid containing from 1 to 12 carbon atoms, inclusive.

2. 7α-methyl-19-nortestosterone acetate.

3. 7α-methyl-19-nortestosterone.

4. 7α-methyl-19-nor-Δ4-androstene-3,17-dione.

5. 7α,17α-dimethyl-19-nortestosterone.

6. 7α-methyl-17α-ethyl-19-nortestosterone.

7. 7α-methyl-17a-ethinyl-19-nortestosterone.

8. 7α - methyl-17α-ethinyl-19-nortestosterone 17-acetate.

References Cited

UNITED STATES PATENTS

2,793,218	5/1957	Herr	260—397.45
2,837,464	6/1958	Nobile	195—51
2,852,511	9/1958	Fried	260—239.55

OTHER REFERENCES

Edwards et al., J.A.C.S. 81, pp. 3156–57 (1959).
Fieser et al., Steroids p. 565, Reinhold Pub. Co., New York, N.Y.

LEWIS GOTTS, *Primary Examiner.*

L. H. GASTON, M. LIEBMAN, *Examiners.*

H. A. FRENCH, *Assistant Examiner.*

CHAPTER NINE

1

2

2,698,855

19-NOR-DELTA-4-ANDROSTENE, 3-ONE, 17-BETA BENZOATE AND METHOD FOR MANUFACTURING SAME

Lawrence Hicks, Chicago, Ill., assignor to Organics, Inc., Chicago, Ill., a corporation of Illinois

No Drawing. Application March 4, 1954,
Serial No. 414,218

2 Claims. (Cl. 260—397.4)

This invention relates to the manufacture of 19-nor-delta-4-androstene, 3-one, 17-beta benzoate (19-nor testosterone benzoate) and it is an object of this invention to produce and to provide a method for producing 19-nor-delta-4-androstene, 3-one, 17-beta benzoate.

In my copending application Ser. No. 353,007, filed May 4, 1953, description is made of the manufacture of 19-Nor-delta-4-androstene, 3-one, 17-beta esters such as the propionate, cyclopentyl propionate, acetate, benzoate and the like and to methods for preparing same where the corresponding 17 ol is reacted for esterification with the corresponding acid anhydride or alkyl halide.

The androstene compounds and their derivatives generally exhibit two types of biological activity—namely, androgenic or male sex hormone activity and myotrophic or protein anabolic activity. In the use for treatment of conditions wherein myothrophic or protein anabolic activity is important, conjoint androgenic activity may not only be undesirable but more often is harmful to the extent that its presence will prohibit use of the particular steroid compound. This is particularly true in pediatrics and in geriatrics.

Many attempts have been made to isolate the desirable mytrophic or protein anabolic activity from the androgenic activity but elimination of the androgenic activity of androstane and androstene compounds generally results also in the lowering or loss also of the protein anabolic activity. The separation of the two types of activity becomes difficult, especially in androstene steroidal compounds of the type described, yet it has been found that the build-up of the steroid molecule with certain groupings as distinguished from others enables such separation in a few instances in the production of a compound which has a high level of a desirable myotrophic activity without objectionable amounts of androgenic activity. A general pattern with respect to the types of groups or their location on the steroid molecule for the development of such results has not, to the present, been established. In the esters of 19-Nor-delta-4-androstene, 3-one, 17-beta ol, it has been found that the aliphatic esters such as the propionate, acetate, cyclopentyl propionate, valerate and the like have a high ratio of the undesirable androgenic activity with respect to the desirable myotrophic or protein anabolic activity. It has been found, however, that the 19-Nor-delta-4-androstene, 3-one, 17-beta benzoate appears unexpectedly to be entirely unrelated to the aliphatic esters in that, unlike the aliphatic esters, the benzoate has a negligible amount of androgenic activity, yet its protein anabolic activity remains high enough so that an unexpectedly high ratio of anabolic activity to androgenic activity is secured.

Aside from these important differences in undesirable androgenic activity of which the benzoate is relatively free, the benzoate ester differs from the aliphatic esters also in the limitations with respect to the methods of manufacture and in the properties of the final compound. Where the aliphatic esters can be formed by reaction of the 17 ol with the corersponding acid anhydride or alkyl halide, the benzoic acid ester cannot be prepared in commercially economical yields by reaction of the 17 ol with the alkyl halide. It seems that the reaction product that is formed comprises a mixture of the corresponding 17 benzoate with the enol dibenzoate from which separation of the 17 benzoate is difficult. With benzoic anhydride as the reactant for esterification, excellent yields of relatively pure benzoate can be secured which requires little, if any, purification as will become apparent

from the following procedure for the preparation of 19-Nor-delta-4-androstene, 3-one, 17-beta benzoate.

The benzoate appears also to differ from the corresponding aliphatic esters such as the acetate, propionate, cyclopentyl propionate and the valerate in the characteristics of the end product which is formed. The aliphatic esters all appear to form as a hydrate containing 1–1.5 moles of water of crystallization. The presence of this water of crystallization appears to make crystallization of the aliphatic esters difficult and they are therefore inclined to exist as amorphous, resinous substances. On the other hand, the benzoate is free of water of crystallization and forms readily into long needle-like crystals having a melting point of 174–175° C. and a specific rotation at 20° in sodium light in 95 percent ethanol of +104.5°.

EXAMPLE 1

Preparation of 19-Nor-delta-4-androstene, 3-one, 17-beta-ol

Three grams of estradiol-17-beta (0.011 mole; M. W. 272.4) was dissolved in 500 ml. of 2.5 N sodium hydroxide solution preferably with warming. To this mixture was added, dropwise at 0.5 degree C., 18.8 ml. (0.2 mole, 25.2 gm., M. W. 126) of dimethylsulfate with good agitation. After all of the dimethylsulfate was added, the mixture was allowed to warm to room temperature with stirring (2–3 hours) and then heated on a water bath (80–90 degrees C.) for one hour. The warm mixture was then diluted with two volumes of water and then cooled with scratching whereby crude methyl ether separated. This is washed well first with water and then by 70 percent methanol. Upon recrystallization from dilute ethanol, it melted at 120–121 degrees C.

17-beta estradiol-3-methyl ether (0.50 g., 0.0017 mole, M. P. 120–121 degrees) was added to the reaction flask, followed by 40 ml. of anhydrous ether. When complete solution of the solid had occurred, 50 ml. of anhydrous liquid ammonia was added with stirring, and 0.50 g. (0.072 mole) of lithium wire was immediately added in small pieces to the homogeneous solution, over a one-minute interval. The blue reaction mixture was stirred an additional ten minutes, then 4.6 g. (0.10 mole) of absolute ethanol was added dropwise over a ten to twenty minute interval with stirring when the foaming subsided. When the blue color had disappeared, most of the ammonia was evaporated by carefully heating on the steam bath, then 100 ml. of cold water was added carefully to decompose the mixture. The aqueous layer was separated and extracted with four 15 ml. portions of ether. The combined solvent layers were washed with two 10 ml. portions of water, one 10 ml. portion of saturated sodium chloride solution, and were then dried over anhydrous potassium carbonate. The drying agent was removed by filtration and the residue obtained after distillation of the solvent was crystallized from thiophene-free benzene to yield 1,4-dihydroestradiol-17-beta-3-methyl ether. M. P. 111–113.5.

To a solution of 220 mg. of the dihydro compound (M. P. 111.5–115.5 degrees) in 15 ml. of boiling methanol, was added over a three-minute period with swirling, a hot solution of 2.5 ml. of concentrated hydrochloric acid and 7.5 ml. of water. The mixture was then allowed to cool slowly in a beaker of hot water over a period of one hour. After heating for a short time, the product was extracted with several portions of ether, the combined extract washed with water, saturated sodium bicarbonate, water and dried over sodium sulfate. Removal of the solvent, recrystallization from methylcyclohexane containing a small amount of ethyl acetate, and drying at 70 degrees (0.05 mm.) for two hours gave 19-nor-delta-4-androstene, 3-one, 17-beta-ol. M. P. 109.5–110.5 degrees.

EXAMPLE 2

Preparation of 19-Nor-delta-4-androstene, 3-one, 17-beta benzoate

27.4 grams (0.1 mole) of 19-Nor-delta-4-androstene, 3-one, 17-beta-ol of Example 1 is dissolved in 500 cc. of anhydrous pyridine and 28.25 grams (0.125 mole) of benzoic anhydride added. The solution is refluxed for about four hours.

3

50. cc. of distilled water is then added and refluxing is continued for an additional four hours to decompose or hydrolyze excess acid anhydride to benzoic acid. This step has been found to be important, otherwise the product will contain excess anhydride which is difficult to eliminate. On the other hand, if the material is hydrolyzed to benzoic acid, the latter is easily separated from the desired product.

The pyridine-water solution containing the steroid ester and free benzoic acid is distilled to a dry residue, and then taken up by solution in benzene. The benzene solution is washed exhaustively with saturated sodium bicarbonate to free it of benzoic acid and it is then washed with 1 N hydrochloric acid to free it of traces of pyridine.

The benzene solution is then exhaustively washed with water to free it of mineral acid and it is then distilled to dryness. The dry residue is dissolved in anhydrous ethanol by boiling under reflux and then sufficient water is added to the alcohol solution to reduce the concentration of the alcohol to 75 percent by volume. Upon cooling, the benzoate crystallizes in long needles. No recrystallization is believed to be necessary since the resulting product indicates substantial purity since the crystals have a melting point of 174–175° C. and a specific rotation of 20° C. at 104.5°.

The yield of the 19-Nor-delta-4-androstene, 3-one, 17-beta benzoate ranges as high as 97 percent of theory.

It has been found that the compound 19-Nor-delta-4-androstene, 3-one. 17-beta benzoate differs materially from the other aliphatic esters both as to activity and use and in the limitations with respect to manufacture and the properties thereof. The differences in reactions available from the benzoate have been unexpected but greatly beneficial in the use of benzoate esters as compared to the propionate or the cyclopentyl propionate or other aliphatic esters of 19-Nor-testosterone. These differences in activity and results which have been clearly established by animal data indicate that the benzoate is practically void of androgenic activity while supplying a high degree of myotrophic or protein anabolic activity whereas the aliphatic esters such as the propionate, cyclopentyl propionate or valerate all show a comparatively high ratio of androgenic activity to myotrophic or protein anabolic activity.

As previously pointed out, high androgenic activity is undesirable in this type of steroid, yet it is, in general, difficult to formulate a steroid which offers a desired protein anabolic activity without supplying at least some amount of androgenic activity. While the aliphatic esters of 19-Nor-testosterone follow the general rule and have a high ratio of androgenic activity to myotrophic or protein anabolic activity, the 19-Nor-testosterone benzoate appears to be non-analogous in that a high degree of protein anabolic activity is secured practically in the absence of any androgenic activity.

This has been established by animal tests performed upon rats in which daily administrations were made to castrated male rats for seven consecutive days by subcutaneous injection to introduce a total of 700 μg. of the various esters contained in corn oil as the diluent.

The following table represents results which were secured as indicated by the growth rates of the various glands. Gain in weight of the ventral prostate gland

4

and seminal vesicles proves androgenic activity and gain in weight of the levator ani proves myotrophic or protein anabolic activity.

No. of Rats	Treatment	Body Weight (gm.)	Ventral Prostate (mg.)	Seminal Vesicles (mg.)	Levator ani (mg.)
5	Oil only	66	11.0	8.6	15.9
5	19-Nor-testosterone benzoate, 700 μg.	70	16.8	12.2	39.1
5	19-Nor-testosterone valerate, 700 μg.	66	46.6	42.8	54.3
5	19-Nor-testosterone propionate resin, 700 μg.	63	52.2	50.4	51.7
5	19-Nor-testosterone propionate crystals, 700 μg.	65	54.8	45.0	48.4
6	Testosterone propionate, 700 μg.	66	89.8	99.9	42.4

For use as a measure in the trade, the important value constitutes the ratio of protein anabolic activity to androgenic activity which can be determined by the growth of the levator ani to the ventral prostate. This ratio from the data secured above is as follows:

19-Nor-testosterone benzoate	4.000
19-Nor-testosterone valerate	1.079
19-Nor-testosterone propionate	0.802
Testosterone propionate	0.336

From these results it will be apparent that the benzoate provides a very desirable amount of activity represented by growth of the levator ani as compared to the relatively negligible growth of the ventral prostate. On the other hand, the growth of the levator ani which is secured by the aliphatic esters is slightly greater in the levator ani with equivalent amounts of injection but the amount of growth in the ventral prostate is even greater which indicates that the aliphatic esters impart a high degree of androgenic activity as compared to the benzoate with a relatively small difference existing in the amount of the protein anabolic activity. This difference is more noticeable in the ratio of the gain in weight of the levator ani as compared to the ventral prostate which indicates that the aliphatic esters impart androgenic activity as high as or greater than the protein anabolic activity whereas the latter is secured in amounts four times greater than the androgenic activity with the benzoate ester.

It will be understood that changes may be made in the details of formulation and application without departing from the spirit of the invention, especially as defined in the following claims.

I claim:

1. The compound 19-Nor-delta-4-androstene, 3-one, 17-beta benzoate.

2. The method of preparing 19-Nor-delta-4-androstene, 3-one, 17-beta benzoate comprising the step of reacting 19-Nor-delta-4-androstene, 3-one, 17-beta-ol with benzoic anhydride.

No references cited.

1

2,891,973

NEW STEROID DERIVATIVE AND METHOD OF PREPARING SAME

Georges Muller, Nogent-sur-Marne, and Leon Velluz, Paris, France, assignors to Les Laboratoires Français de Chimiotherapie, Paris, France, a body corporate of France

No Drawing. Application November 20, 1956
Serial No. 623,296

Claims priority, application France December 6, 1955

1 Claim. (Cl. 260—397.4)

The present invention relates to 19-nortestosterone hexahydrobenzoate and to the method of preparing the same.

The importance of the angular methyl group at the 19-position of non-aromatic steroid hormones is well known. It is also known that the removal of this angular methyl group by aromatization of the A ring followed by partial reduction leads to substantial changes of the physiological activity of the products treated in this manner. For example, 19-nor-testosterone possesses a high anti-folliculin activity with a greatly reduced virilizing activity in comparison to that of testosterone. This important property permits the prolonged use of the compound in women, for example, in treating syndromes of hyperfolliculinaemia, without any danger of causing virilism.

Since 19-nor-testosterone is not as readily available as testosterone, it would be highly desirable to obtain a similarly active product which could be administered at smaller and more widely spaced doses so as to compensate for the difficulties in preparation by using proportionally less thereof. These applicants have found that 19-nor-testosterone hexahydrobenzoate fulfills these conditions, since it has not only a delayed action, but constitutes a product having particularly favorable properties.

It is, therefore, one object of the present invention to provide a method of producing 19-nor-testosterone hexahydrobenzoate.

This and other objects and advantages of this invention will appear more clearly from the herein following detailed description and from the claims.

The process of preparing 19-nor-testosterone hexahydrobenzoate according to the invention consists in reacting, in the presence of a suitable condensing agent, a hexahydrobenzoyl halide with a solution of 19-nor-testosterone and isolating the 19-nor-testosterone hexahydrobenzoate obtained in this manner by centrifuging or filtering.

A preferred method of carrying out the process of the invention consists in operating in a solvent which also acts as condensing agent. This permits to react a hexahydrobenzoyl halide with 19-nor-testosterone in the presence of a tertiary base such as pyridine, which acts by fixing the hydracide that develops. This operation is carried out at a temperature between 0° C. and the refluxing temperature of the solvent used, but preferably at about room temperature. Upon completion of the

2

reaction, the resulting product is extracted and washed to eliminate the condensing agent, and the 19-nor-testosterone hexahydrobenzoate is recovered by centrifuging, filtering or evaporating to dryness.

The 19-nor-testosterone used for the process of the invention may be prepared, for example, according to Wilds and Nelson (J. Am. Chem. Soc., 1953, 75, 5366), by reducing the 3-methyl ether of estradiol, followed by a hydrolysis of the resulting 3-methyl ether of 1,4-di-hydro 3,17β-estradiol.

The following example is presented to illustrate the present invention, without intent however to thereby limit the scope of the appended claims.

EXAMPLE

Preparation of 19-nor-testosterone hexahydrobenzoate

3 g. of 19-nor-testosterone prepared according to Wilds and Nelson (J. Am. Chem. Soc., 1953, 75, 5366) are dissolved in 30 cc. of anhydrous pyridine. 3 cc. of hexahydrobenzoyl chloride are added, and the solution is left undisturbed for sixteen hours at room temperature. The reaction mixture is taken up with 150 cc. of chloroform, washed with water, normal hydrochloric acid, sodium bicarbonate and again with water, and is then dried over magnesium sulfate and vacuum evaporated to dryness. The residue is taken up with 100 cc. of petroleum ether (boiling point: 40–50° C.) and the solution obtained in this manner is filtered, concentrated to a small volume and left in the refrigerator for three hours. After separation and drying in vacuo, 2.8 g. (67%) of 19-nor-testosterone hexahydrobenzoate are obtained, having a melting point of 88–89° C., $[\alpha]_D^{20}=+50°\pm5$ (c.=0.5%, chloroform). The mother liquor left after crystallization produces, upon refrigeration, another 0.95 g. (23%) of the product. This new 19-nor-testosterone hexahydrobenzoate appears in the form of small, elongated prisms that are insoluble in water, but are soluble in organic solvents.

Analysis: $C_{25}H_{36}O_3=384.5$—
    Calculated: 78.1% C; 9.4% H.
    Found: 77.9% C; 9.3% H.

We claim:

The process of producing 19-nor-testosterone hexahydrobenzoate consisting in dissolving 19-nor-testosterone in anhydrous pyridine, adding hexahydrobenzoylchloride at room temperature to the resulting solution, allowing the mixture to stand at room temperature until esterification is completed, extracting the reaction mixture with chloroform, washing the chloroform extract with water, N hydrochloric acid, sodium bicarbonate solution, and water, drying the washed extract, evaporating the extract to dryness in a vacuum, dissolving the evaporation residue in petroleum ether, filtering off undissolved, concentrating the solution by evaporation, allowing the highly concentrated solution to crystallize at refrigerator temperature, and filtering off the crystals of 19-nor-testosterone hexahydrobenzoate.

References Cited in the file of this patent

UNITED STATES PATENTS

2,785,189   Hicks ---------------- Mar. 12, 1957

1

2

2,891,974

SUBSTITUTED 2,5-ANDROSTADIENES

Percy L. Julian, Oak Park, and Helen C. Printy, Chicago,
Ill., assignors to The Julian Laboratories, Inc., Franklin
Park, Ill., a corporation of Illinois

No Drawing. Application March 13, 1958
Serial No. 721,101

12 Claims. (Cl. 260—397.4)

This invention relates to the preparation of a new series of anabolic steroids. More particularly, this invention relates to substituted 2,5-androstadienes, especially 17β-hydroxy-3-acyloxy-2,5-androstadien-4-one derivatives, and to the processes for making them.

The compounds of this invention have growth stimulating or tissue building activity (anabolic) with a minimum of virilizing (androgenic) or feminizing (estrogenic) activity. These 2,5-androstadienes, therefore, have a particularly favorable anabolic/androgenic ratio when compared to the standard drug in this field, testosterone. An additional feature of this invention is the preparation of these 2,5-androstadienes from easily obtainable starting materials.

The anabolic steroids of this invention are represented by the following general formula:

Formula I

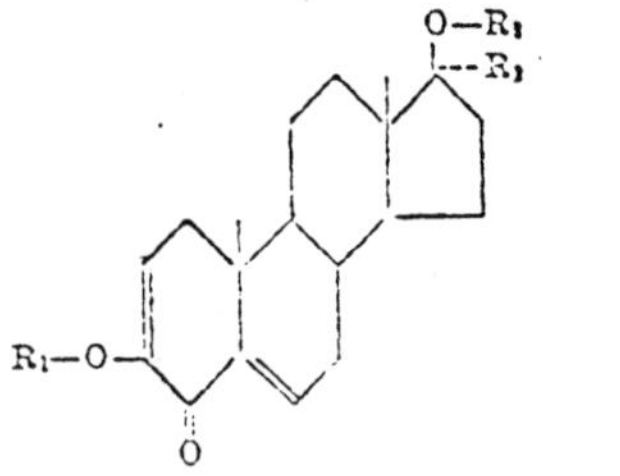

when:

R_1 represents an acyl moiety, for instance, formyl, a lower alkanoyl of from 2 to 6 carbons, benzoyl or hexahydrobenzoyl;

R_2 represents a hydrogen or an alkyl of 1 to 3 carbons; and

R_3 represents a hydrogen or an acyl moiety, for instance, a lower alkanoyl of from 2 to 6 carbons such as acetyl, benzoyl or hexahydrobenzoyl.

Preferred compounds are represented by Formula I when R_1 represents acetyl or formyl, R_2 represents a hydrogen or α-methyl and R_3 represents a hydrogen or acetyl.

In practice, R_1 and R_3 may represent any acyl derivatives which possess activity as such or upon hydrolysis to the active hydroxylated compound in vivo. Illustrative of such acyl derivatives are oleate, palmitate, isobutyrate, stearate, benzoate, hemiphthalate, nicotinate, β-naphthoate, glycolate, cyclopentylpropionate, phenylacetate, hemimaleate and hemisuccinate. Of course the acyl moiety must be one which is derived from a nontoxic, stable and pharmaceutically acceptable acid.

The compounds of this invention are prepared by shifting the 3-keto-Δ⁴ unsaturated system of the corresponding testosterone derivative of the novel 4-keto-Δ⁵ system of Formula I. For example, the testosterone derivative is dibrominated at the 2 and 6 positions with two moles of bromine in inert solvent such as ether, methylene chloride or acetic acid at ice bath temperature, from about —5 to 10° C., usually with a trace of hydrogen

bromide. The resulting 2,6-dibrominated testosterone then serves as starting material in the novel process which also is an object of this invention:

Formula II

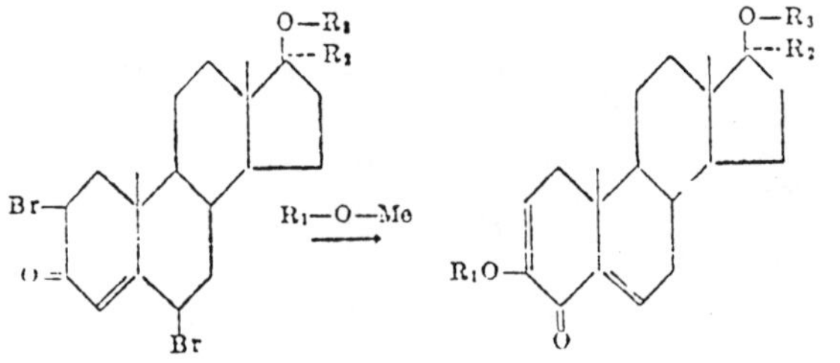

The dibromo derivative of Formula II in which R_1, R_2 and R_3 are as previously described, is purified or used as a crude mixture isolated from the bromination reaction.

The rearrangement of the unsaturated system is accomplished by reacting the brominated derivative with an excess of an alkaline salt of a lower aliphatic acid in a low boiling solvent in which the ingredients are at least partially soluble. The acid salt is preferably an alkali metal salt, advantageously sodium or potassium, of a lower aliphatic acid of from 1 to 8 carbons. In practice, a wide range of acid salts may be used, for instance, those with benzoate, hexahydrobenzoate, oleate or palmitate anions or those with lithium, calcium or magnesium cations.

As a convenience, a large excess of the metal salt ingredient is used, such as 1 to 5 times by weight of the dibromo derivative. The metal salt can be used in as little as two molar equivalents but advantageous results are obtained by using a large excess of the acid salt. The medium for the reaction is usually a low boiling solvent, in which the reactants are partially soluble, such as low boiling alcohols, ketones, chlorinated hydrocarbons or mixtures thereof. Exemplary of the solvents used are those boiling below about 120° C., such as methyl ethyl ketone, methanol, propanol, isobutanol, isopropanol, butanol, methylene chloride or mixtures thereof. Preferred are anhydrous ethanol, acetone and methyl ethyl ketone.

The reaction is run advantageously at the boiling point of the solvent employed. The temperature is not, however, allowed to go above the thermal decomposition point of the dibromo starting material and may be run at room temperature, i.e. 25° C. The reaction is advantageously run as a slurry with stirring at the boiling point of the solvent. The time for substantially complete rearrangement varies with the reaction conditions as well as with the structures of the dibromo intermediates but is normally from about 1 to about 18 hours at reflux temperature.

The novel compounds of this invention are isolated by concentrating the reaction mixture, dissolving the metal salts by washing with water and extracting into a water-immiscible solvent, such as ether or methylene chloride. The organic extracts are washed with water, dried and concentrated to give the desired product.

The rearrangement is preferably run on the 17-acyl derivatives with retention of the 17-acyl group, however, the 17-ol analogue is rearranged with equally good yields and may be 17-acylated by conventional reactions thereafter.

The following examples will serve to illustrate the preparation of the novel compounds as well as variations of the processes of this invention. The scope of this invention is not to be limited by these examples since it will be obvious to one skilled in the art that these ex-

3

amples are merely illustrative of this invention and that modifications thereof are possible.

Example 1

A solution of 3.3 g. (0.01 mole) of testosterone acetate in 110 ml. of anhydrous ether is cooled in an ice bath to 0–2° C. Two drops of 30% HBr in acetic acid are added, followed by a solution of 3.2 g. (0.02 mole) of bromine in 25 ml. of acetic acid, added over a seven minute period. The colorless brominated solution is kept at 0–2° C. for an additional ten minutes, then is concentrated in vacuo with gentle warming to a volume of 20 ml. The voluminous white crystalline precipitate, which is obtained, is filtered, washed with cold ethanol, and dried at room temperature. A first crop of 2,6-dibromotestosterone acetate, M.P. 170–172° C. is obtained.

A suspension of 1.0 g. of the dibromide and 4.0 g. of dry potassium acetate in 40 ml. of distilled acetone is stirred and refluxed for one hour. The reaction mixture is concentrated to a thick slush, water added to dissolve the potassium salts, and the organic material extracted with methylene chloride. The methylene chloride is washed with water and concentrated to a solid, halogen-free crystalline mass. The residue crystallized from ether in glistening prisms gives 3,17β-diacetoxy-2,5-androstadien-4-one, M.P. 173–174° C., [α]$_D^{22}$—11.9° (ethanol).

Example 2

One gram of 2,6-dibromotestosterone acetate (Example 1) is stirred and refluxed with 4.0 g. of fused potassium acetate and 25 ml. of anhydrous ethanol for four hours. Concentration to a slush, addition of water and filtration of the insoluble residue gives 3,17β-diacetoxy-2,5-androstadien-4-one, M.P. 169–173° C.

Example 3

A solution of 3.3 g. of testosterone acetate in 33 ml. of methylene chloride is brominated at 10° C. with 3.2 g. of bromine in 20 ml. of methylene chloride. The brominated solution is concentrated in vacuo with gentle heating, and the total residue refluxed with 15.0 g. of sodium acetate in 150 ml. of acetone for 12 hours. Working up as described in Example 1, the reaction mixture gives 3,17β-diacetoxy-2,5-androstadien-4-one.

Example 4

Testosterone (2.88 g., 0.01 mole) is dissolved in 200 ml. of anhydrous ether and brominated with 3.2 g. (0.02 mole) of bromine in 20 ml. of acetic acid. The ethereal bromination solution is washed with 5% sodium bicarbonate solution to remove acids, dried over sodium sulfate, and concentrated in vacuo to dryness. The residue is stirred and refluxed for 15 hours with 15 g. of potassium acetate in 150 ml. of methyl ethyl ketone. The reaction is worked up as in Example 1 to give 3-acetoxy-17β-hydroxy-2,5-androstadien-4-one, M.P. 128–134° C.

A solution of 500 mg. of this product in 10 ml. of pyridine is reacted with 250 mg. of benzoyl chloride. Quenching in water and extracting with ether gives 3-acetoxy-17β-benzoyloxy-2,5-androstadien-4-one.

Example 5

A mixture of 9.2 g. of 2,6-dibromotestosterone acetate, 35 g. of potassium formate and 350 ml. of acetone is stirred and refluxed for 15 hours. The reaction is worked up as described in Example 1, to give 3-formoxy-17β-acetoxy-2,5-androstadien-4-one, M.P. 195–205° C.

Example 6

A solution of 3.46 g. of 17α-methyltestosterone acetate in 35 ml. of methylene chloride is converted to the 2,6-dibromide by treatment with 3.2 g. of bromine in 20 ml. of methylene chloride. The methylene chloride solution

4

is washed with 5% sodium bicarbonate solution to remove acid and concentrated to dryness. The total brominated product is refluxed for three hours with 12.0 g. of potassium acetate in 120 ml. of acetone. The reaction mixture is worked up as described in Example 1 to give a residue which yields, upon crystallization from acetone, 3,17β-diacetoxy-17α-methyl - 2,5 - androstadien - 4 - one, M.P. 170–176° C.

Example 7

Fifteen grams of 2,6-dibromo-17α-methyltestosterone is stirred and refluxed for 15 hours with 60.0 g. of fused potassium acetate and 150 ml. of acetone. The reaction is worked up as described in Example 2. Crystallization of the product from acetone gives 3-acetoxy-17β-hydroxy-17α-methyl-2,5-androstadien-4 - one, M.P. 190–194° C.

Example 8

A solution of 5.6 g. of testosterone stearate in 50 ml. of methylene chloride is converted to the dibromo derivative with 1.6 g. of bromine in 25 ml. of methylene chloride. After reaction at reflux with 10.0 g. of potassium acetate in 150 ml. of acetone-ethanol mixture for five hours as in Example 6, a solid product 3-acetoxy-17β-stearoyloxy-2,5-androstadien-4-one, is obtained.

Example 9

A solution of 3.6 g. of 17α-ethyltestosterone acetate in 45 ml. of methylene chloride is reacted with 1.6 g. of bromine. The resulting dibromo derivative is purified and reacted with 12.0 g. of sodium acetate in 150 ml. of acetone at reflux for two hours. The reaction mixture is worked up as in Example 1 to give 17α-ethyl-3,17β-diacetoxy-2,5-androstadien-4-one.

Example 10

A solution of 3.9 g. of testosterone isocaproate in 75 ml. of methylene chloride is reacted with 1.6 g. of bromine in 25 ml. of methylene chloride. The dibromo derivative is then heated at reflux in 75 ml. of methyl ethyl ketone with 10.0 g. of sodium isocaproate for three hours. After working up the reaction mixture as in Example 1, the product, 3,17β-di-isocaproyloxy-2,5-androstadien-4-one, is obtained.

Example 11

A suspension of 1.0 g. of 2,6-dibromotestosterone acetate and 5.0 g. of sodium benzoate in 50 ml. of acetone is heated at reflux with stirring for two hours. The reaction mixture is quenched in water and worked up as in Example 1, to give 17β-acetoxy-3-benzoyloxy-2,5-androstadien-4-one.

What is claimed is:

1. A chemical compound having the following formula:

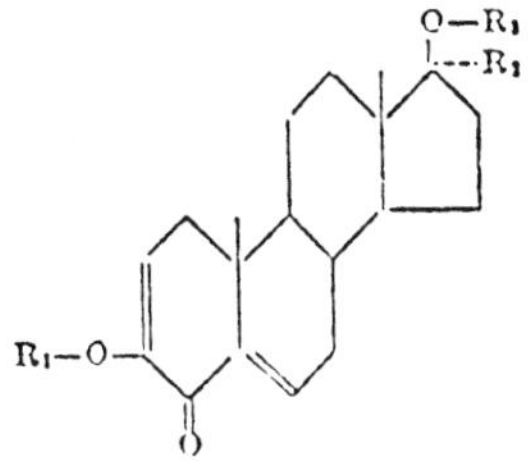

in which R$_1$ is acyl derived from a nontoxic, stable and pharmaceutically acceptable acid; R$_2$ is a member selected from the group consisting of hydrogen and lower alkyl; and R$_3$ is a member selected from the group consisting of hydrogen and acyl derived from a nontoxic, stable and pharmaceutically acceptable acid.

5

2. The method of forming compounds having the following formula:

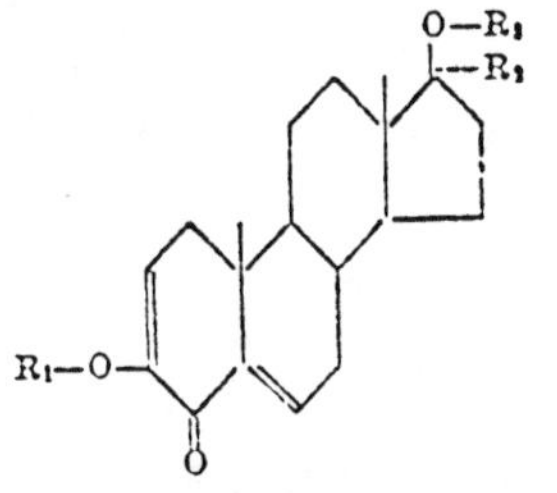

in which R_1 is acyl derived from a nontoxic, stable and pharmaceutically acceptable acid; R_2 is a member selected from the group consisting of hydrogen and lower alkyl; and R_3 is a member selected from the group consisting of hydrogen and acyl derived from a nontoxic, stable and pharmaceutically acceptable acid, which comprises reacting with at least two molar equivalents of the alkali metal salt of a carboxylic acid in a solvent of boiling point less than about 120° C. in which the reactants have substantial solubility at from about 25° C. to about 120° C. a compound having the following formula:

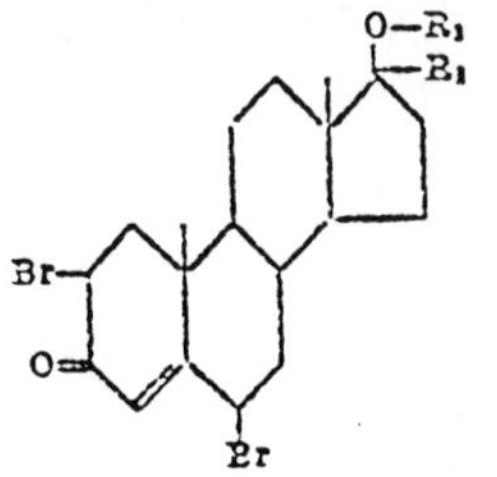

in which R_2 is a member selected from the group consisting of hydrogen and lower alkyl and R_3 is a member selected from the group consisting of hydrogen and acyl derived from a nontoxic, stable and pharmaceutically acceptable acid.

3. The method of claim 2 characterized in that the reaction is run at the boiling point of the solvent.

6

4. The method of claim 2 characterized in that the carboxylic acid is a lower aliphatic acid of from 1 to 8 carbons.

5. The method of claim 2 characterized in that a large excess of the alkali metal salt reactant is used.

6. A chemical compound having the following formula:

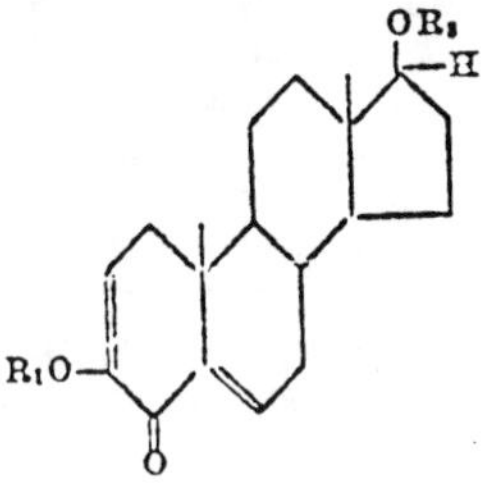

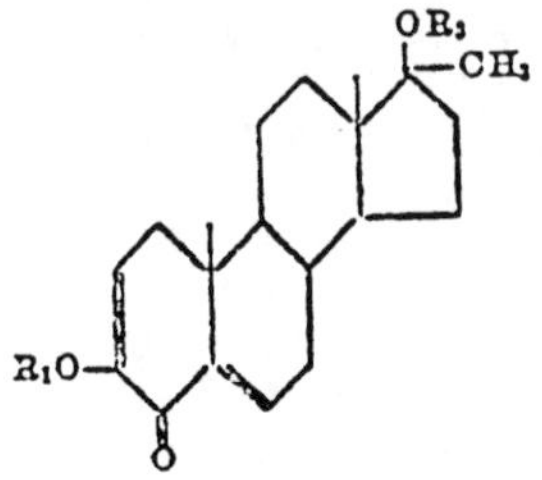

in which R_1 and R_3 are lower alkanoyl moieties of from 2 to 6 carbons.

7. A chemical compound having the following formula:

in which R_1 and R_2 are lower alkanoyl moieties of from 2 to 6 carbons.

8. 3,17β-diacetoxy-2,5-androstadien-4-one.

9. 3-formoxy-17β-acetoxy-2,5-androstadien-4-one.

10. 3,17β-diacetoxy-17α-methyl-2,5-androstadien-4-one.

11. 17α-ethyl-3,17β-diacetoxy-2,5-androstadien-4-one.

12. 3-acetoxy-17β-hydroxy-2,5-androstadien-4-one.

No references cited.

CHAPTER TEN

1

2

2,721,871

17-ALKYL DERIVATIVES OF 19-NORTESTOS-TERONE

Frank B. Colton, Chicago, Ill., assignor to G. D. Searle & Co., Chicago, Ill., a corporation of Illinois

No Drawing. Application September 13, 1954,
Serial No. 455,751

4 Claims. (Cl. 260—397.4)

The present invention relates to a new group of hypotensive and anabolic agents with low androgenic activity and, more particularly, to 19-nortestosterone derivatives substituted in the 17-position by a lower alkyl radical containing 2–8 carbon atoms.

These compounds can be represented by the general structural formula

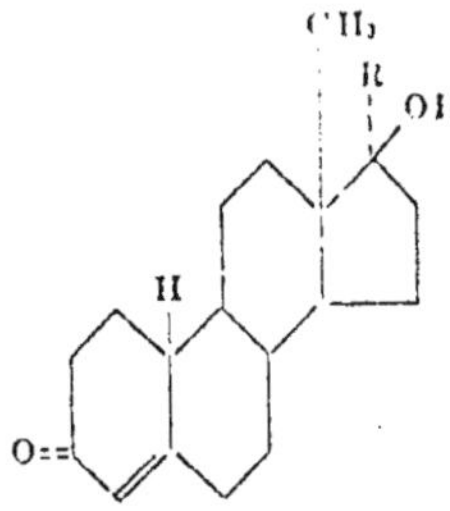

wherein R is a lower alkyl radical containing 2–8 carbon atoms such as ethyl, straight and branched propyl, butyl, pentyl, hexyl, heptyl, and octyl.

The compounds of my invention are valuable anabolic agents, i. e. they promote nitrogen retention. They produce this effect at a dosage which causes only a very low degree of androgenic activity. It is well known that testosterone propionate is an effective anabolic agent but its clinical utility for that purpose is greatly limited because in many patients the androgenic effects are undesirable. In the case of the claimed compounds the effective anabolic doses are so small that prolonged administration becomes practical without undesirable side effects.

Another important field of utility of these compounds is their anti-hypertensive effect, an effect which is not shared by 19-nortestosterone or its 17-methyl derivative. The compounds of this invention are particularly effective in overcoming the hypertension produced by the mineralocorticoid hormone desoxycorticosterone.

These compounds are conveniently obtained by the treatment of the methyl ether of esterone with an organo-metallic compound of the type RLi or RMgBr (R being a lower alkyl group as defined hereinabove) and a Birch type reduction of the 3-methoxy-17α-alkyl-1,3,5-estratrien-17-ol thus formed.

An alternative source for the preparation of the 17-ethyl-19-nortestosterone is the 3-methoxy-13-methyl-17α - ethynyl - 1,4,6,7,8,9,11,12,13,14,16,17-dodecahydro-15H-cyclopenta[a]phenanthren-17-ol of my U. S. Patent No. 2,691,028, issued October 5, 1954, which is converted by treatment with hydrochloric acid in aqueous methanol to 17α-ethynyl-19-nortestosterone; the latter is then hydrogenated over a noble metal catalyst to reduce the ethynyl to an ethyl group. An alternative procedure is also available for the preparation of the 17-propyl derivative. The methyl ether of estrone is treated with allyl magnesium bromide and successive hydrogenation of the allyl group in the presence of a noble metal catalyst and of the aromatic ring by the Birch process, followed by

treatment with hydrochloric acid in aqueous methanol yields 17-propyl-19-nortestosterone.

The compounds which constitute my invention and the methods for their preparation will appear more fully from the consideration of the following examples which are given for the purpose of illustration only and are not to be construed as limiting the invention in spirit or in scope. In these examples quantities are indicated in parts by weight.

Example 1

To a refluxing solution of 47.5 parts of 3-methoxy-13-methyl - 17α-ethynyl-1,4,6,7,8,9,11,12,13,14,16,17-dodecahydro-15H-cyclopenta[a]phenanthren-17-ol in 3200 parts of methanol and 1000 parts of water are added 240 parts of concentrated hydrochloric acid. Refluxing is continued for an additional 5 minutes after which the solution is maintained at room temperature for 15 minutes. Then 13,000 parts of water are added and the mixture is cooled to 0° C. After standing for several hours at that temperature, the mixture is filtered and the precipitate is dried and crystallized from ethyl acetate. The 17-ethynyl-19-nortestosterone thus obtained melts at about 202–204° C.

Through a mixture of 11 parts of charcoal containing 5% palladium and 2000 parts of dioxane a stream of hydrogen is passed for 60 minutes. Then 86 parts of 17-ethynyl-19-nortestosterone in 1500 parts of dioxane are added and the mixture is hydrogenated until 2 moles of hydrogen are absorbed. The catalyst is then removed by filtration and the solvent is evaporated under vacuum. The crystalline residue is dissolved in 2700 parts of benzene and thus applied to a chromatography column containing 5000 parts of silica gel. The column is washed with 2700 parts of benzene, 4500 parts of a 10% solution of ethyl acetate in benzene and 27,000 parts of a 20% solution of ethyl acetate in benzene and is then eluted with 30,000 parts of a 30% solution of ethyl acetate in benzene. The resulting eluate is concentrated under vacuum and the residue is recrystallized from methanol and dried to constant weight at 75° C. The 17-ethyl-19-nortestosterone thus obtained melts at about 140–141° C. Its ultraviolet absorption spectrum shows a maximum at 240 millimicrons with a molecular extinction coefficient of 16,500.

Example 2

To a stirred mixture of 8.5 parts of magnesium in 140 parts of ether there are added 5 parts of allyl bromide in 15 parts of ether. Then, in the course of 45 minutes, a mixture of 20 parts of the methyl ether of esterone and 95 parts of allyl bromide in 630 parts of ether are added. After 3 hours of refluxing the mixture is cooled to 0° C., washed repeatedly with 10% ammonium chloride solution and then with water, dried over anhydrous sodium sulfate, filtered and evaporated. The residue is taken up in ether. The ether solution is partially concentrated and diluted with petroleum ether. The crystalline 17α-allyl-3-methoxy-1,3,5(10)-estratrien-17-ol thus obtained melts at about 91–91.5° C.

A mixture of 11.5 parts of 17α-allyl-3-methoxy-1,3,5-(10)-estratrien-17-ol, 3 parts of charcoal containing 5% palladium and 160 parts of ethanol is hydrogenated until one mole of hydrogen has been absorbed. The mixture is then filtered through filter aid and the filtrate is evaporated under vacuum. The residue is crystallized from a mixture of ether and methanol to yield 17α-propyl-3-methoxy-1,3,5(10)-estratrien-17-ol melting at about 93–94° C.

To a stirred mixture of 6 parts of 17α-propyl-3-methoxy-1,3,5(10)-estratrien-17-ol in 500 parts of ammonia and 140 parts of ether, 7 parts of lithium are added in the course of 20 minutes. The mixture is stirred for 30 minutes after which 46 parts of ethanol are added dropwise in the course of an hour. Stirring is continued until all of the ammonia has disappeared. Then water is added and the ether layer is separated, washed with water, dried over anhydrous sodium sulfate, filtered and evaporated. Crystallization from a mixture of ether in methanol yields 17α-propyl-3-methoxy-2,5(10)-estradien-17-ol melting at about 150–152° C.

A mixture of 18 parts of 17α-propyl-3-methoxy-2,5-(10)-estradien-17-ol, 320 parts of methanol, 80 parts of water, and 18 parts of concentrated hydrochloric acid is refluxed for 5 minutes and then permitted to stand for 15 minutes in hot water. A sufficient amount of hot water is added until the mixture becomes turbid. Upon standing 17-propyl-19-nortestosterone precipitates which, crystallized from a mixture of acetone and petroleum ether, melts at 120–122° C.

Example 3

To a stirred suspension of 16.5 parts of the methyl ether of estrone in 300 parts of ether there is added a solution of butyl lithium prepared from 115 parts of 1-bromobutane and 6.7 parts of lithium in 600 parts of ether. Stirring is continued for an hour after which the mixture is decomposed with methanol and dilute sulfuric acid and extracted with ether. This extract is washed with saturated sodium chloride solution, dried over anhydrous sodium sulfate, filtered and evaporated under nitrogen. The residue is crystallized from methanol and water and then applied in benzene solution to a chromatography column containing 1000 parts of alumina. The column is washed with 1800 parts of a 10% solution of petroleum ether in benzene and then eluted with 9000 parts of a 10% solution of petroleum ether in benzene. This eluate is evaporated and the residue is recrystallized from aqueous methanol to yield 3-methoxy-17α-butyl-1,3,5(10)-estratrien-17β-ol.

To a solution of 37.2 parts of this compound in 500 parts of ether and 500 parts of liquid ammonia are added 3.5 parts of short strips of lithium wire with stirring. The dark blue solution is stirred for 10 minutes after which 32 parts of methanol are added dropwise in the course of 15 minutes to decolorize the solution. Then 56 additional parts of methanol are slowly added and, after most of the ammonia has been evaporated, 1100 parts of ether and 700 parts of water are added with stirring. The organic layer is separated, washed with saturated sodium chloride solution, dried over sodium sulfate, filtered and concentrated under vacuum. To the oily residue are added 1110 parts of methanol and 500 parts of water and the mixture is heated to reflux. Then 240 parts of concentrated hydrochloric acid are added and refluxing is continued for 6 minutes. The mixture is then extracted

with ether. The ether solution is washed with a saturated solution of sodium chloride, dried over sodium sulfate, filtered and evaporated under vacuum. The residue is applied in benzene to a chromatography column containing 350 parts of silica gel. The column is washed with 500 parts of benzene and then with 3000 parts of a 10% solution of ethyl acetate in benzene. Elution with 2000 parts of a 20% solution of ethyl acetate in benzene, concentration of the eluate and crystallization from aqueous methanol then yields 17-butyl-19-nortestosterone which melts at about 127–128° C.

Example 4

Substitution of an equivalent amount of 1-bromooctane for the 1-bromobutane in the process of the preceding example yields 17-octyl-19-nortestosterone. The infrared absorption spectrum of that compound shows maxima at 2.8 and 6.05 microns. The ultraviolet absorption spectrum shows a maximum at 240.5 millimicrons with a molecular extinction coefficient of 17,000.

I claim:

1. A compound of the structural formula

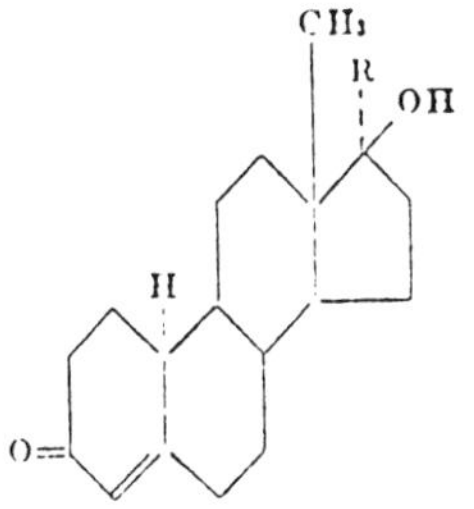

wherein R is a lower alkyl radical containing 2–8 carbon atoms.

2. 17-ethyl-19-nortestosterone.

3. 17-propyl-19-nortestosterone.

4. 17-butyl-19-nortestosterone.

References Cited in the file of this patent

UNITED STATES PATENTS

2,308,835	Ruzicka	Jan. 19, 1943
2,374,369	Miescher	Apr. 24, 1945
2,698,855	Hicks	Jan. 4, 1955

FOREIGN PATENTS

| 211,488 | Switzerland | Dec. 2, 1940 |
| 211,653 | Switzerland | Jan. 16, 1941 |

OTHER REFERENCES

Jones et al.: Jour. Am. Chem. Soc., 72, 956–61 (1950).
Birch: Jour. Chem. Soc. 1950, 367–68.

CHAPTER ELEVEN

1

3,128,283
17-OXYGENATED OXA-STEROIDS AND
INTERMEDIATES THERETO
Raphael Pappo, Skokie, Ill., assignor to G. D. Searle &
Co., Chicago, Ill., a corporation of Delaware
No Drawing.   Filed Dec. 11, 1961, Ser. No. 158,577
Claims priority, application Mexico May 10, 1961
20 Claims.   (Cl. 260—343.2)

The present invention is concerned with novel steroidal lactones and, more particularly, with 17-oxygenated androstane and estrane derivatives in which the A ring contains a lactone structure. These lactones can be represented by the structural formula

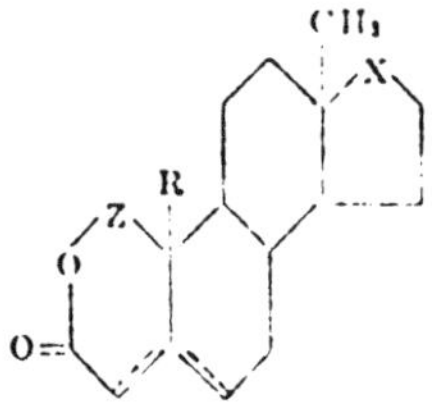

in which R can be hydrogen or a methyl radical, Z can be a

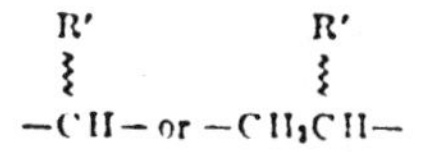

radical, wherein R' is hydrogen or a lower alkyl radical attached to the carbon atom adjacent to the oxygen atom, and the wavy line indicates the alternative α or β stereochemical configuration, X is a carbonyl, β-hydroxymethylene, β-(lower alkanoyl)-oxymethylene, α-(lower alkyl)-β-hydroxymethylene, or α-(lower alkyl)-β-(lower alkanoyl)oxymethylene radical, and the dotted lines indicate the optional presence of a 4,5 or 5,6 double bond.

The lower alkyl radicals included in the foregoing structural representation are exemplified by methyl, ethyl, propyl, butyl, pentyl, hexyl, and the branched-chain isomers thereof. Lower alkanoyl radicals comprehended in the X term of that formula are, for example, formyl, acetyl, propionyl, butyryl, valeryl, caproyl, and the branched-chain radicals isomeric therewith.

This application is a continuation-in-part of my copending application, Serial No. 29,594, filed May 17, 1960, now abandoned.

A preferred object of this invention is to provide compounds of the structural formula

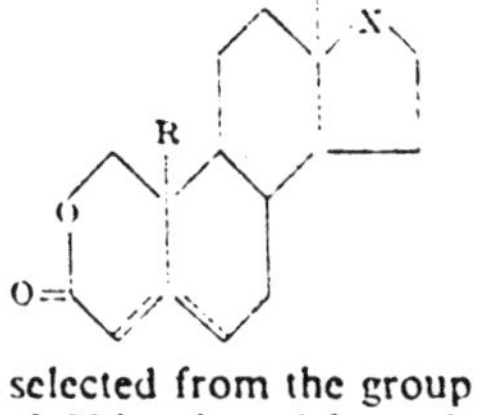

wherein R is selected from the group consisting of hydrogen and methyl, X is selected from the group consisting of carbonyl, β-hydroxymethylene, β-(lower alkanoyl)oxymethylene, α-(lower alkyl)-β-hydroxymethylene, and α-(lower alkyl)-β-(lower alkanoyl)oxymethylene, and the dotted lines indicate the optional presence of a 4,5 or 5,6 double bond.

A further object of this invention is to provide com-

2

pounds of the structural formula

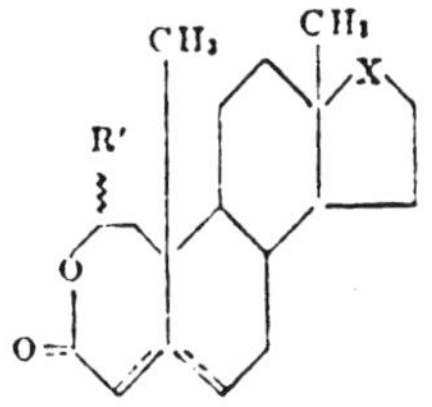

wherein X, R', and the dotted lines have the identical meanings defined supra.

A further object of this invention is to provide compounds of the structural formula

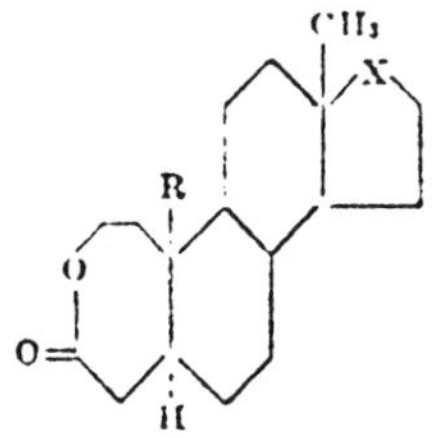

wherein R and X have the identical meanings described supra.

A further object of this invention is to provide compounds of the structural formula

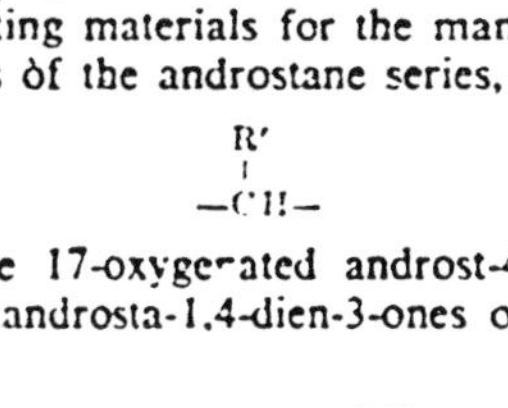

wherein X and the dotted lines have the identical meanings defined supra.

Suitable starting materials for the manufacture of the instant lactones of the androstane series, wherein Z is a

radical, are the 17-oxygenated androst-4-en-3-ones and 17-oxygenated androsta-1,4-dien-3-ones of the structural formula

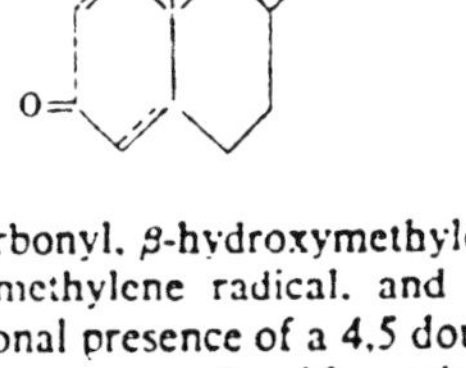

wherein X is a carbonyl, β-hydroxymethylene, or α-(lower alkyl)-β-hydroxymethylene radical, and the dotted line indicates the optional presence of a 4,5 double bond. Reaction of the latter compounds with a mixture of osmium tetroxide and lead tetracetate results in cleavage of the 1,2-double bond to produce the 1,2-seco-A-nor compounds of the structural formula

Instead of lead tetracetate, other similar reagents such as sodium periodate or potassium chlorate can be used. The latter process is preferably conducted in an aqueous medium containing a water-miscible alkanoic acid such as acetic, propionic, butyric, isobutyric, valeric, or isovaleric. Reaction temperatures of 0–80° and reaction times of ½–48 hours are satisfactory for this process, although the preferred ranges are 15–35° and 2–24 hours. The reaction times and temperatures are, of course, interdependent so that a higher operating temperature will, in general, result in a shorter reaction time.

Specific examples of the aforementioned novel process are the reaction of 5α-androst-1-ene-3,17-dione, 17β-hydroxy-17α-methyl-5α-androst-1-en-3-one, or 17β-hydroxy-17α-methylandrosta-1,4-dien-3-one in aqueous acetic acid with osmium tetroxide and lead tetracetate to afford 1,17-dioxo-1,2-seco-A-nor-5α-androstan-2-oic acid, 17β-hydroxy - 17α-methyl-1-oxo-1,2-seco-A-nor-5α-androstan-2-oic acid, and 17β-hydroxy-17α-methyl-1-oxo-1,2-seco-A-norandrost-3-en-2-oic acid, respectively.

The novel intermediate 1,2-seco-A-nor compounds are converted to the corresponding instant lactones by reaction with a suitable reducing agent. Typically, the aforementioned 17β-hydroxy-17α-methyl-1-oxo-1,2-seco-A-nor-5α-androstan-2-oic acid and 17β-hydroxy-17α-methyl-1-oxo-1,2-seco-A-norandrost-3-en-2-oic acid are converted to 17β-hydroxy-17α-methyl-2-oxa-5α-androstan-3-one and 17β-hydroxy-17α-methyl-2-oxaandrost-4-en-3-one, respectively, by reduction with sodium borohydride in aqueous sodium hydroxide.

The aforementioned 1,2-seco-A-nor intermediates are converted to the instant 1-alkyl lactones by reaction with the appropriate alkyl organometallic reagent. For example, the instant 17β-hydroxy-17α-methyl-1-oxo-1,2-seco-A-nor-5α-androstan-2-oic acid is allowed to react with ethereal methyl magnesium bromide in tetrahydrofuran, and the resulting adduct is treated with aqueous hydrochloric acid to yield a mixture of the 1α-methyl and 1β-methyl isomers of 17β-hydroxy-1,17α-dimethyl-2-oxa-5α-androstan-3-one, which are separable by virtue of the difference in ease of lactonization of the corresponding hydroxy acids.

The instant lactones of the 5α-estrane series are produced by processes analogous to those aforementioned, utilizing as starting materials 17-oxygenated 5α-estr-1-en-3-ones of the structural formula

Typically, 17β-hydroxy-17α-methyl-5α-estr-1-en-3-one is treated with osmium tetroxide and lead tetracetate in aqueous acetic acid to yield 17β-hydroxy-17α-methyl-1-oxo-1,2-seco-A-nor-5α-estran-2-oic acid, which is reduced with sodium borohydride in aqueous sodium hydroxide to produce 17β-hydroxy-17α-methyl-2-oxa-5α-estran-3-one.

The instant lactones of the estr-4-ene and estr-5-ene series are manufactured by a sequence of reactions utilizing as the starting material, 6β-19-epoxy-5α-androstane-3β,

17β-diol 3,17-diacetate, the preparation of which is described by Bowers et al., Chem. and Ind., 1299 (1960). Hydrolysis of this diester in methanol with aqueous sodium hydroxide followed by chromic acid oxidation of the diol results in 6β,19-epoxy-5α-androstane-3-17-dione. Bromination in tetrahydrofuran followed by dehydrobromination by heating with magnesium oxide in dimethylformamide affords 6β,19-epoxy-5α-androst-1-ene-3,17-dione. Chromic acid oxidation followed by treatment of the resulting 6β-hydroxy-10β-carboxy lactone with aqueous potassium carbonate in methanol followed by acetylation with acetic anhydride in pyridine results in 6β-hydroxy-5α-estr-1-ene-3,17-dione 6-acetate. Reaction of the latter substance with osmium tetroxide and lead tetracetate in aqueous acetic acid produces 6β-hydroxy-1,17-dioxo-1,2-seco-A-nor-5α-estran-2-oic acid 6-acetate. Reduction of this substance with aqueous sodium borohydride followed by chromic acid oxidation yields 6β-hydroxy-2-oxa-5α-estrane-3,17-dione 6-acetate. The latter substance is treated with aqueous alkali to afford the corresponding 6β-ol, which is dehydrated, suitably by heating with phosphorus oxychloride in pyridine or, alternatively, by conversion to the methanesulfonate followed by heating in pyridine, to afford 2-oxaestr-4-ene-3,17-dione. Treatment of this diketone with sodium borohydride and aqueous sodium hydroxide followed by acidification with dilute aqueous hydrochloric acid results in 17β-hydroxy-2-oxaestr-4-en-3-one. The corresponding 17α-alkyl-17β-hydroxy lactones are obtained by treating the aforementioned 6β,19-epoxy-5α-androstane-3,17-dione with methanol in the presence of p-toluenesulfonic acid to yield the corresponding 3-dimethyl ketal, which is treated with an alkyl Grignard reagent, then with aqueous hydrochloric acid to afford a 17α-alkyl-17β-hydroxy-6β,19-epoxy-5α-androstan-3-one. The latter substances are subjected to the aforementioned processes to afford the instant 17α-alkyl-17β-hydroxy lactones of the estr-4-ene series. By those processes, for example, 6β-19-epoxy-17β-hydroxy-17α-methyl-5α-androstan-3-one is converted to 17β-hydroxy-17α-methyl-2-oxaestr-4-en-3-one.

The A-ring saturated lactones of this invention, wherein Z is an ethylene group, are obtained by a process utilizing as starting materials compounds of the structural formula

wherein R is hydrogen or a methyl radical, X is β-hydroxymethylene or α-(lower alkyl)-β-hydroxymethylene. Reaction of these substances with isopropenyl acetate affords the corresponding 3-enol acetate, which is treated with ozone, then with zinc dust and finally with sodium hydroxide to afford the intermediate 17-oxygenated-2-oxo-2,3-seco-3-oic acids. Reduction with sodium borohydride in aqueous sodium hydroxide affords the corresponding 2-hydroxy-3-oic acid, which is cyclized by heating at an elevated temperature in a suitable inert solvent to afford the instant 3-oxa-4-ones. These processes are exemplified by the reaction of 17β-hydroxy-17α-methyl-5α-androstan-3-one with isopropenyl acetate and p-toluenesulfonic acid to afford 17α-methyl-5α-androst-2-ene-3,17β-diol 3,17-diacetate. Treatment of this enol acetate with ozone, zinc dust and finally with sodium hydroxide affords 17β-hydroxy-17α-methyl-2-oxo-2,3-seco-5α-androstan-3-oic acid 17-acetate. Reduction with sodium borohydride in aqueous sodium hydroxide produces 2,17β-dihydroxy-17α-methyl-2,3-seco-5α-androstan-3-oic acid, and cyclization of this hydroxy acid by refluxing in tertiary-butylbenzene

5

results in the instant 17β-hydroxy-17α-methyl-3-oxa-A-homo-5α-androstan-4-one.

The compounds of this invention, wherein Z is a

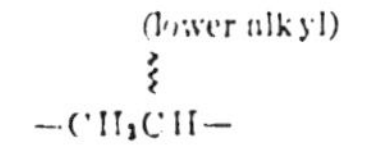

$$\overset{\text{(lower alkyl)}}{\underset{\;}{-CH_2CH-}}$$

radical are obtained by subjecting starting materials of the structural formula

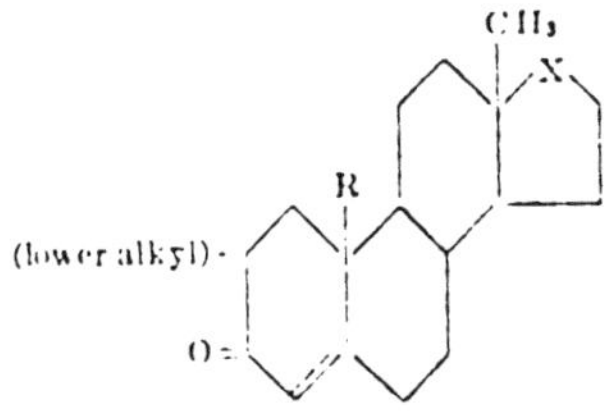

wherein R, X, and the dotted line have the identical meanings defined supra, to treatment with a peracid. The resulting lactones are converted to the corresponding hydroxy-acid by heating with aqueous alkali, followed by acidification. Typically, 17β-hydroxy-2α,17α-dimethyl-5α-androstan-3-one in methylene chloride is treated with peracetic acid in the presence of sodium acetate to afford 17β - hydroxy-2α,17α-dimethyl-3-oxa-A-homo-5α-androstan-4-one. Heating this lactone in methanol with aqueous sodium hydroxide, followed by acidification with dilute hydrochloric acid results in 2β,17β-dihydroxy-2α,17α-dimethyl-2,3-seco-5α-androstan-3-oic acid.

A preferred procedure for the manufacture of the instant compounds of the structural formula

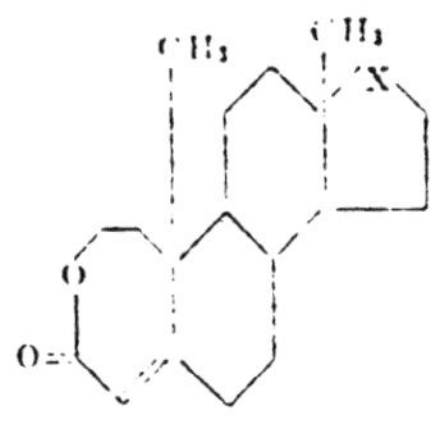

involves reaction of starting materials of the structural formula

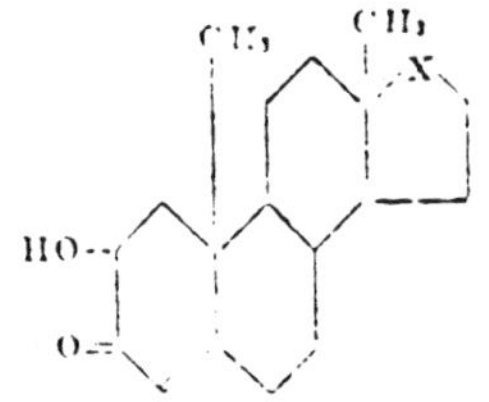

the preparations of which are described by J. S. Baran, J.A.C.S., 80, 1687 (1958), with an oxidizing agent such as lead tetraacetate or periodic acid to afford the corresponding 2-oxo-2,3-seco-androst-4-en-3-oic acids. These 2-oxo-3-oic acids are reduced to the corresponding 2-hydroxy-3-oic acids, which are converted to the instant 3-oxaandrost-4a-en-4-ones by refluxing in an inert solvent. For example, 2α,17β-dihydroxy-17α-methylandrost-4-en-3-one in aqueous acetic acid is treated with lead tetraacetate to afford 17β - hydroxy-17α-methyl-2-oxo-2,3-seco-androst-4-en-3-oic acid. Reduction with sodium borohydride yields 2,17β-dihydroxy-17α-methyl-2,3-seco-androst-4-en-3-oic acid, which is cyclized by heating in benzene to produce 17β-hydroxy-17α-methyl-3-oxa-A-homo-androst-4a-en-4-one.

The instant compounds of the structural formula

6

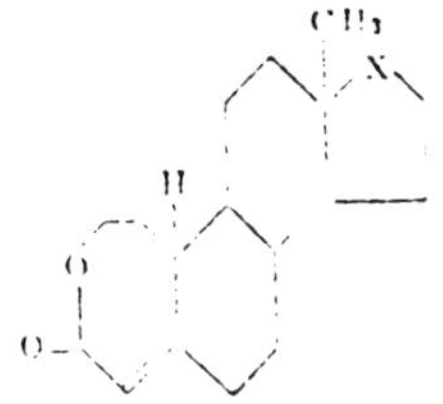

can be manufactured from the corresponding aforementioned 6β-acetoxy-19-nor compounds of the structural formula

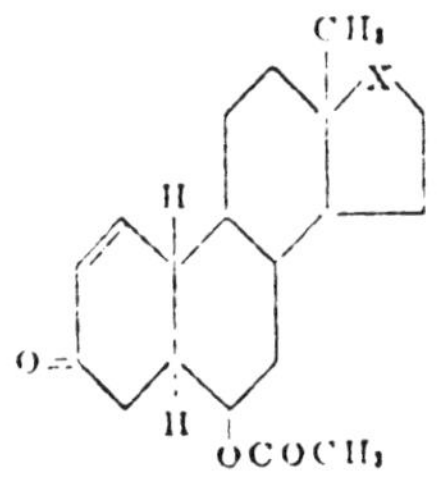

Hydrogenation of the 1,2-double bond of the latter substances followed by reaction with a peracid such as peracetic acid results in the corresponding 3-oxa-4-ones. The latter substances are then treated with dilute alkali to afford the free 6β-ol, which is converted to the methanesulfonate by the aforementioned process. The methanesulfonates upon heating in pyridine afford the corresponding 3-oxa-androst-4a-en-4-ones, which are converted to the corresponding 3-oxa-5α-androstan-4-ones and 3-oxa-5β-androstan-4-ones by catalytic hydrogenation. Specifically, 6β,17β-dihydroxy-17α-methyl-5α-estr-1-en-3-one 6-acetate is reduced with 5% palladium-on-carbon catalyst to yield 6β,17β-dihydroxy-17α-methyl-5α-estran-3-one 6-acetate. Reaction of this substance in methylene dichloride with aqueous peracetic acid affords 6β,17β-dihydroxy - 17α-methyl-3-oxa-A-homo-5α-estran-4-one 6-acetate. This ester is heated with dilute aqueous sodium hydroxide in methanol to yield the corresponding 6β-ol, which is converted to the 6β-methanesulfonate by reaction with methanesulfonyl chloride in pyridine. Heating the latter substance in pyridine results in 17β-hydroxy-17α-methyl-3-oxa-A-homo-estr-4a-en-4-one. Reduction of the latter substance with hydrogen and 5% palladium-on-carbon catalyst results in 17β-hydroxy-17α-methyl-3-oxa-A-homo-5α-estran-4-one and 17β-hydroxy-17α-methyl-3-oxa-A-homo-5β-estran-4-one.

The 5,6-dehydro lactones of this invention can be manufactured by heating the corresponding 4,5-dehydro compounds with aqueous alkali in methanol, followed by acidification with dilute acid. For example, 17β-hydroxy-17α-methyl-2-oxaandrost-4-en-3-one in methanol is heated at the reflux temperature with 5% aqueous sodium hydroxide, and this mixture is acidified with 10% aqueous acetic acid to produce a mixture of 17β-hydroxy-17α-methyl-2-oxaandrost-5-en-3-one and the Δ⁴ isomer, which are separated chromatographically.

The instant 17-oxo-lactones are obtained by oxidation of the corresponding 17β-hydroxy compounds. Typically, 17β-hydroxy-2-oxa-5α-androstan-3-one in acetone is treated with aqueous chromic acid to yield 2-oxa-5α-androstane-3,17-dione.

Acylation of the secondary hydroxy group of the instant 17β-ols with a lower alkanoic acid anhydride in pyridine produces the corresponding 17β-(lower alkanoates). Typically, 17β-hydroxy-2-oxa-5α-androstan-3-one is treated with acetic anhydride to produce 17β-acetoxy-2-oxa-5α-androstan-3-one.

The instant 17α-(lower alkyl)-17β-(lower alkanoyl)-oxy compounds are obtained by acylation of the corresponding alcohol with an isopropenyl-(lower alkanoate) in the presence of an acidic catalyst. For example 17β-hydroxy-17α-methyl-2-oxaandrostan-3-one is treated with isopropenyl acetate and p-toluenesulfonic acid, resulting in 17β-acetoxy-17α-methyl-2-oxa-5α-androstan-3-one.

Reduction of the instant 4,5-dehydro lactones, suitably with hydrogen in the presence of a hydrogenation catalyst such as palladium results in the corresponding 5α and 5β compounds.

Equivalent to the lactones of this invention are the corresponding hydroxy-acids, with which they are in equilibrium in aqueous solution, and also the alkali metal salts derived therefrom. These relationships are illustrated as follows:

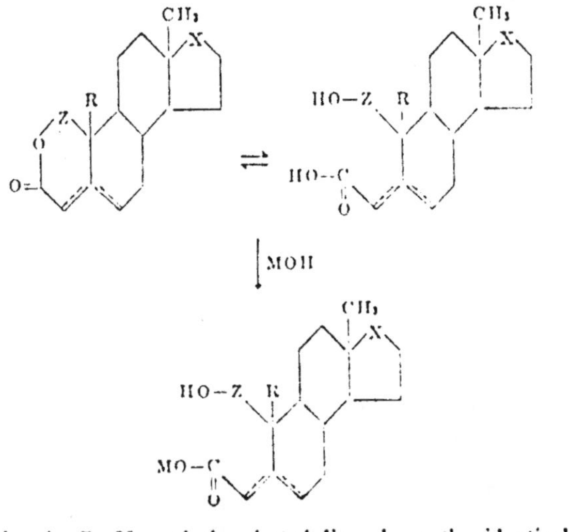

wherein R, X, and the dotted lines have the identical significance as defined supra, and M is the ion of an alkali metal such as sodium or potassium.

Although the instant novel intermediates are represented in the form of an aldehydo-acid, it will be apparent to those skilled in the art that these derivatives actually exist as an equilibrium mixture containing also the corresponding lactol form. This relationship is shown below:

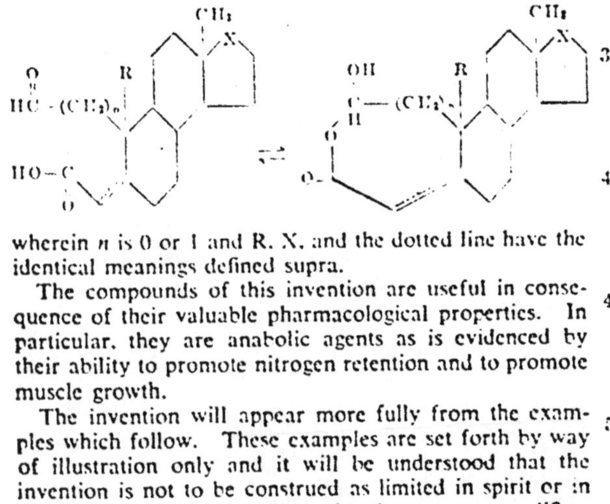

wherein n is 0 or 1 and R, X, and the dotted line have the identical meanings defined supra.

The compounds of this invention are useful in consequence of their valuable pharmacological properties. In particular, they are anabolic agents as is evidenced by their ability to promote nitrogen retention and to promote muscle growth.

The invention will appear more fully from the examples which follow. These examples are set forth by way of illustration only and it will be understood that the invention is not to be construed as limited in spirit or in scope by the details contained therein, as many modifications in materials and methods will be apparent from this disclosure to those skilled in the art. In these examples, temperatures are given in degrees centigrate (° C.). Quantities of materials are expressed in parts by weight unless otherwise noted.

Example 1

A mixture of 2.45 parts of 17β-hydroxy-5α-estran-3-one, 2.2 parts of acetic anhydride, and 20 parts of pyridine is allowed to stand at room temperature for about 16 hours, then is diluted with ice water. The resulting precipitate is collected by filtration, washed successively with water, dilute hydrochloric acid, dilute aqueous sodium bicarbonate, dried, and crystallized from aqueous methanol to yield 17β-acetoxy-5α-estran-3-one. M.P. about 104–106°.

A solution of 8 parts of 17β-acetoxy-5α-estran-3-one in 63 parts of glacial acetic acid is cooled by means of an ice bath. To this solution is added portionwise, under nitrogen with stirring, 25 parts of a 2 N bromine in acetic acid solution, and agitation is continued for about 15 minutes longer. The reaction mixture is diluted with

water, and the resulting precipitate is collected by filtration, washed successively with dilute aqueous sodium bicarbonate and water, then dried. This solid, containing 17β-acetoxy-2-bromo-5α-estran-3-one, is refluxed in 30 parts of collidine for about 15 minutes, and the mixture is cooled and diluted with 175 parts of ether. The ether solution is washed successively with water, dilute hydrochloric acid, aqueous sodium bicarbonate, and saturated aqueous sodium chloride, dried over anhydrous magnesium sulfate, and evaporated to dryness at reduced pressure. The residue is dissolved in benzene and adsorbed on silica gel. Elution of the chromatographic column with 4% ethyl acetate in benzene affords 17β-acetoxy-5α-estr-1-en-3-one. M.P. 133.5–135.5°.

To a solution of 2 parts of 17β-acetoxy-5α-estr-1-en-3-one in 7.9 parts of methanol is added one part of potassium hydroxide dissolved in 2 parts of water, and the resulting solution is heated at reflux for about one hour. The reaction mixture is cooled, then poured slowly into ice water, and the resulting mixture is extracted with ether. The ether solution is washed with water, dried over anhydrous potassium carbonate and evaporated to dryness in vacuo. Recrystallization of the residue from acetone-petroleum ether affords 17β-hydroxy-5α-estr-1-en-3-one, which displays infrared maxima at about 2.75, 3.4, and 5.95 microns and a maximum in the ultraviolet at 229 millimicrons with an extinction coefficient of about 9800.

Example 2

To a solution of 14.5 parts of 17β-hydroxy-17α-methyl-5α-estran-3-one in 150 parts of dimethylformamide is added 0.2 part of p-toluenesulfonic acid monohydrate. The resulting mixture is stirred and treated dropwise with a solution of 8 parts of bromine and 250 parts of dimethylformamide at room temperature over a period of about 12 hours. This reaction mixture is allowed to stand at room temperature for about 12 hours, then is poured slowly into ice water. The resulting precipitate is collected by filtration, washed with water, and dissolved in ether. This ether solution is dried over anhydrous potassium carbonate, then concentrated to dryness to afford 2-bromo-17β-hydroxy-17α-methyl-5α-estran-3-one. This substance is dissolved in 100 parts of dimethylformamide; then 3.9 parts of lithium chloride and 2.3 parts of lithium carbonate are added to the solution. The resulting mixture is heated at reflux with stirring in an atmosphere of nitrogen for about 6 hours, then is cooled and extracted with ether. The ether extract is washed successively with water, dilute hydrochloric acid, aqueous sodium carbonate, and water; dried over anhydrous potassium carbonate, and evaporated to dryness in vacuo. The residue is dissolved in benzene and adsorbed on silica gel. Elution with 15% ethyl acetate in benzene followed by recrystallization from acetone-heptane affords 17β-hydroxy-17α-methyl-5α-estr-1-en-3-one. M.P. 141–142.5°; $[\alpha]_D = +87°$ (chloroform).

Example 3

To a solution of 15.2 parts of 17α-ethyl-17β-hydroxy-5α-estran-3-one in 750 parts of dimethylformamide is added 0.5 part of p-toluenesulfonic acid monohydrate, and the resulting mixture is treated dropwise with a solution of 8 parts of bromine in 200 parts of dimethylformamide over a period of about 24 hours. The reaction mixture is poured into a mixture of ice and water, and the resulting precipitate is collected by filtration, washed successively with aqueous sodium bicarbonate and water, and dried to afford 2-bromo-17α-ethyl-17β-hydroxy-5α-estran-3-one. To a solution of the latter substance in 90 parts of dimethylformamide is added 3.9 parts of lithium chloride and 2.25 parts of lithium carbonate, and the resulting mixture is heated at reflux, under nitrogen, for about 6 hours. This reaction mixture is cooled, treated with water, and extracted with ether. The ether solution is washed successively with dilute hydrochloric acid and water, dried over anhydrous potassium carbonate, and concentrated to dryness in vacuo. The residue is dissolved in benzene and adsorbed on silica gel. Elution of the chromatographic column with 8% ethyl acetate in benzene followed by recrystallization from ethyl acetate-heptane results in 17α-ethyl-17β-hydroxy-5α-estr-1-en-3-one, M.P. 170–173°; $[\alpha]_D = +42.4°$.

Example 4

To a solution of 8 parts of 5α-androst-1-ene-3,17-dione in 120 parts of acetic acid containing 15 parts of water is added 50 parts of lead tetraacetate and 0.75 part of osmium tetroxide. This reaction mixture is stirred for about 4 hours at room temperature, then is stored at room temperature for about 16 hours, and finally is extracted with benzene. The benzene solution is washed with water, and extracted with aqueous potassium bicarbonate. The aqueous extracts are acidified with dilute hydrochloric acid, then extracted with a mixture of ethyl acetate and benzene. This organic extract is washed with water, dried over anhydrous sodium sulfate, and evaporated to dryness at reduced pressure. The resulting residue is dissolved in 20 parts of pyridine, then treated with 10 parts of 20% aqueous sodium bisulfite. This mixture is stirred for about 20 minutes at room temperature, then is diluted with water and extracted with ethyl acetate. The aqueous layer is separated and acidified by means of dilute sulfuric acid, and this acidic mixture is extracted with benzene. The benzene solution is washed with water, dried over anhydrous sodium sulfate, and concentrated to dryness in vacuo to afford 1,17-dioxo-1,2-seco-A-nor-androstan-2-oic acid.

To a solution of 2 parts of 1,17-dioxo-1,2-seco-A-nor-androstan-2-oic acid in 20 parts of water containing 4 parts of 20% aqueous sodium hydroxide is added a solution of 10 parts of sodium borohydride in 80 parts of water. This mixture is stored at room temperature for about 24 hours, then it is washed with ether and acidified with aqueous hydrochloric acid. The resulting mixture is extracted with ethyl acetate-ether, and the organic layer is separated, washed successively with aqueous potassium carbonate and water, dried over anhydrous sodium sulfate, then evaporated to dryness at reduced pressure. The crystalline residue is triturated with ether, then recrystallized from butanone to afford pure 17β-hydroxy-2-oxa-5α-androstan-3-one, M.P. about 198–203°.

Example 5

To a solution of 6.36 parts of 17β-hydroxy-17α-methyl-5α-androst-1-en-3-one in 95 parts of acetic acid and 12 parts of water is added 40 parts of lead tetraacetate and 0.6 part of osmium tetroxide. This mixture is stored at room temperature for about 24 hours, then is treated with 2 parts of lead tetraacetate. Evaporation to dryness at reduced pressure affords a residue, which is extracted with benzene. The benzene extract is washed with water, and extracted with aqueous potassium bicarbonate. The aqueous extract is washed with ether, acidified with dilute sulfuric acid, then extracted with ethyl acetate-benzene. This organic extract is washed with water, dried over anhydrous sodium sulfate, and concentrated to dryness in vacuo. To a solution of the residual crude product in 20 parts of pyridine is added 10 parts of 20% aqueous sodium bisulfite and the mixture is stirred for about 20 minutes at room temperature. This mixture is then diluted with water, washed with ethyl acetate, acidified with dilute sulfuric acid, and finally extracted with benzene. The benzene extract is washed with water, dried over anhydrous sodium sulfate, and evaporated to dryness at reduced pressure to produce crude 17β-hydroxy-17α-methyl-1-oxo-1,2-seco-A-nor-5α-androstan-2-oic acid, which after recrystallization from aqueous isopropyl alcohol, melts at about 166–173° (dec.).

An aqueous slurry of 6 parts of 17β-hydroxy-17α-methyl-1-oxo-1,2-seco-A-nor-5α-androstan-2-oic acid in 200 parts of water is made alkaline to pH 10 by the addition of dilute aqueous sodium hydroxide, then is treated with 6 parts of sodium borohydride. This mixture is allowed to react at room temperature for about 3 hours. Benzene is added and the resulting mixture is acidified carefully with dilute hydrochloric acid. The benzene layer is separated, and the aqueous layer is further extracted with benzene. The combined benzene extracts are washed successively with aqueous potassium bicarbonate and water, dried over anhydrous sodium sulfate, then evaporated to dryness in vacuo. The resulting residue is triturated with ether to afford pure 17β-hydroxy-17α-methyl-2-oxa-5α-androstan-3-one, M.P. about 235–238°; $[\alpha]_D = -23°$ (chloroform). It is represented by the structural formula

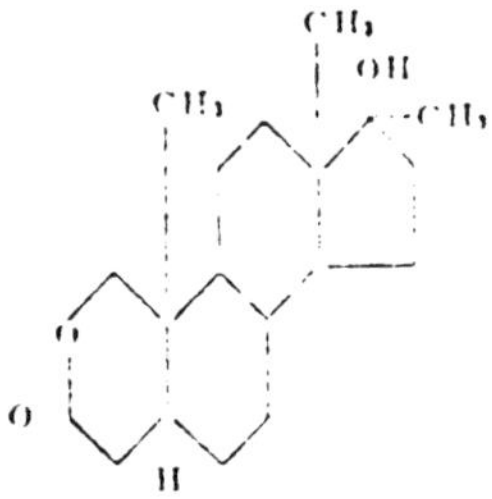

Example 6

The substitution of an equivalent quantity of 17α-ethyl-17β-hydroxy-5α-androst-1-en-3-one in the process of Example 5 results in 17α-ethyl-17β-hydroxy-1-oxo-1,2-seco-A-nor-5α-androstan-2-oic acid and 17α-ethyl-17β-hydroxy-2-oxa-5α-androstan-3-one, M.P. about 192–195°. The latter compound is represented by the structural formula

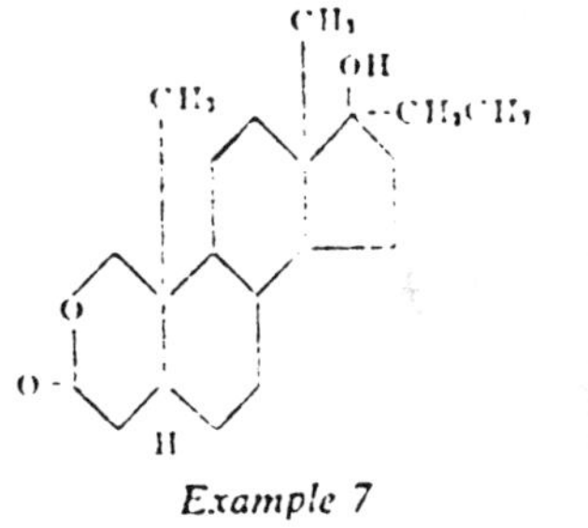

Example 7

To a solution of 3 parts of 17β-hydroxy-2-oxa-5α-androstan-3-one in 40 parts of acetone is added dropwise, 3 parts by volume of an aqueous solution, 8 N in chromium trioxide and 8 N in sulfuric acid. The mixture is allowed to stand at room temperature for about 3 minutes, then it is treated with isopropyl alcohol to destroy excess oxidizing agent, and is finally evaporated to dryness under nitrogen. The resulting residue is extracted with ether-benzene, and this extract is washed successively with water, dilute hydrochloric acid, dilute aqueous sodium hydroxide, and water, then dried over anhydrous sodium sulfate, and concentrated to dryness in vacuo to afford crystals of 2-oxa-5α-androstane-3,17-dione, M.P. about 172–173°. Recrystallization from methylcyclohexane-benzene affords a sample which melts at about 173–174°.

Example 8

To a solution of 50 parts of androsta-1,4-diene-3,17-dione in 546 parts of tertiary-butyl alcohol and 700 parts of water is added 9 parts of potassium chlorate and 4.5 parts of osmium tetroxide, and the resulting mixture is stored at room temperature for about 15 days, then is concentrated at reduced pressure to afford a dark-colored oil. This oil is extracted with benzene, and the benzene solution is separated, clarified by filtration, washed successively with 5% aqueous sodium hydroxide and water, dried over anhydrous sodium sulfate, and concentrated in vacuo to yield a crystalline residue consisting of a mixture of the isomeric 1,2- and 4,5-glycols. Fractional crystallization of this mixture, first from benzene-ether, then from benzene produces pure 4,5-dihydroxyandrost-1-ene-3,17-dione, which melts at about 203–208° and displays infrared maxima at about 2.80, 2.87, 3.40, 5.74, 5.90, and 6.22 microns and also an ultraviolet maximum at about 229 millimicrons with a molecular extinction coefficient of about 9,500, and 1,2-dihydroxyandrost-4-ene-3,17-dione, melting at about 206–210° and characterized by infrared maxima at about 2.80, 2.87, 3.40, 5.74, 5.94, and 6.18 microns, and also an ultraviolet maximum at about 238 millimicrons with a molecular extinction coefficient of about 14,000.

To a solution of 8.4 parts of the latter crude mixture of isomeric glycols in 130 parts of acetic acid and 25 parts of water is added 35 parts of lead tetracetate, and this mixture is stirred at 50–60° for about 1¼ hours, then is diluted with water and is extracted with benzene. The benzene layer is separated, washed successively with water, an aqueous solution 1 molar in potassium carbonate and 1 molar in potassium bicarbonate, and water, dried over anhydrous sodium sulfate, and concentrated to dryness in vacuo. The crystalline residue is recrystallized from benzene to yield 1,17-dioxo-1,2-seco-A-nor-androst-3-en-2-oic acid, M.P. about 245–253°. This compound is characterized by an ultraviolet maximum at about 225.5 millimicrons with a molecular extinction coefficient of about 13,700.

To a solution of 4.75 parts of 1,17-dioxo-1,2-seco-A-norandrost-3-en-2-oic acid in 12 parts of chloroform is added successively a solution of 5 parts of sodium borohydride in 60 parts of water and 5 parts of 10% aqueous sodium hydroxide. This mixture is stirred at room temperature for about 4 hours, after which time the organic layer is separated by decantation, washed successively with aqueous sodium hydroxide and water, and dried over anhydrous sodium sulfate. The solvent is distilled at reduced pressure to afford the crude product. Recrystallization from isopropyl alcohol results in pure 17β-hydroxy-2-oxaandrost-4-en-3-one, M.P. about 205–207°. It is characterized by an ultraviolet absorption maximum at about 223.5 millimicrons with a molecular extinction coefficient of about 14,000, and is represented by the structural formula

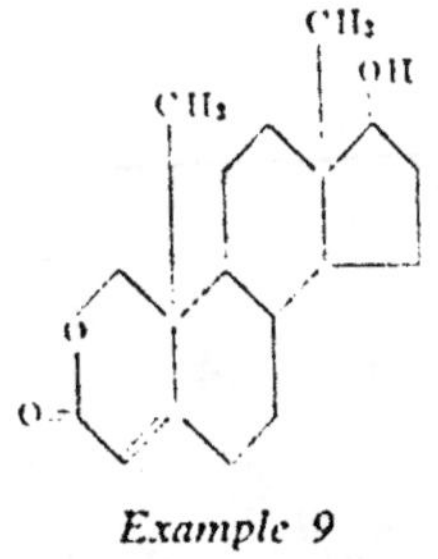

Example 9

A solution of 50 parts of 17β-hydroxy-17α-methyl-androsta-1,4-dien-3-one in 546 parts of tertiary-butyl alcohol and 700 parts of water is treated with 8.5 parts of potassium chlorate and 4.25 parts of osmium tetroxide. This reaction mixture is stored at room temperature for about 7 days, then is concentrated in vacuo at room temperature to produce a dark-colored residual oil. Extraction of this oil with chloroform affords an organic solution, which is washed successively with aqueous sodium hydroxide and water, dried over anhydrous sodium sulfate, and evaporated to dryness at reduced pressure to afford a mixture of the isomeric 1,2- and 4,5-glycols. Fractional crystallization from ether-benzene affords 4,5,17β-trihydroxy-17α-methylandrost-1-en-3-one, M.P. about 187–193°, which yields a pure sample melting at about 199–201° after recrystallization from isopropyl alcohol, and exhibits an ultraviolet maximum at about 229.5 milli-

microns with a molecular extinction coefficient of about 9,350 and also infrared maxima of about 2.79, 2.87, 3.40, 3.47, 5.91, and 6.18 microns, and 1,2,17β-trihydroxy-17α-methylandrost-4-en-3-one, M.P. about 193–195.5°, which displays an ultraviolet maximum at about 239 millimicrons with a molecular extinction coefficient of about 13,300 and also characteristic infrared maxima at about 5.94 and 6.18 microns.

To 1.338 parts of the latter crude mixture of isomeric glycols in 21 parts of acetic acid and 4 parts of water is added 5.6 parts of lead tetracetate, and this reaction mixture is stirred at 50–60° for about 1¼ hours. Dilution with water followed by extraction with chloroform yields an organic solution, which is washed with an aqueous solution 1 M in potassium carbonate and 1 M in potassium bicarbonate, then is dried over anhydrous sodium sulfate. Evaporation of this solution to dryness and trituration of the resulting residue with benzene produces 17β-hydroxy - 17α - methyl-1-oxo-1,2-seco-A-nor-androst-3-en-2-oic acid, M.P. about 250–265°. It displays infrared maxima at about 2.80, 3.00, 3.35, 3.41, 5.84, and 6.10 microns and an ultraviolet maximum at about 226.5 millimicrons with a molecular extinction coefficient of about 13,100.

To a solution of 2.18 parts of 17β-hydroxy-17α-methyl-1-oxo-1,2-seco-A-norandrost-3-en-2-oic acid in 60 parts of chloroform is added successively a solution of 2.18 parts of sodium borohydride in 30 parts of water and 2.5 parts of 10% aqueous sodium hydroxide. This reaction mixture is stirred at room temperature for about 4 hours, and the organic layer is separated by decantation, then washed successively with aqueous sodium hydroxide and water, dried over anhydrous sodium sulfate, and concentrated to dryness at reduced pressure to yield the crude product. Recrystallization from benzene affords pure 17β-hydroxy-17α-methyl - 2 - oxaandrost-4-en-3-one, M.P. about 230–240° (dec.). It displays an ultraviolet absorption maximum at about 223.5 millimicrons with a molecular extinction coefficient of about 12,500, and is represented by the structural formula

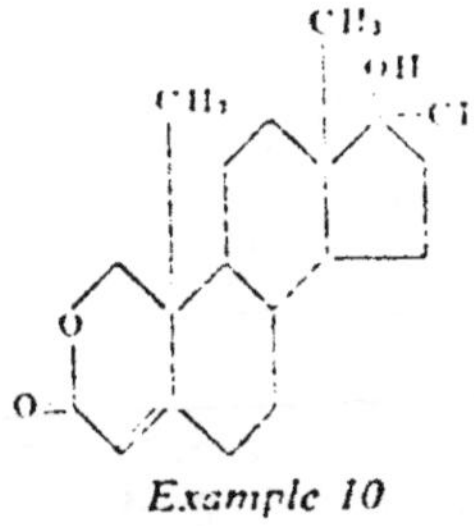

Example 10

The substitution of an equivalent quantity of 17α-ethyl-17β-hydroxyandrosta-1,4-dien-3-one in the procedure of Example 9 results in 17α-ethyl-17β-hydroxy-1-oxo-1,2-seco-A-nor-androst-3-en-2-oic acid, which is converted, by the processes of that example, to 17α-ethyl-17β-hydroxy-2-oxaandrost-4-en-3-one. The latter substance is represented by the structural formula

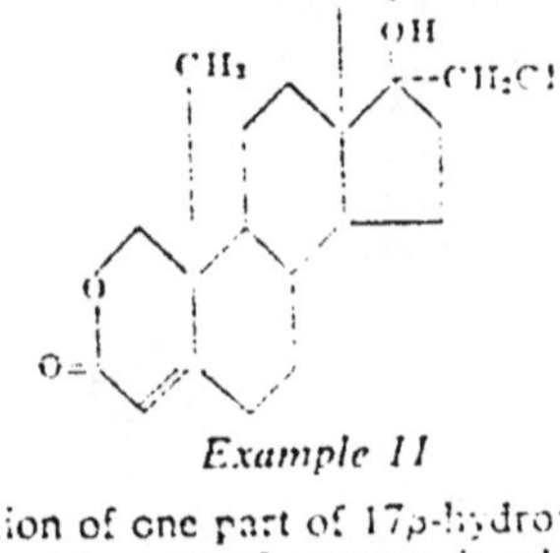

Example 11

To a solution of one part of 17β-hydroxy-2-oxaandrost-4-en-3-one in 16 parts of acetone is added one part by volume of an aqueous solution, 8 N in chromium trioxide and 8 N in sulfuric acid. This reaction mixture is allowed to stand at room temperature for about 5 minutes,

13

then is treated with one part of isopropyl alcohol and is diluted with water. Extraction with benzene affords an organic solution, which is washed with dilute sodium hydroxide, dried over anhydrous sodium sulfate, and concentrated to dryness to yield 2-oxaandrost-4-ene-3,17-dione, M.P. about 178–183°.

Example 12

The substitution of an equivalent quantity of 17β-hydroxy-5α-estr-1-en-3-one in the procedure of Example 4 results in 17β-hydroxy-1-oxo-1,2-seco-A-nor-5α-estran-2-oic acid and 17β-hydroxy-2-oxa-5α-estran-3-one.

Example 13

The substitution of an equivalent quantity of 17β-hydroxy-2-oxa-5α-estran-3-one in the procedure of Example 7 results in 2-oxa-5α-estrane-3,17-dione.

Example 14

By substituting an equivalent quantity of 17β-hydroxy-17α-methyl-5α-estr-1-en-3-one and otherwise proceeding according to the processes of Example 5, 17β-hydroxy-17α-methyl-1-oxo-1,2-seco-A-nor-5α-estran-2-oic acid and 17β-hydroxy-17α-methyl-2-oxa-5α-estran-3-one are obtained.

Example 15

The substitution of an equivalent quantity of 17α-ethyl-17β-hydroxy-5α-estr-1-en-3-one in the procedure of Example 4 results in 17α-ethyl-17β-hydroxy-1-oxo-1,2-seco-A-nor-5α-estran-2-oic acid and 17α-ethyl-17β-hydroxy-2-oxa-5α-estran-3-one.

Example 16

A mixture of one part of 6β,19-epoxy-5α-androstane-3β,17β-diol 3,17-diacetate, 80 parts of methanol, and 10 parts of 10% aqueous sodium hydroxide is heated at reflux for about 2 hours. The solution is cooled, concentrated to a small volume under reduced pressure, then diluted with water and extracted with benzene. The benzene solution is concentrated to dryness at reduced pressure. The resulting residue is dissolved in 80 parts of acetone, and this solution is treated dropwise with a small excess of an aqueous solution, 8 N in chromium trioxide and 8 N in sulfuric acid. The excess oxidant is destroyed by the addition of a small quantity of isopropyl alcohol. This mixture is concentrated under nitrogen, then diluted with water and extracted with benzene. The benzene extract is washed successively with aqueous sodium hydroxide and water, dried over anhydrous sodium sulfate, and concentrated at reduced pressure to afford 6β,19-epoxy-5α-androstane-3,17-dione.

Example 17

To a solution of one part of 6β,19-epoxy-5α-androstane-3,17-dione in 80 parts of methanol is added 0.2 part of p-toluenesulfonic acid, and the resulting mixture is stored at room temperature for about 16 hours. The mixture is then treated with 0.2 part of sodium methoxide and concentrated to a small volume in vacuo. Water is added and the resulting aqueous mixture is extracted with benzene. The benzene solution is dried over anhydrous sodium sulfate and concentrated to dryness to afford 6β,19-epoxy-5α-androstane-3,17-dione 3-dimethyl ketal.

To a solution of one part of 6β,19-epoxy-5α-androstane-3,17-dione 3-dimethyl ketal in 35 parts of ether is added dropwise 3 parts of volume of 3 M ethereal methyl magnesium bromide. This reaction mixture is kept at room temperature for about 4 hours, then is cooled by means of an ice bath and treated with about 20 parts of 5% aqueous hydrochloric acid. This two-phase mixture is stirred at room temperature for about 2 hours, after which time the organic layer is separated, washed successively with water, 5% aqueous potassium bicarbonate, and water, then dried over anhydrous sodium sulfate and concentrated at reduced pressure to yield 17β-hydroxy-17α-methyl-6β,19-epoxy-5α-androstan-3-one. This substance

14

is characterized by infrared maxima at about 2.85 and 5.85 microns.

Example 18

To a solution of 2 parts of 6β,19-epoxy-5α-androstane-3,17-dione in 26.4 parts of tetrahydrofuran is added, at −5° over a period of about 15 minutes, a solution of 1.05 parts of bromine in 3.2 parts of methylene chloride. The reaction mixture is then diluted with water and extracted with benzene. The benzene solution is washed successively with 5% aqueous bicarbonate and water, dried over anhydrous sodium sulfate, and concentrated to dryness under reduced pressure to afford a residue. To 0.08 part of magnesium oxide suspended in 7 parts of dimethylformamide is added, at the reflux temperature, 0.8 part of the latter residue. Refluxing is continued for about 30 minutes, after which time the mixture is poured into about 20 parts of ice water containing one part of concentrated sulfuric acid. This mixture is extracted with benzene, and the benzene solution is washed with water, dried over anhydrous sodium sulfate, and concentrated to dryness in vacuo, to yield 6β,19-epoxy-5α-androst-1-ene-3,17-dione.

To a solution of one part of 6β,19-epoxy-5α-androst-1-ene-3,17-dione in 35 parts of acetone is added 4 parts by volume of an aqueous solution, 8 N in chromium trioxide and 8 N in sulfuric acid. After standing at room temperature for about 2 hours, this mixture is treated with isopropyl alcohol to destroy any excess reagent, then is diluted with water, and extracted with benzene. The benzene solution is concentrated to dryness. A solution of one part of the latter residue in 80 parts of methanol is treated with 10 parts of 10% aqueous potassium carbonate, and this mixture is heated at reflux for about 2 hours. This solution is acidified with excess aqueous hydrochloric acid, then concentrated to a small volume at reduced pressure. Extraction of the resulting residue with benzene affords an organic solution which is washed with water, dried over anhydrous sodium sulfate and concentrated to dryness under reduced pressure to yield 6β-hydroxy-5α-estr-1-ene-3,17-dione.

A mixture of one part of 6β-hydroxy-5α-estr-1-ene-3,17-dione, 10 parts of acetic anhydride, and 20 parts of pyridine is kept at room temperature for about 16 hours, then is diluted with water and extracted with benzene. The organic solution is washed with water, dried over anhydrous sodium sulfate, and evaporated to dryness to yield 6β-hydroxy-5α-estr-1-ene-3,17-dione 6-acetate.

A mixture of one part of 6β-hydroxy-5α-estr-1-ene-3,17-dione 6-acetate, 20 parts of acetic acid, 2 parts of water, 7 parts of lead tetraacetate, and 0.1 part of osmium tetroxide is stirred at room temperature for about 24 hours, then is extracted with benzene. The organic extract is washed with water and extracted with aqueous potassium bicarbonate. This alkaline aqueous extract is acidified with dilute hydrochloric acid, then is extracted with ethyl acetate-benzene. This organic solution is evaporated to dryness, then is dissolved in 3 parts of pyridine and treated with 1.5 parts of 20% aqueous sodium bisulfite. The resulting mixture is stirred for about 30 minutes, then is diluted with water and extracted with ethyl acetate. The aqueous layer is acidified with dilute sulfuric acid, then is extracted with benzene. The benzene solution is washed with water, dried over anhydrous sodium sulfate, and evaporated to dryness to yield a residue containing 6β-acetoxy-1,17-dioxo-1,2-seco-A-nor-5α-estran-2-oic acid. To the latter residue is added a solution of one part of sodium borohydride in 50 parts of water, and the resulting mixture is stirred at room temperature for about 4 hours, then is acidified to pH 3 with dilute hydrochloric acid, and is extracted with benzene. The benzene extract is washed successively with aqueous potassium carbonate and water, dried over anhydrous sodium sulfate, and evaporated to dryness to afford 6β-acetoxy-17β-hydroxy-2-oxa-5α-estran-3-one.

15

To a solution of one part of 6β-acetoxy-17β-hydroxy-2-oxa-5α-estran-3-one in 50 parts of acetone is added a slight excess of an aqueous solution, 8 N in chromium trioxide and 8 N in sulfuric acid. The excess oxidant is destroyed by the addition of isopropyl alcohol, and the mixture is concentrated to dryness. The residue is extracted with benzene, and the benzene extract is washed with water, dried over anhydrous sodium sulfate, and concentrated to dryness to yield 6β-acetoxy-2-oxa-5α-estrane-3,17-dione.

A mixture of one part of 6β-acetoxy-2-oxa-5α-estrane-3,17-dione, 50 parts of methanol, and 10 parts of 10% aqueous sodium hydroxide is heated at reflux for about 5 hours, then is cooled, concentrated to a small volume, and diluted with water. The resulting mixture is extracted with benzene, and the benzene extract is washed with water, dried over anhydrous sodium sulfate, and evaporated to dryness to yield 6β-hydroxy-2-oxa-5α-estrane-3,17-dione.

Example 19

To a solution of 10 parts of 6β-hydroxy-2-oxa-5α-estrane-3,17-dione in 100 parts of pyridine is added, at 0°, 7.4 parts of methanesulfonyl chloride. This reaction mixture is stored at room temperature for about 16 hours, then is diluted with water and extracted with benzene. The benzene extract is washed with water, dried over anhydrous sodium sulfate, and evaporated to dryness at reduced pressure. The latter residue is dissolved in 20 parts of pyridine, and the resulting solution is heated at reflux for about 3 hours. The cooled mixture is diluted with water and extracted with benzene. The organic solution is separated, washed with water, dried over anhydrous sodium sulfate, and evaporated to dryness at reduced pressure to yield 2-oxaestr-4-ene-3,17-dione.

Example 20

A mixture of one part of 2-oxaestr-4-ene-3,17-dione, 0.3 part of sodium hydroxide, 1 part of sodium borohydride, 40 parts of methanol, and 50 parts of water is stirred at room temperature for about 4 hours, then is acidified with dilute hydrochloric acid and extracted with benzene. The benzene extract is washed successively with aqueous potassium carbonate and water, dried over anhydrous sodium sulfate and evaporated to dryness to yield 17β-hydroxy-2-oxaestr-4-en-3-one.

Example 21

By substituting an equivalent quantity of 17β-hydroxy-17α-methyl-6β,19-epoxy-5α-androstan-3-one and otherwise proceeding according to the processes of Example 18, 6β,17β-dihydroxy-17α-methyl-2-oxa-5α-estran-3-one is obtained.

Example 22

The substitution of an equivalent quantity of 6β,17β-dihydroxy-17α-methyl-2-oxa-5α-estran-3-one in the procedure of Example 19 results in 17β-hydroxy-17α-methyl-2-oxaestra-4-en-3-one.

Example 23

A mixture containing one part of 17β-hydroxy-17α-methyl-2-oxaandrost-4-en-3-one, 10 parts of 5% aqueous sodium hydroxide, and 50 parts of methanol is heated at reflux for about 10 minutes, then is cooled to 0–5° and treated at that temperature with 10 parts of cold 10% aqueous acetic acid. The acidic mixture is diluted with water and extracted with benzene. The organic solution is washed successively with cold 5% aqueous potassium bicarbonate and water, dried over anhydrous sodium sulfate, and concentrated to dryness. The residue is dissolved in benzene and chromatographed on silica gel. Elution with 50% ether in benzene affords 17β-hydroxy-17α-methyl-2-oxaandrost-5-en-3-one.

Example 24

The substitution of an equivalent quantity of 17α-ethyl-

16

17β-hydroxy-2-oxaandrost-4-en-3-one in the procedure of Example 23 results in 17α-ethyl-17β-hydroxy-2-oxaandrost-5-en-3-one.

Example 25

The substitution of an equivalent quantity of 17β-hydroxy-2-oxaandrost-4-en-3-one in the procedure of Example 23 affords 17β-hydroxy-2-oxaandrost-5-en-3-one.

Example 26

The substitution of an equivalent quantity of 2-oxaandrost-4-ene-3,17-dione in the procedure of Example 23 results in 2-oxaandrost-5-ene-3,17-dione.

Example 27

By substituting an equivalent quantity of 2-oxaestr-4-ene-3,17-dione and otherwise proceeding according to the processes of Example 23, 2-oxaestr-5-ene-3,17-dione is obtained.

Example 28

By substituting an equivalent quantity of 17β-hydroxy-2-oxaestr-4-en-3-one and otherwise proceeding according to the processes of Example 23, 17β-hydroxy-2-oxaestr-5-en-3-one is obtained.

Example 29

The substitution of an equivalent quantity of 17β-hydroxy-17α-methyl-2-oxaestr-4-en-3-one in the procedure of Example 23 results in 17β-hydroxy-17α-methyl-2-oxaestr-5-en-3-one.

Example 30

A mixture of 2.5 parts of 17β-hydroxy-17α-methyl-5α-androstan-3-one, 25 parts of isopropenyl acetate, and 0.2 part of concentrated sulfuric acid is distilled slowly over a period of about 3 hours. The mixture is then cooled, treated with 0.5 part of sodium acetate, and concentrated to dryness. This residue is extracted with methylene chloride, and the extract is concentrated to dryness at reduced pressure to afford 17α-methyl-5α-androst-2-ene-3,17β-diol 3,17-diacetate.

A solution of 17α-methyl-5α-androst-2-ene-3,17β-diol 3,17-diacetate in 180 parts of ethyl acetate is cooled to −70° and saturated with ozone. The reaction mixture is purged with nitrogen, then is treated with 15 parts of zinc dust and 18 parts of acetic acid containing 15 parts of water. The resulting mixture is stirred at −70° for one hour, at room temperature for one hour, then is diluted with 50 parts of water and stirred for about 30 minutes. The mixture is filtered to remove zinc, and the organic layer is separated, washed successively with water, dilute aqueous sodium bicarbonate, and water, dried over anhydrous sodium sulfate, and evaporated to dryness.

A solution of the latter residue in 150 parts of chloroform is added to a solution of 10 parts of sodium borohydride and 2 parts of sodium hydroxide in 200 parts of water, and the resulting mixture is stirred for about 6 hours. The organic layer is separated, then acidified with dilute hydrochloric acid, and the resulting precipitate is collected by filtration, washed with water, and dried to afford crude 2,17β-dihydroxy-17α-methyl-2,3-seco-5α-androstan-3-oic acid.

This crude product is dissolved in a solution of 10 parts of sodium hydroxide in 200 parts of water, and the resulting solution is heated on the steam bath for about 7 hours, then is cooled and acidified with dilute hydrochloric acid. The crystalline precipitate is collected by filtration, washed with water, dried, then stirred with benzene for about 30 minutes. The crystalline material is collected by filtration, then crystallized as the sodium salt from an aqueous sodium hydroxide solution. The crystalline sodium salt is dissolved in water, and the resulting solution is acidified with dilute hydrochloric acid. The precipitate which forms is collected by filtration and recrystallized from acetone to produce pure 2,17β-dihydroxy-17α-methyl-2,3-seco-5α-androstan-3-oic acid, M.P. about 214–215°.

A mixture of one part of 2,17β-dihydroxy-17α-methyl-2,3-seco-5α-androstan-3-oic acid and 175 parts of tertiary-butylbenzene is stirred and distilled slowly over a period of about 3 hours. The mixture is then concentrated to dryness and the residue is extracted with chloroform. The chloroform extract is washed successively with aqueous potassium carbonate and water, dried over anhydrous sodium sulfate, and evaporated to dryness at reduced pressure. Recrystallization of this residue from benzene yields 17β-hydroxy-17α-methyl-3-oxa-A-homo-5α-androstan-4-one, M.P. about 241–245°, which is represented by the structural formula

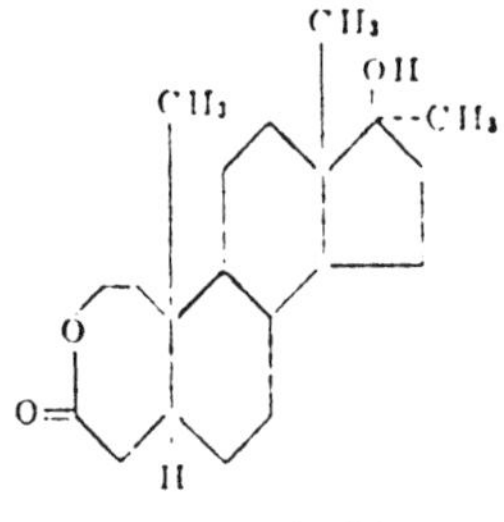

Example 31

The substitution of an equivalent quantity of 17β-hydroxy-5α-androstan-3-one in the procedure of Example 30 affords 2,17-dihydroxy-2,3-seco-5α-androstan-3-oic acid and 17β-hydroxy-3-oxa-A-homo-5α-androstan-4-one.

Example 32

The substitution of an equivalent quantity of 17β-hydroxy-3-oxa-A-homo-5α-androstan-4-one in the procedure of Example 7 results in 3-oxa-A-homo-5α-androstane-4,17-dione.

Example 33

A mixture of one part of 2α,17β-dihydroxy-17α-methyl-androst-4-en-3-one, 0.8 part of periodic acid dihydrate, 10 parts of pyridine, and 8 parts of water is stored at room temperature for about 24 hours. The resulting crystalline product is collected by filtration, washed with 50% aqueous pyridine, and dried to yield 17β-hydroxy-17α-methyl-2-oxo-2,3-seco-androst-4-en-3-oic acid, M.P. about 219–223° (dec.).

A mixture of one part of 17β-hydroxy-17α-methyl-2-oxo-2,3-seco-androst-4-en-3-oic acid, one part of sodium borohydride, and 10 parts of water is stirred at room temperature for about 16 hours, then is acidified with cold dilute hydrochloric acid. The acidic mixture is extracted with chloroform, and the organic extract is washed with water, dried over anhydrous sodium sulfate, and concentrated to dryness at room temperature under reduced pressure, resulting in 2,17β-dihydroxy-17α-methyl-2,3-seco-androst-4-en-3-oic acid, which melts at 155–162° with decomposition, resolidifies and melts at 182–184°.

A mixture of one part of 2,17β-dihydroxy-17α-methyl-2,3-seco-androst-4-en-3-oic acid and 80 parts of benzene is heated at the reflux temperature for about 15 minutes. The solvent is distilled at reduced pressure to afford 17β-hydroxy-17α-methyl-3-oxa-A-homo-androst-4a-en-4-one, M.P. about 182–184°, which is represented by the structural formula

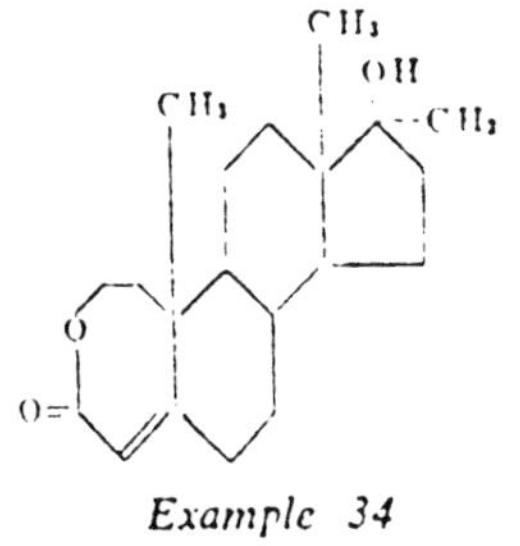

Example 34

The substitution of an equivalent quantity of 2α,17β-dihydroxyandrost-4-en-3-one in the procedure of Example

33 results in 17β-hydroxy-2-oxo-2,3-seco-androst-4-en-3-oic acid, 2,17β-dihydroxy-2,3-seco-androst-4-en-3-oic acid, and 17β-hydroxy-3-oxa-A-homo-androst-4a-en-4-one.

Example 35

The substitution of an equivalent quantity of 17β-hydroxy-3-oxa-A-homo-androst-4a-en-4-one in the procedure of Example 7 results in 3-oxa-A-homo-androst-4a-ene-4,17-dione.

Example 36

The substitution of an equivalent quanity of 17β-hydroxy-17α-methyl-3-oxa-A-homo-androst-4a-en-4-one in the procedure of Example 23 results in 17β-hydroxy-17α-methyl-3-oxa-A-homo-androst-5-en-4-one.

Example 37

The substitution of an equivalent quantity of 17β-hydroxy-3-oxa-A-homo-androst-4a-en-4-one in the procedure of Example 23 results in 17β-hydroxy-3-oxa-A-homo-androst-5-en-4-one.

Example 38

The substitution of an equivalent quantity of 17β-hydroxy-3-oxa-A-homo-androst-5-en-4-one in the procedure of Example 7 affords 3-oxa-A-homo-androst-5-ene-4,17-dione.

Example 39

A mixture of 1 part of 6β,17β-dihydroxy-17α-methyl-5α-estr-1-en-3-one, 80 parts of ethanol and 0.5 part of 5% palladium-on-carbon catalyst is stirred in a hydrogen atmosphere at atmospheric pressure until one molecular equivalent of hydrogen is absorbed. The catalyst is removed by filtration, and the filtrate is concentrated to dryness to afford 6β,17β-dihydroxy-17α-methyl-5α-estran-3-one.

To a solution of 1 part of 6β,17β-dihydroxy-17α-methyl-5α-estran-3-one in 30 parts of methylene chloride is added 2 parts by volume of 40% peracetic acid in acetic acid and 0.5 parts of dry sodium acetate, and this reaction mixture is stirred at room temperature for about 7 days, then is washed successively with water, aqueous potassium carbonate, and water, dried over anhydrous sodium sulfate, and evaporated to dryness. The residue is dissolved in benzene, chromatographed on silica gel, then eluted with 50% ether in benzene to afford 6β,17β-dihydroxy-17α-methyl-3-oxa-A-homo-5α-estran-4-one.

A mixture of 1 part of 6β,17β-dihydroxy-17α-methyl-3-oxa-A-homo-5α-estran-4-one, 0.74 part of methanesulfonyl chloride and 30 parts of pyridine is stored at 0° for about 16 hours, then is diluted with ice and water. Extraction with benzene affords an organic solution, which is washed with water, dried over anhydrous sodium sulfate, and concentrated to dryness. This residue is dissolved in 50 parts of pyridine, and the resulting solution is heated at reflux for about 3 hours, then is cooled, diluted with water, and extracted with benzene. The benzene layer is separated, washed with water, dried over anhydrous sodium sulfate, and evaporated to dryness to yield 17β-hydroxy-17α-methyl-3-oxa-A-homo-estr-4a-en-4-one.

Example 40

A mixture of 1 part of 17β-hydroxy-17α-methyl-3-oxa-A-homo-estr-4a-en-4-one, 50 parts of ethanol, and 7.5 parts of 5% palladium-on-carbon catalyst is stirred with hydrogen at atmospheric pressure until one molecular equivalent of hydrogen is absorbed. The catalyst is removed by filtration, and the filtrate is concentrated to dryness. The residue is dissolved in benzene, chromatographed on silica gel, and eluted with 50% ether in benzene to yield 17β-hydroxy-17α-methyl-3-oxa-A-homo-5β-estran-4-one and 17β-hydroxy-17α-methyl-3-oxa-A-homo-5α-estran-4-one.

Example 41

To a solution of 7.5 parts of 17β-hydroxy-2α,17α-dimethyl-5α-androstan-3-one in 15 parts of methylene chloride is added 3.3 parts by volume of a solution, prepared by dissolving 1 part of dry sodium acetate in 20 parts by volume of 40% peracetic acid in acetic acid. The mixture is stored at room temperature for about 4 days, then is diluted with benzene, washed successively with 5% aqueous potassium carbonate and water, dried over anhydrous sodium sulfate, and evaporated to dryness. The crystalline residue is triturated with benzene to yield 17β-hydroxy-2α,17α-dimethyl-3-oxa-A-homo-5α-androstan-4-one, M.P. about 214–230°.

Example 42

To a solution of one part of 17β-hydroxy-2α,17α-dimethyl-3-oxa-A-homo-5α-androstan-4-one in 16 parts of methanol is added 5% aqueous sodium hydroxide to pH 10, and this reaction mixture is heated on a steam bath for about 5 minutes, then is diluted with 30 parts of water, and is heated for about 30 minutes longer. This mixture is cooled, washed with chloroform, and acidified with dilute hydrochloric acid. The resulting precipitate is collected by filtration, washed with water, dried, and recrystallized from acetone to yield pure 2β-17β-dihydroxy-2α,17α-dimethyl-2,3-seco-5α-androstan-3-oic acid, M.P. about 190° (dec.).

Example 43

To a cooled solution of 4.2 parts of 17β-hydroxy-17α-methyl-1-oxo-1,2-seco-A-nor-5α-androstan-2-oic acid in 133 parts of tetrahydrofuran is added dropwise with stirring 28 parts by volume of 3 M ethereal methyl magnesium bromide. The mixture is stirred for about 30 minutes longer, then is treated dropwise with excess ethanol. This solution is treated with excess dilute hydrochloric acid, then is extracted with chloroform. The organic solution is concentrated to dryness, and the residue is dissolved in 24 parts of methanol, is treated with 30 parts of 10% aqueous sodium hydroxide. This mixture is heated on the steam bath for about 30 minutes, diluted with water, cooled, and washed with chloroform. The aqueous solution is cooled with ice, then is acidified with acetic acid to pH 5–6. The resulting acidic mixture is immediately extracted with chloroform. The organic layer is washed with aqueous sodium hydroxide, then is concentrated to dryness. Recrystallization from benzene affords 17β-hydroxy-1β,17α-dimethyl-2-oxa-5α-androstan-3-one, M.P. about 190–201°.

The foregoing aqueous sodium hydroxide washings are combined and acidified to pH 2–3 with cold dilute hydrochloric acid. The mixture is extracted with chloroform, and the organic extract is washed successively with aqueous sodium hydroxide and water, dried over anhydrous sodium sulfate, and concentrated to dryness at reduced pressure. The crystalline residue is recrystallized from benzene to yield 17β-hydroxy-1α,17α-dimethyl-2-oxa-5α-androstan-3-one, M.P. about 200–205°.

Example 44

The substitution of an equivalent quantity of 17β-hydroxy-17α-methyl-1-oxo-1,2-seco-A-norandrost-3-en-2-oic acid in the procedure of Example 43 results in -17β-hydroxy-1,17α-dimethyl-2-oxaandrost-4-en-3-one.

Example 45

The substitution of an equivalent quantity of 17β-hydroxy-1,17α-dimethyl-2-oxaandrost-4-en-3-one in the procedure of Example 23 results in 17β-hydroxy-1,17α-dimethyl-2-oxaandrost-5-en-3-one.

Example 46

The substitution of an equivalent quantity of ethyl magnesium bromide in the procedure of Example 43 affords the 1β-ethyl and 1α-ethyl isomers of 1-ethyl-17β-hydroxy-17α-methyl-2-oxa-5α-androstan-3-one.

Example 47

A mixture of 1 part of 17β-hydroxy-2-oxa-5α-androstan-3-one, 10 parts of acetic anhydride, and 20 parts of pyridine is allowed to stand at room temperature for about 15 hours, then is diluted with water. This aqueous mixture is extracted with benzene, and the benzene extract is washed successively with dilute hydrochloric acid and water, dried over anhydrous sodium sulfate, and concentrated to dryness in vacuo to yield 17β-acetoxy-2-oxa-5α-androstan-3-one, which displays characteristic infrared maxima at about 5.80 and 8.00 microns.

Example 48

The substitution of an equivalent quantity of 17β-hydroxy-2-oxa-5α-estran-3-one in the procedure of Example 47 results in 17β-acetoxy-2-oxa-5α-estran-3-one.

Example 49

The substitution of an equivalent quantity of 17β-hydroxy-2-oxaandrost-4-en-3-one in the procedure of Example 47 results in 17β-acetoxy-2-oxaandrost-4-en-3-one.

Example 50

The substitution of an equivalent quantity of propionic anhydride in the procedure of Example 47 results in 17β-propionoxy-2-oxa-5α-androstan-3-one, M.P. about 163°.

Example 51

A mixture of 1 part of 17β-hydroxy-17α-methyl-2-oxa-5α-androstan-3-one, 100 parts of isopropenyl acetate, and 0.1 part of p-toluenesulfonic acid monohydrate is stirred for about 5 hours, then is diluted with ether, washed with aqueous sodium bicarbonate, and evaporated to dryness in vacuo to afford 17β-acetoxy-17α-methyl-2-oxa-5α-androstan-3-one.

Example 52

The substitution of an equivalent quantity of 17β-hydroxy-17α-methyl-2-oxaandrost-4-en-3-one in the procedure of Example 51 results in 17β-acetoxy-17α-methyl-2-oxaandrost-4-en-3-one.

Example 53

The substitution of an equivalent quantity of 17β-hydroxy-17α-methyl-2-oxa-5α-estran-3-one in the procedure of Example 51 results in 17β-acetoxy-17α-methyl-2-oxa-5α-estran-3-one.

Example 54

The substitution of an equivalent quantity of isopropenyl propionate in the procedure of Example 51 results in 17α-methyl-17β-propionoxy-2-oxa-5α-androstan-3-one.

What is claimed is:

1. A compound of the formula

wherein R is selected from the group consisting of hydrogen and methyl, X is selected from the group of radicals consisting of carbonyl, β-hydroxymethylene, α-(lower alkyl)-β-hydroxymethylene, β-(lower alkanoyl)oxymethylene, and α-(lower alkyl)-β-(lower alkanoyl)oxymethylene, and the dotted lines indicate the optional presence of a double bond between carbon atom 5 and an adjacent secondary carbon atom.

2. A compound of the formula

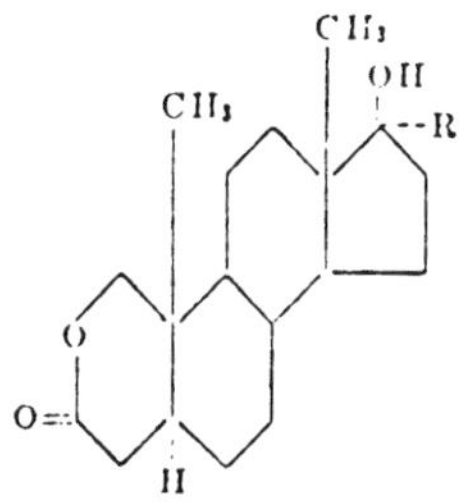

wherein R is an unsubstituted lower alkyl radical.

3. A compound of the formula

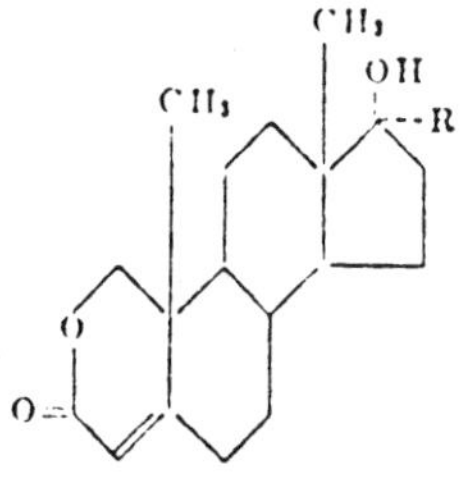

wherein R is an unsubstituted lower alkyl radical.

4. A compound of the formula

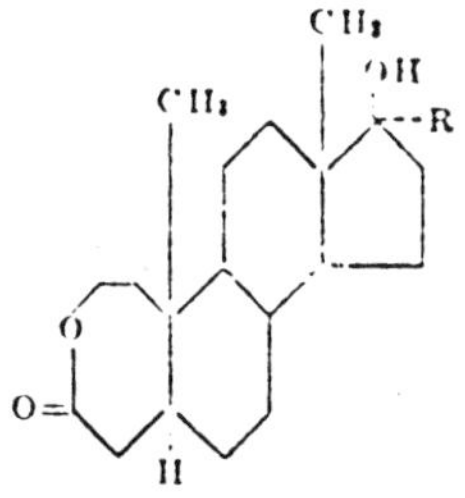

wherein R is an unsubstituted lower alkyl radical.

5. 17β-hydroxy-2-oxa-5α-androstan-3-one.

6. 17β-hydroxy-17α-methyl-2-oxa-5α-androstan-3-one.

7. 17α-ethyl-17β-hydroxy-2-oxa-5α-androstan-3-one.

8. 2-oxa-5α-androstane-3,17-dione.

9. 17β-hydroxy-2-oxaandrost-4-en-3-one.

10. 17β-hydroxy-17α-methyl-2-oxaandrost-4-en-3-one.

11. 2-oxaandrost-4-ene-3,17-dione.

12. 17β-hydroxy-1α,17α-dimethyl-2-oxa-5α-androstan-3-one.

13. 17β-hydroxy-1β,17α-dimethyl-2-oxa-5α-androstan-3-one.

14. 17β-hydroxy-17α-methyl-3-oxa-A-homo-5α-androstan-4-one.

15. 17β-hydroxy-2α,17α-dimethyl-3-oxa-A-homo-5α-androstan-4-one.

16. A compound of the formula

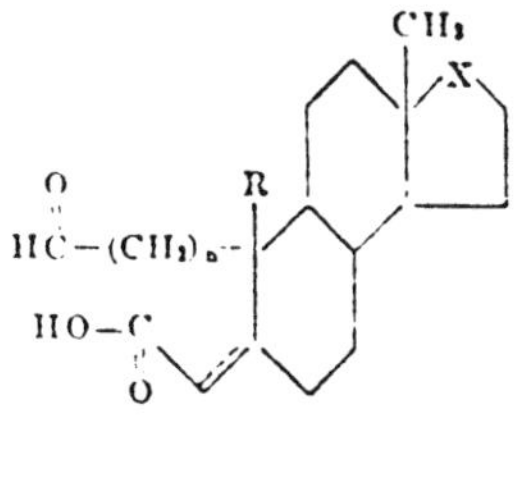

wherein R is selected from the group consisting of hydrogen and methyl, X is selected from the group of radicals consisting of carbonyl, β-hydroxymethylene, and α-(lower alkyl)-β-hydroxymethylene, n is selected from the group consisting of 0 and 1, and the dotted line indicates the optional presence of a 4,5-double bond.

17. 17β-hydroxy-17α-methyl-3-oxa-A-homo-androst-4a-en-4-one.

18. A compound of the formula

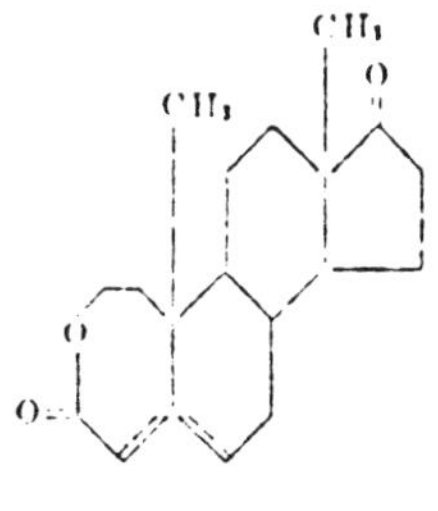

wherein the dotted lines indicate the presence of a double bond between carbon atom 5 and an adjacent carbon atom.

19. A compound of the formula

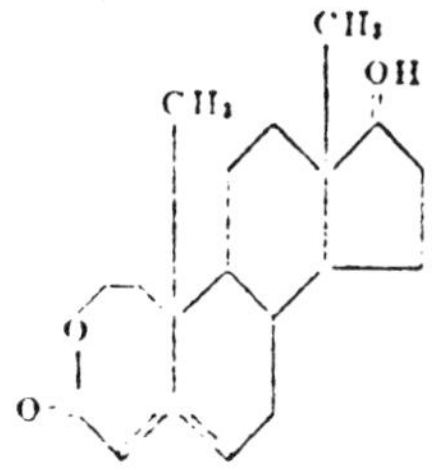

wherein the dotted lines indicate the presence of a double bond between carbon atom 5 and an adjacent carbon atom.

20. A compound of the formula

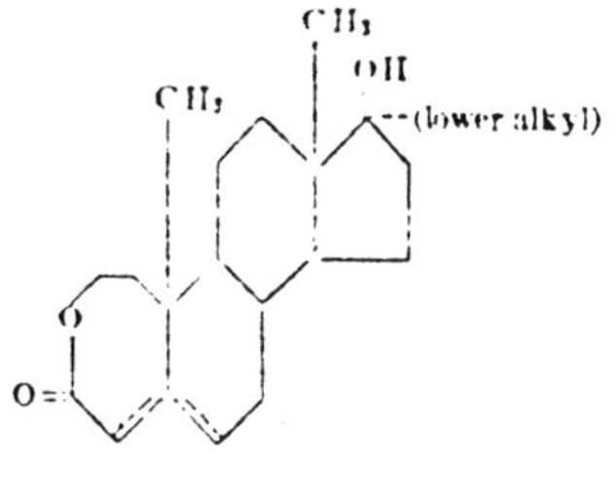

wherein the dotted lines indicate the presence of a double bond between carbon atom 5 and an adjacent carbon atom.

References Cited in the file of this patent

Rull et al.: Bull. Soc. Chim., Fr. (July-December 1958), p. 1579.

UNITED STATES PATENT OFFICE
CERTIFICATE OF CORRECTION

Patent No. 3,128,283   April 7, 1964

Raphael Pappo

It is hereby certified that error appears in the above numbered patent requiring correction and that the said Letters Patent should read as corrected below.

Column 22, lines 26 to 39, for that portion of the formula reading

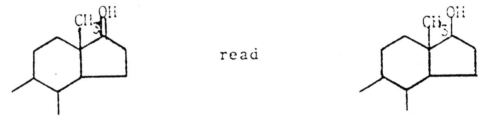

read

Signed and sealed this 19th day of October 1965.

CHAPTER TWELVE

1

3,060,201
4-HYDROXY-17α-METHYL-3-KETO - Δ⁴ - STEROIDS OF ANDROSTANE AND 19-NOR-ANDROSTANE SERIES AND ESTERS THEREOF
Bruno Camerino, Milan, Bianca Patelli, Stradella, and Giovanni Sala, Milan, Italy, assignors to Società Farmaceutici Italia, Milan, Italy, a corporation of Italy
No Drawing. Filed June 3, 1959, Ser. No. 817,744
Claims priority, application Great Britain June 6, 1958
18 Claims. (Cl. 260—397.4)

This invention relates to new steroid compounds, and their process of preparation.

This application is a continuation-in-part of our co-pending or co-filed application Serial No. 817,743, filed June 3, 1959, subsequently abandoned.

The new steroids are of the following general types:

Compounds A of the general formula:

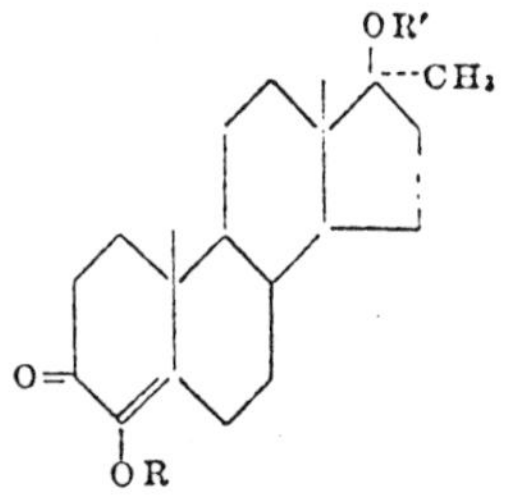

in which R and R' are hydrogen atoms or acyl groups each containing not more than 9 carbon atoms, R and R' being the same or different.

Compounds B, namely 4,11-beta-dihydroxy-17-alpha-methyl-testosterone and esters thereof, of the general formula:

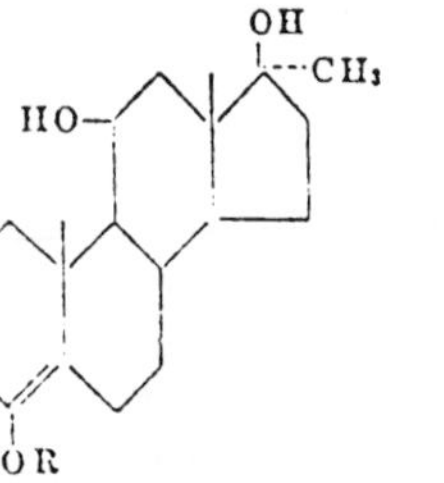

wherein R is hydrogen or an acyl group derived from an aliphatic, cyclic or partly cyclic carboxylic acid containing not more than 9 carbon atoms, for example from cyclo-pentane-propionic acid or benzoic acid.

Compounds C, namely 4-hydroxy-17-alpha-methyl-19-nortestosterone and esters thereof of the general formula:

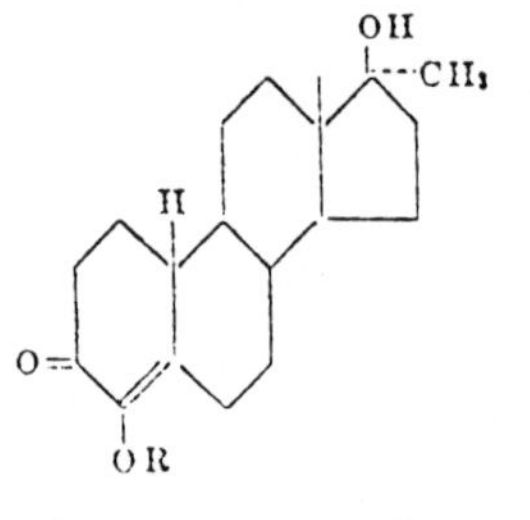

wherein R is hydrogen or an acyl group derived from an aliphatic, cyclic or partly cyclic carboxylic acid con-

2

taining not more than 9 carbon atoms, for example from cyclopentane-propionic acid or benzoic acid.

The preparation of the compounds of the types A, B, and C will be described in that order.

Preferred compounds of type A provided by the invention are 4-hydroxy - 17 - alpha-methyltestosterone, 4-hydroxy-17-alpha-methyltestosterone - 4 - acetate and 4-hydroxy-17-alpha-methyltestosterone - 4 - cyclopentylpropionate, 4-hydroxy-17-alpha - methyltestosterone-4-succinate, 4-hydroxy-17-alpha-methyltestosterone-4,17-diacetate, 4-hydroxy-17-alpha-methyltestosterone-17-acetate and 4-hydroxy-17-alpha-methyltestosterone-17-propionate.

The steroids of the present invention may be prepared according to the following reaction scheme:

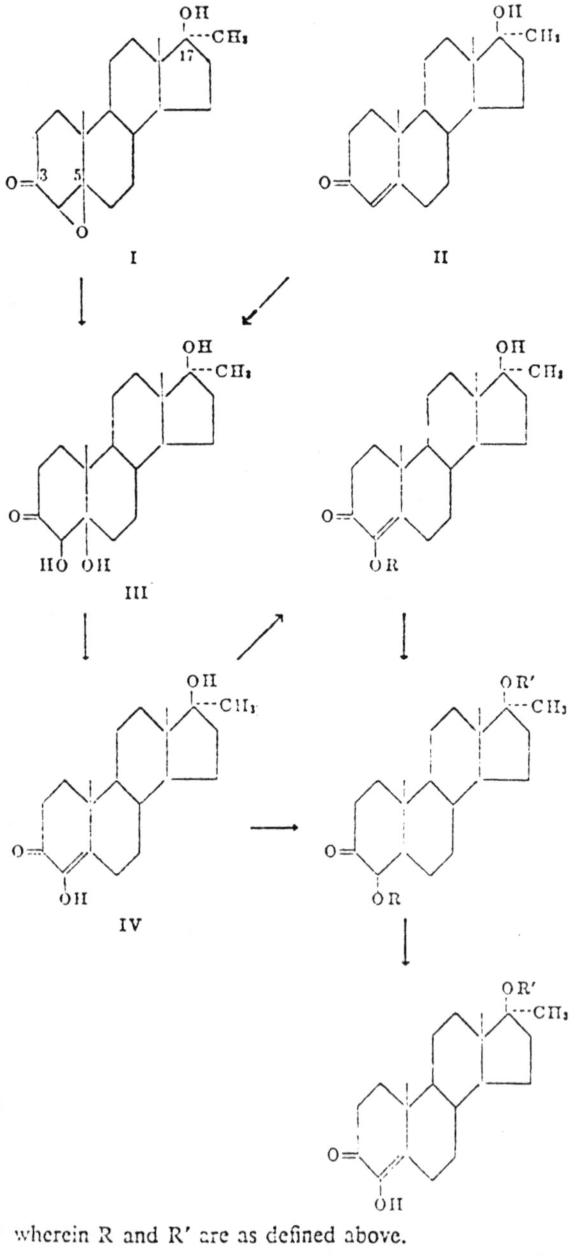

wherein R and R' are as defined above.

Thus the invention further provides a method of preparing 4-hydroxy-17-alpha-methyltestosterone which comprises selectively dehydrating 4,5-dihydroxy-17-alpha-methyltestosterone (III) in position 5 in alkaline solution. It is noted that said compound III is also, and perhaps preferably, named 17-alpha-methyl-androstane-4-beta,5-alpha,17-beta-triol-3-one.

In practising the process of the present invention, the said compound (III) may be obtained either from the corresponding 4,5-epoxide by reaction with dilute sulfuric acid in methanol solution at room temperature, or from 17-alpha-methyltestosterone. Preferably it is dehydrated with potassium hydroxide in water and methanol.

The dehydration, in which only the hydroxy group in position 5, and not the hydroxy group in position 17, is eliminated, is the most surprising part of the process of this invention.

It is known that the hydroxy group in position 17 of 17-alpha-methyltestosterone is eliminated very easily. Thus, by reacting the 4,5-diol with sulfuric and acetic acid mixture, sulfuric acid in benzene, formic acid or boron trifluoride in ether, compounds are obtained lacking the hydroxy group in position 17.

Only dehydration in alkaline solution causes selective elimination of the hydroxy group in position 5, the hydroxy group in position 17 remaining unaffected.

The hydroxy group in position 4 of 4-hydroxy-17-alpha-methyltestosterone (IV) may then be esterified by reaction with the chloride or anhydride of a carboxylic acid containing up to and including nine carbon atoms. The esterification of 4-hydroxy-17-alpha-methyltestosterone with the chloride or anhydride of a carboxylic acid in the presence of pyridinium chloride, provides the 4,17-diesters. The 17-monoesters of 4-hydroxy-17-alpha-methyltestosterone may be obtained by selective alkaline hydrolysis in 4-position of the 4,17-diesters.

The compounds of the invention provide highly active pharmacological agents. For example 4-hydroxy-17-alpha-methyltestosterone is a strong protein anabolic steroid, having a high myotrophic and low androgenic effect.

Its myotrophic activity is about three times higher than that of 17-alpha-methyltestosterone and at least 5 times higher than that of 17-alpha-ethyl-19-nortestosterone. Its androgenic activity is lower than that of 17-alpha-methyltestosterone.

It is also notable that while 4-hydroxy-testosterone acetate is devoid of oral activity, 4-hydroxy-17-alpha-methyltestosterone, one of the compounds provided by the present invention, is highly effective orally. Therefore, 4-hydroxy-17-alpha-methyltestosterone is useful for treatment of protein depletion, preparation for surgery, recovery from surgery, recovery from severe illness, nutritional care of carcinomatosis and chronic diseases, premature infants, wound healing, bone fracture and osteoporosis.

The following examples illustrate preferred embodiments of the invention.

EXAMPLE 1

4-Hydroxy-17-Alpha-Methyltestosterone (IV)

A solution of 1 g. of crude 4,5-oxido-17-alpha-methyltestosterone (I) in 50 ml. of methanol is allowed to stand at room temperature overnight with 10 ml. of water and 1 ml. of concentrated sulfuric acid. It is then poured into water containing sodium chloride and extracted three times with ethyl acetate. The solvent is washed with water, then with 10% sodium bicarbonate solution and again with water to neutrality. The residue remaining after evaporation of the solvent is crystallized from methanol, giving 17-alpha-methyl-androstane-4-beta,5-alpha,17-beta-triol-3-one with a melting point of 203–205° C.

A solution of 0.220 g. of 17-aipha-methyl-androstane-4-beta,5-alpha,17-beta-triol-3-one in 100 ml. of methanol is allowed to stand at room temperature for 22 hours, under nitrogen, with 0.300 g. of potassium hydroxide in 4 ml. of water and 20 ml. of methanol. The solution is

then neutralized with acetic acid, concentrated in vacuo, diluted with water and extracted three times with ethyl acetate. The extract is washed with water and the solvent removed by distillation. The remaining residue is chromatographed over Florisil 30–60 mesh. The fractions eluted with benzene and benzene-ether (10:1) are combined and by crystallization from ether-petroleum ether give 4-hydroxy-17-alpha-methyltestosterone (IV) (0.120 g.) melting at 168–170° C. and having an ultraviolet absorption maximum at 277 mμ, with a molecular extinction coefficient of 12,920.

EXAMPLE 2

4-Hydroxy-17-Alpha-Methyltestosterone (IV)

A solution of 20 g. of 17-alpha-methyltestosterone (II) in 500 ml. of trimethylcarbinol is treated by addition of 56 ml. of 30% hydrogen peroxide and 1 g. of osmium tetroxide in 80 ml. of trimethylcarbinol.

After the mixture has stood at room temperature for 22 hours, 12 ml. of hydrogen peroxide are added. The reaction mixture is allowed to stand at room temperature for an additional 20 hours, then concentrated in vacuo to one-third of its original volume, diluted with water, and the reaction product extracted with ethyl acetate. The extract is washed with water, several times with 10% sodium bisulphite solution, then with 4% sodium bicarbonate solution and finally with water to neutrality. The residue remaining after evaporation of the solvent does not show ultraviolet absorption. 1 g. of this crude substance, by crystallization from methanol, gives 17-alpha-methyl-androstane-4,5,17-beta-triol-3-one (0.400 g.) melting at 192–194° C.

A solution of 20 g. of crude 17-alpha-methyl-androstane-4,5,17-beta-triol-3-one in 1 liter of methanol is heated under reflux in a stream of nitrogen for 20 minutes; then 20 g. of potassium hydroxide in 40 ml. of water and 200 ml. of methanol are added. 5 minutes after the addition, the solution is treated by addition of 20 ml. of acetic acid and concentrated in vacuo. The residue is diluted with water containing sodium chloride and extracted three times with ethyl acetate. The extract is washed with 10% sodium bicarbonate solution and then with water to neutrality. The residue remaining after evaporation of the solvent is dissolved in acetone; addition of petroleum ether gives 4-hydroxy-17-alpha-methyltestosterone (8 g.) (IV) melting at 168–170° C. The mother liquors chromatographed over Florisil 30–60 mesh yield an additional 5 g. of the same substance melting at 168–170° C.

EXAMPLE 3

The 4-Acetate of 4-Hydroxy-17-Alpha-Methyltestosterone

A solution of 0.5 g. of 4-hydroxy-17-alpha-methyltestosterone in 3 ml. of pyridine is treated by addition of 0.5 ml. of acetic anhydride and allowed to stand at room temperature overnight; then ice is added, and after standing in an ice-bath for one hour, the mixture is extracted three times with ethyl acetate; the extract is washed with a 2-N hydrochloric acid solution, then with water, 10% sodium bicarbonate solution and again with water to neutrality. The residue (0.560) remaining after evaporation of the solvent is dissolved in ether, yielding, by addition of petroleum ether, 4-hydroxy-17-alpha-methyltestosterone-4-acetate (0.350 g.) melting at 138–140° C. and having an ultraviolet absorption maximum at 246 mμ, with a molecular extinction coefficient of 13,740.

EXAMPLE 4

The 4-Cyclopentylpropionate of 4-Hydroxy-17-Alpha-Methyltestosterone

In the same manner as Example 3, 4-hydroxy-17-alpha-methyltestosterone-4-cyclopentylpropionate is prepared by reacting 4-hydroxy-17-alpha-methyltestosterone

5

with more than one equivalent of cyclopentylpropionyl chloride in pyridine.

EXAMPLE 5

4-Hydroxy-17-Alpha-Methyltestosterone-4-Succinate

A mixture of 2 g. of 4-hydroxy-17-alpha-methyltestosterone, dissolved in 10 ml. of pyridine, and 2 g. of succinic anhydride is heated on a water bath for 1 hour and then allowed to stand at room temperature for two days.

After adding water and 2 N HCl, the solution is extracted with ethyl acetate. The extract is washed with water and 2 N NaOH. The alkaline solution is acidified with 2 N HCl and extracted again with ethyl acetate.

The extract which has been washed to neutrality is evaporated and the residue is crystallized from acetone/petroleum ether.

The product, melting at 161–163° C., has an ultraviolet absorption maximum at 247 mμ, with a molecular extinction coefficient of 14,650.

EXAMPLE 6

4-Hydroxy-17-Alpha-Methyltestosterone-4,17-Diacetate

A mixture of 5 g. of 4-hydroxy-17-alpha-methyltestosterone, 10 ml. acetic anhydride, 2.5 ml. pyridine and 1 g. pyridinium chloride, dissolved in 10 ml. of chloroform is heated to boiling for three hours.

The solvent is removed and the residue is treated with ice. The product is extracted with ethyl acetate. the extract is washed with 2 N HCl, water, 10% aqueous solution of NaHCO$_3$ and finally with water. After removing the solvent, ether is added. 3.5 g. of product, melting at 152–156° C., are obtained having an ultraviolet absorption maximum at 246 mμ, and a molecular extinction coefficient of 15,470.

EXAMPLE 7

4-Hydroxy-17-Alpha-Methyltestosterone-17-Acetate

500 mg. of 4-hydroxy-17-alpha-methyltestosterone-4,17-diacetate dissolved in 20 ml. of methanol, are treated with 500 mg. of KHCO$_3$ dissolved in 5 ml. of water, at 40° C. for 1 hour. The solution is cooled, neutralized with acetic acid, concentrated to a small volume and extracted with ethyl acetate. The neutral extract is evaporated and the residue crystallized from methanol.

The product (200 mg.) melts at 178–180° C., and has an ultraviolet absorption maximum at 277 mμ, with a molecular extinction coefficient of 12,450.

EXAMPLE 8

4-Hydroxy-17-Alpha-Methyltestosterone-17-Propionate

A mixture of 2 g. of 4-hydroxy-17-alpha-methyltestosterone-4-acetate, 10 ml. of pyridine, 4 ml. propionic anhydride, 400 mg. of pyridinium chloride in 2 ml. of chloroform, is heated to boiling for three hours and then allowed to stand at room temperature for a night. Ice is added to the solution with stirring. After stirring for 1 hour the product is extracted with ethyl acetate and the extract is washed with 2 N HCl, water, an aqueous 10% solution of NaHCO$_3$ and finally with water.

The solvent is evaporated and the residue (2.4 g.) dissolved in 80 ml. of methanol, is treated with 2.4 g. of KHCO$_3$ in 20 ml. of water, at 40° C. for 1 hour. The cooled solution is neutralized with acetic acid, concentrated to a small volume and extracted with ethyl acetate. The extract is evaporated to dryness.

The residue is crystallized from methanol.

The product (500 mg.) melts at 172–174° C. and has an ultraviolet absorption maximum at 277 mμ, with a molecular extinction coefficient of 11,860.

Pharmacological Activities—Anabolic Activity

Myotrophic and androgenic activity of 4-hydroxy-17-

6

alpha-methyltestosterone per os were determined according to the method of Herschberger, Shipley and Meyer (Proc. Soc. Exp. Biol. and Med. 83, 175 (1953)). The results are shown in Table I.

TABLE I.—MYOTROPHIC AND ANDROGENIC ACTIVITY OF 4-HYDROXY-17-ALPHA-METHYLTESTOSTERONE AND OTHER STEROIDS. ALL THE STEROIDS ARE APPLIED "PER OS"

Steroid	Animals No.	Dose, mg./die/7 days	Levator ani, mg.	Ventral prostate, mg.	Therapeutic index
Controls	174		8.6±0.33	9.3±0.41	
17-alpha-methyltestosterone	41	1	13.4	36.3	0.38
	77	2	17.7	43.9	0.29
	6	4	25.5	73.7	0.26
17-alpha-ethyl-19-nortestosterone	10	1	12.5	15.4	0.64
	10	2	16.2	19.2	0.77
	9	4	20.5	31.5	0.54
4-hydroxytestosterone acetate	6	2	8.01	10.8	
4-hydroxy-17-alpha-methyltestosterone	10	0.5	22.6	32.4	0.61
	9	1	22.8	29.7	0.66
	9	2	30.7	48.1	0.57
4-hydroxy-17-alpha-methyltestosterone-4-acetate	7	1	25.3	37.8	0.58
4-hydroxy-17-alpha-methyltestosterone-4-cyclopentyl-propionate	7	1	23.3	34.8	0.57

The results show that 4-hydroxy-17-alpha-methyltestosterone per os possesses a high myotrophic and low androgenic effect. Its myotrophic activity is about 3 times higher than that of 17-alpha-methyltestosterone, and at least 5 times higher than that of 17-alpha-ethyl-19-nortestosterone. Its androgenic activity is definitely lower than that of 17-alpha-methyltestosterone. Therefore 4-hydroxy-17-alpha-methyltestosterone presents a good therapeutic index (levator ani weight increase/ ventral prostate weight increase) definitely higher than 17-alpha-methyltestosterone and comparable with 17-alpha-ethyl-19-nortestosterone.

It is worth mentioning that while 4-hydroxytestosterone acetate is devoid of oral activity, its 17-alpha-methyl derivative is orally highly effective.

Other Hormonal Effects

4-hydroxy-17-alpha-methyltestosterone is devoid of progestational activity; in fact it does not stimulate the uterine proliferation in immature rabbits primed with estradiol.

At a dosage 4 times higher than desoxycorticosterone acetate it does not present Na-retaining activity in adrenal-ectomized rats.

Other alkaline reagents soluble in a lower alkanol can be used in the dehydration of the 4,5-dehydroxy compound, viz. sodium and ammonium hydroxides.

Since our principal purpose is to make steroids of high anabolic activity by oral administration, our principal present interest, in respect to the esters, is in the type described above, and especially in the acetate and cyclopropionate. However, it is obvious to chemists, and is within the broader purview of this invention, to prepare esters of other types such as of polycarboxylic acids, and of carboxylic acids generally, containing substituents such as halo, sulphonyl, amino, nitro, and also esters of inorganic acids.

The carbon skeleton of the 4,5-dihydroxy-17-alpha-methyltestosterone is preferably unsubstituted, but the dehydration step described above is also considered generally applicable, i.e. to compounds in which said skeleton contains substituents.

The preparation of the compounds of type B will now be described.

The invention further provides a method of preparing 4,11-beta-dihydroxy-17-alpha-methyltestosterone which comprises dehydrating 4,5,11-beta-trihydroxy-17-alpha-

7

methyltestosterone (IIIA) in position 5 only, said dehydration being effected in alkaline solution, preferably by employing a methanolic solution of potassium hydroxide. Said compound IIIA is also termed 17-alpha-methyl-androstane,4,5,11-beta,17-beta-tetrol-3-one.

To obtain the esters, 4,11-beta-dihydroxy-17-alpha-methyltestosterone is reacted with a chloride or anhydride of a carboxylic acid as defined above. The esterification may be effected in the presence of a tertiary amine.

The essence of the method of this aspect of the invention is the dehydration whereby only the hydroxy group in position 5 and not that in position 17 is eliminated.

It is known in fact, that the hydroxy group in the 17-position of 17-alpha-methyltestosterone and 17-alpha-methyl-19-nortestosterone can be eliminated very easily. By reaction of the 4,5-diol-compound with a mixture of sulfuric and acetic acids, sulfuric acid in benzene, formic acid, borontrifluoride in ether, compounds are obtained lacking the 17-hydroxy group.

Only dehydration in alkaline solution causes selective elimination of the hydroxy group in the 5-position, the hydroxy group in 17-position remaining unaffected.

It has been found that 4,11-beta-dihydroxy-17-alpha-methyltestosterone is a strong protein anabolic steroid, having a high myotrophic and low androgenic effect. It possesses a strong myotrophic activity, 6–10 times higher than that of 17-alpha-methyltestosterone and the same androgenic effect as 17-alpha-methyltestosterone.

Therefore 4,11-beta-dihydroxy-17-alpha-methyltestosterone, orally highly effective, is useful in the treatment of protein depletion, preparation for surgery, recovery from surgery, recovery from severe illness, nutritional care of carcinomatosis and chronic diseases, premature infants, wound healing, bone fractures and osteoporosis.

The following example is given to illustrate the invention.

EXAMPLE 9

4,11-Beta-Dihydroxy-17-Alpha-Methyltestosterone

A solution of 1.35 g. of 11-beta-hydroxy-17-alpha-methyltestosterone in 40 ml. of trimethylcarbinol is treated by addition of 4.2 ml. of 36% H_2O_2, 0.8 ml. of water and 0.084 g. of OsO_4 dissolved in 6.7 ml. of trimethylcarbinol.

The solution is allowed to stand for 42 hours at room temperature, then concentrated to one third of its original volume and diluted with water. A 10% aqueous solution of sodium bisulphite is added up to precipitation and then an aqueous solution of sodium bicarbonate to neutrality. The osmium salt is filtered off and the solution is concentrated to a small volume under vacuum.

The residue is treated with 20 ml. of hot methanol and boiled with 1 g. of KOH dissolved in 10 ml. of methanol for 5 minutes in a nitrogen atmosphere. The solution is neutralized with acetic acid, concentrated to a small volume under reduced pressure and extracted with ethyl acetate. The extract is washed with water and evaporated.

The residual product (0.75 g.) is chromatographed over Florisil (30–60 mesh). The fractions eluted with benzene-ether (3:1) yield 4,11-beta-dihydroxy-17-alpha-methyltestosterone melting at 183–185° C. and having an ultraviolet absorption maximum at 278 mμ with a molecular extinction coefficient of 12,040.

Treatment of 4,11-beta-dihydroxy-17-alpha-methyl-testosterone with an acylating agent such as an acyl halide or acyl anhydride in a tertiary amine such as pyridine, at room temperature, causes selective acylation of the hydroxy group in the 4-position, the hydroxy group in the 17-position remaining unaffected. In this way the 4-esters such as the acetate, propionate, cyclopentylpropionate, benzoate, phenylpropionate can be obtained.

Myotrophic and Androgenic Activity

Oral myotrophic and androgenic activity of 4,11-beta-dihydroxy-17-alpha-methyltestosterone has been examined

8

on the castrated immature rat according to levator ani muscle and ventral prostate test (L. G. Herschberger, E. G. Shipley, R. K. Meyer, Proc. Soc. Exp. Biol. Med. 83, 1953, p. 175).

The results are shown in Table II.

TABLE II.—ORAL MYOTROPHIC AND ANDROGENIC ACTIVITY OF 4,11-BETA-DIHYDROXY - 17 - ALPHA-METHYLTESTOSTERONE (THE FIGURES IN PARENTHESIS INDICATE THE NUMBER OF THE ANIMALS)

Steroid	Daily dose, mg.	Levator ani, mg.	Ventral prostate, mg.	Therapeutic index
Controls		8.6	9.3	
17-alpha-methyltestosterone (41)	1	13.4	25.3	0.13
17-alpha-methyltestosterone (77)	2	17.7	43.9	0.21
17-alpha-methyltestosterone (9)	4	25.5	73.7	0.25
4,11-beta-dihydroxy-17-alpha-methyltestosterone (8)	0.1	21.2	22.7	0.04
Do	0.25	21.6	21.1	1.21
Do	0.5	24.2	27	0.88
Do	2	31.9	48.4	0.53

The data summarized in Table II demonstrate that 4,11-beta-dihydroxy-17-alpha-methyltestosterone possesses a strong myotrophic activity, 6–10 times higher than that of 17-alpha-methyltestosterone and the same androgenic effect as 17-alpha-methyltestosterone.

The preparation of the compounds of type C will now be described.

The invention further provides a method of preparing 4-hydroxy-17-alpha-methyl-19-nortestosterone which comprises dehydrating 4,5-dihydroxy-17-alpha-methyl-19-nortestosterone (IIIB) in position 5 only, said dehydration being effected in alkaline solution, preferably by employing a methanolic solution of potassium hydroxide, at room temperature (15 to 35° C.). Said compound IIIB is also termed 17-alpha-methyl-19-norandrostane, 4,5,17-triol-3-one.

To obtain the esters, 4-hydroxy-17-alpha-methyl-19-nortestosterone is reacted with a chloride or anhydride of a carboxylic acid as defined above. The esterification may be effected in the presence of a tertiary amine.

The essence of the method of the invention is the dehydration whereby only the hydroxy group in position 5 and not that in position 17 is eliminated. It is known in fact that the hydroxy group in the 17-position of 17-alpha-methyl-19-nortestosterone can be very easily eliminated. By reaction of the 4,5-diol-compound with a mixture of sulfuric and acetic acid, sulfuric acid in benzene, formic acid, borontrifluoride in ether, compounds are obtained lacking the 17-hydroxy group.

Only dehydration in alkaline solution at room temperature causes selective elimination of the hydroxy group in 5-position, the hydroxy group in 17-position remaining unaffected.

4-hydroxy-17-alpha - methyl - 19 - nortestosterone possesses high myothrophic and androgenic properties. Its myotrophic activity is about 27 times higher than that of 17-alpha-methyltestosterone and its androgenic activity is 5 times higher than that of the same product, when both the steroids are administered per os. Therefore 4-hydroxy-17-alpha-methyl-19-nortestosterone is useful as androgen in the treatment of symptoms of male climacteric, male hypogondaism, menopausal symptoms, menorrhagia, metrorrhagia, and as anabolic in the treatment of protein carency.

The following example is given to illustrate the invention.

EXAMPLE 10

4-Hydroxy-17-Alpha-Methyl-19-Nortestosterone

A solution of 1 g. of 17-alpha-methyl-19-nortestosterone in 26 ml. of trimethyl-carbinol is treated by addition of 2.8 ml. of 30% hydrogen peroxide and 0.050 g. of osmium tetroxide in 4.5 ml. of trimethylcarbinol.

After the reaction mixture has stood at room temperature for 20 hours, an additional 0.5 ml. of hydrogen peroxide is added. The solution is allowed to stand for 22 hours, then concentrated to one third of its original volume, diluted with water and extracted four times with ethyl acetate. The extract is washed with water, several times with 10% sodium bisulphite solution, then with 4% sodium bicarbonate solution and finally with water to neutrality. The crude 17-alpha-methyl-19-nortestosterone-4,5-diol remaining after distillation of the solvent does not show ultraviolet absorption. It is then dissolved in 500 ml. of methanol and treated by addition of 1.5 g. of KOH in 20 ml. of water, and 100 ml. of methanol in a nitrogen atmosphere. The solution is allowed to stand at room temperature overnight, then neutralized with acetic acid and concentrated to a small volume; it is then diluted with water containing NaCl and extracted with ethyl acetate.

The extract is washed with water and the solvent removed. The residual product is chromatographed over Florisil 30–60 mesh. The fraction eluted with benzene and benzene-ether (9:1) yield the 4-hydroxy-17-alpha-methyl-19-nortestosterone melting at 168–170° C. and having an ultraviolet absorption maximum at 277 mμ, with a molecular extinction coefficient of 12,750.

Treatment of 4-hydroxy-17-alpha-methyl-19-nortestosterone with an acylating agent such as an acyl halide or acyl anhydride in a tertiary amine such as pyridine, at room temperature, causes selective acylation of the hydroxy group in 4-position, the 17-position remaining unaffected. In this way the 4-esters such as the acetate, propionate, cyclopentylpropionate, benzoate and phenylpropionate can be obtained.

Pharmacological Activities

(1) Oral myotrophic and androgenic activity of 4-hydroxy-17-alpha-methyl-19-nortestosterone were examined according to the levator ani muscle and the ventral prostate test in the castrated male rat (L. G. Herschberger, E. G. Shipley, R. K. Meyer, Proc. Soc. Exp. Biol. Med., 83, 1953, p. 175).

The results are summarized in Table III.

TABLE III.—MYOTROPHIC AND ANDROGENIC ACTIVITY IN CASTRATED RATS (THE FIGURES IN PARENTHESIS INDICATE THE NUMBER OF ANIMALS)

Steroid	Daily dose, mg.	Method of administration	Levator ani, mg.	Ventral prostate, mg.	Therapeutic index
Controls (174)			8.6	9.3	
17 - alpha - methyltestosterone (41)	1	Oral	13.4	36.3	0.18
17 - alpha - methyltestosterone (77)	2	do	17.7	43.9	0.26
17 - alpha - methyltestosterone (6)	4	do	25.5	73.7	0.26
17 - alpha - etyl - 19 - nortestosterone (10)	1	do	12.5	15.4	0.64
Do	2	do	16.2	19.2	0.77
17 - alpha - ethyl - 19 - nortestosterone (9)	4	do	20.5	31.5	0.54
4 - hydroxy - 17 - alpha - methyltestosterone (10)	0.5	do	22.6	32.4	0.61
4 - hydroxy - 17 - alpha - methyltestosterone (9)	1	do	22.8	30.7	0.66
Do	2	do	30.7	48.1	0.57
4 - hydroxy - 17 - alpha - methyl - 19 - nortestosterone (8)	0.1	do	18.6	23.7	0.69
Do	0.25	do	27.3	34.1	0.77
Do	0.5	do	37.1	49.3	0.71

The data of Table III show that 4-hydroxy-17-alpha-methyl-19-nortestosterone possesses strong myotrophic and androgenic properties, respectively 27 and 5 times more valuable than those of 17-alpha-methyltestosterone, when both the steroids are administered per os.

(2) Androgenic activity of 4-hydroxy-17-alpha-methyl-19-nortestosterone was also tested on the chick's comb test (Munson R.L., Shops M.C., Endocrinol. 62, 1958, p. 173). The results are shown in Table IV.

TABLE IV.—ANDROGENIC ACTIVITY (CHICK'S COMB TEST-LOCAL APPLICATION)

Steroid	Daily dose γ	Comb growth index
Androsterone	0.1	65.6
Do	0.4	76.7
Do	1.6	95.4
17-alpha-methyltestosterone	0.1	62.4
Do	0.4	81.4
Do	1.6	92
4 - hydroxy - 17 - alpha - methyl - 19 - nortestosterone		83.6
Do	0.4	85.6
Do	0.8	92.1
Do	1.6	

The results summarized in Table IV demonstrate that 4-hydroxy-17-alpha-methyl-19-nortestosterone possesses the same androgenic activity as 17-alpha-methyl-testosterone and androsterone, when locally tested on the chick's comb.

(3) Other hormonal activities: 4-hydroxy-17-alpha-methyl-19-nortestosterone possesses a strong antiestrogenic activity (Edgren and Calhoun: Proc. Soc. Exp. Biol. Med., 94, 1957, p. 537). It does in fact inhibit the uterotrophic effect of oestrone in immature female mice. Its potency is about 2.5 times that of testosterone propionate.

4-hydroxy-17-alpha-methyl-19-nortestosterone does not present progestational activity (McPhail, J. Physiol. 83, 1955, p. 145); estrogenic activity (Rubin et al. Endrocinol., 49, 1951, p. 429); liver glycogen deposition (Stafford et al., Proc. Soc. Exp. Biol. Med., 89, 1955, p. 371) and antiinflammatory effect (Singer, Borman: Fed. Proc., 14, 1955, p. 281).

We claim:

1. A compound of the general formula

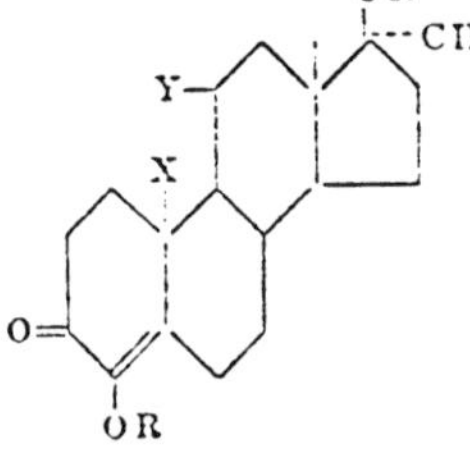

in which R and R' are taken from the group consisting of hydrogen and the same or different acyl radicals each containing not more than 9 carbon atoms, the acyl group being of the formula R_3CO— and being the acyl radical of an acid taken from the group consisting of aliphatic, aromatic, and alicyclic and aromatic substituted aliphatic acids, R_3 being a hydrocarbon group, X being taken from the class consisting of hydrogen and methyl, Y being taken from the class consisting of hydrogen and hydroxy.

2. The compounds of the formula:

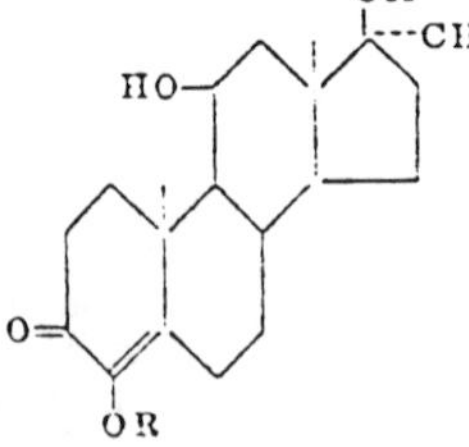

in which R is taken from the group consisting of H and acyl radicals containing not more than 9 carbon atoms, of the formula R_3CO— in which R_3 is a hydrocarbon group.

3. The compound, 4,11 - beta - dihydroxy - 17 - alpha - methyltestosterone.

11

4. The compounds of the formula:

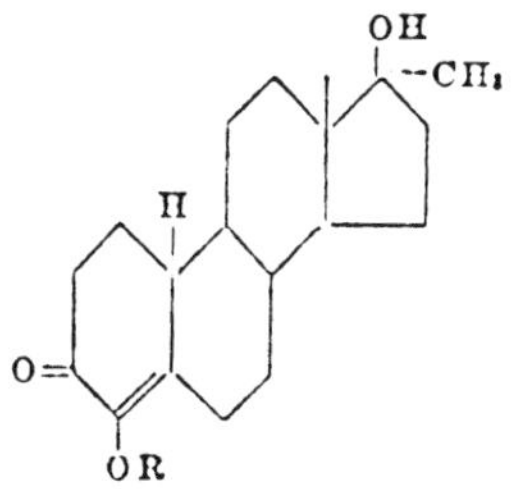

in which R is taken from the group consisting of H and acyl radicals containing not more than 9 carbon atoms, of the formula R₃CO in which R₃ is a hydrocarbon group.

5. The compound, 4-hydroxy-17-alpha-methyl-19-nor-testosterone.

6. A compound of the formula:

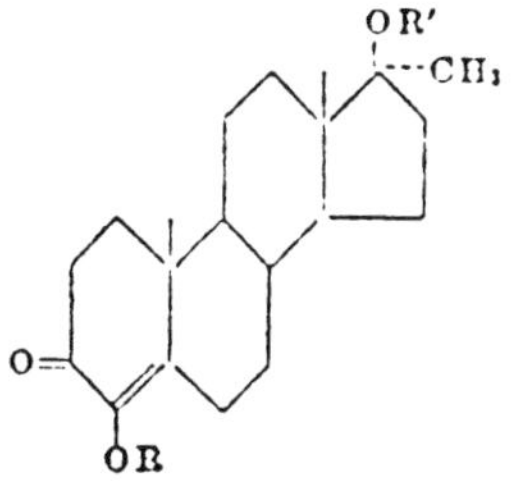

wherein R and R′ are taken from the group consisting of hydrogen and —COR″, in which R″ is a hydrocarbon radical having no more than 9 carbon atoms.

7. 4-hydroxy-17-alpha-methyltestosterone.

12

8. 4-acetoxy-17-alpha-methyltestosterone.

9. The 4-cyclopentylpropionate of 4-hydroxy-17-alpha-methyltestosterone.

10. 4-hydroxy-17-alpha-methyltestosterone-4-succinate.

11. 4 - hydroxy - 17-alpha-methyltestosterone-4,17-diacetate.

12. 4-hydroxy-17-alpha-methyltestosterone-17-acetate.

13. 4 - hydroxy-17-alpha-methyltestosterone-17-propionate.

14. A process of making 4-hydroxy-17-alpha-methyltestosterone comprising allowing a compound of the group consisting of 17-alpha-methylandrostane-4-beta,5-alpha.17-beta-triol-3-one and the corresponding 5-beta compound to stand for at least several hours at about room temperature, in a gas atmosphere inert to the reaction, in an aqueous methanol solution of KOH.

15. 4,11-beta-dihydroxy-17-alpha-methyl-testosterone-4-acetate.

16. 4,11 - beta-dihydroxy-17-alpha-methyl-testosterone-4-cyclopentylpropionate.

17. 4 - hydroxy-17-alpha-methyl-19-nortestosterone-4-acetate.

18. 4 - hydroxy-17-alpha-methyl-19-nortestosterone-4-cyclopentylpropionate.

References Cited in the file of this patent

UNITED STATES PATENTS

2,908,682   Bible et al. _____ Oct. 13, 1959

OTHER REFERENCES

"Journal of American Chemical Society" (1956), vol. 78, article by Camerino et al., page 3541 relied on.

CHAPTER THIRTEEN

1

2,927,921

PROCESS FOR THE MANUFACTURE OF 3-KETALS OF POLYKETO STEROIDS AND PRODUCTS OBTAINED THEREBY

Eugene P. Oliveto, Bloomfield, and Emanuel B. Hershburg, West Orange, N.J., assignors to Schering Corporation, Bloomfield, N.J., a corporation of New Jersey

No Drawing. Application May 19, 1954
Serial No. 430,998

16 Claims. (Cl. 260—239.55)

The present invention relates to an improved procedure for selectively blocking the 3-keto group of polyketic steroids having one of their keto groups in the 3-position, whereby various chemical operations can be conducted on the unprotected keto group or groups, or on certain of them, after which the protected keto group or groups can be regenerated, and to certain products obtained by such procedure.

This application is a continuation-in-part of our copending application Serial No. 322,354, filed November 24, 1952, now U.S. Patent 2,773,888.

It is the general object of the present invention to provide an improved procedure for the preparation of various 3-keto-hydroxy steroids and their esters and other functional derivatives from the corresponding polyketo compounds.

A further object of the invention is to produce new 3-keto-hydroxy steroids and their functional derivatives which possess physiological activity or can serve as intermediates for the preparation of other compounds of therapeutic value.

A more specific object of the invention is to convert polyketo steroids wherein one of the keto groups is in the 3-position, into 3-ketals, while the other keto group or groups remain free and so can be operated on to alter them chemically, or even to remove them, after which the 3-keto group can be regenerated.

Other objects and advantages of the invention will become apparent as the more detailed description thereof proceeds.

The 3-keto group is one of the more reactive of the keto groups present in steroid compounds, so that it is generally impossible to operate on the other keto groups without at the same time altering the 3-keto group. However, in many instances it is necessary to preserve, in the final product, the 3-keto group of the starting or of an intermediate compound. A procedure whereby the 3-keto group is selectively blocked in the presence of one or more other keto groups, whereby such other keto groups can be chemically transformed, after which the 3-keto group can be easily regenerated, accordingly presents a highly advantageous and commercially valuable manipulation in the field of steroid synthesis.

We have found that in the presence of certain catalysts the 3-keto group, provided that it is not conjugated to a double bond, can be selectively ketalized with alcohols and thereby protected against reagents employed to alter the remaining keto group or groups, provided further that such reagents do not operate to hydrolyze the 3-ketal group. After the chemical operations on the free keto groups are completed, the ketal group is hydrolyzed to regenerate the keto group. By such proce-

2

which heretofore have baffled synthesis, while known compounds can be obtained in a simpler manner and/or in greater yield.

According to our invention, relatively stable ketals can be produced by reacting alcohols in the presence of an anhydride of a relatively weak inorganic acid with 3-keto steroids having one or more additional keto groups, there being no double bond in the 1,2 or 4,5-positions. The inorganic anhydride should be one which combines chemically with the water formed by the resulting ketalization, so that such water is removed from the reaction mixture and the reaction thereby caused to proceed in the desired direction. It may at this point be mentioned that while the invention is of particular advantage in the selective blocking of the 3-keto group of polyketo steroids, whereby chemical operations on the other keto groups are made possible without affecting the 3-keto group, it will be obvious that our process is applicable also to 3-keto steroids having no other keto group but instead being susceptible at other points in the molecule, for example, to reduction, as for the saturation of nuclear double bonds in rings B, C and D, or the reduction of an ester group to an alcohol group, etc., which would cause simultaneous reduction, in whole or in part, of the 3-keto group were it left free. However, since the commercially most valuable form of our invention at the present time is in connection with the selective reduction of certain keto groups of polyketo steroids while protecting the 3-keto group against reduction, the invention will be further described in connection with polyketo steroids (of which one keto group is always in the 3-position) and the chemical conversion or elimination of keto groups other than the 3-keto group.

While various inorganic anhydrides capable of stably binding the water that is liberated during the ketalization can be employed, such as B_2O_3 and SO_2, we have obtained best results with selenium dioxide (SeO_2) and the most satisfactory embodiments of our invention will accordingly be described with the use of such compound as the catalyst. Also, although various alcohols can be employed for the manufacture of the corresponding ketals, such as benzyl and β-phenethyl alcohols, we prefer to employ the lower aliphatic alcohols (i.e. those having from 1 to 5 carbon atoms) and, in particular, methyl alcohol, which will accordingly be employed by way of illustration in the more detailed disclosure hereinafter. The primary alcohols are preferred although some secondary alcohols can be utilized, like isobutyl alcohol. Tertiary alcohols, like tertiary butyl alcohol, are generally unsatisfactory, as is isopropyl alcohol. Ethyl, n-propyl, n-butyl and n-amyl alcohols are suitable for our process, as are polyhydric alcohols like ethylene and propylene glycols.

While our invention will operate with any saturated 3-ketone, the yield of ketal drops markedly when the starting compound is substituted at the 2 and/or 4 position, as by relatively large atoms or groups, such as chlorine, bromine, or iodine atoms. However, we have found a way to increase the yields of these ketal compounds by adding to the reaction mixture (containing the steroid, an alcohol or glycol, and selenium dioxide) a small amount of a strong acid, e.g. p-toluene sulfonic acid, benzene sulfonic acid, trichloracetic acid, or perchloric acid. While in such case the strong acid alone gives none of the desired ketal, and selenium dioxide mixture of the two gives excellent yields of 3-ketals containing substituents at positions 2 and/or 4. The strong acid may be present also during the ketalization of 3-keto steroids which are not substituted in the 2 and/or 4 positions, but generally will not then markedly affect the yield of ketal.

In carrying out our process, the polyketo steroid is reacted with the alcohol, preferably methanol, in the presence of a selenium dioxide at room or at moderately elevated temperature to form the 3-ketal. The so formed ketal can then be subjected to a variety of reactions which may or may not involve the other keto groups present. Thus, the ketal can be pyrolyzed to yield a 3-methoxy-Δ^3-steroid, which can then be brominated to produce the 3-keto-4-bromo compound. Upon dehydrobromination, the Δ^4-unsaturation characteristic of cortisone and other steroid hormones can be produced. On the other hand, the 3-ketal can be reacted with a reducing agent to effect reduction of, for example, a 20-keto group, after which the 3-keto group can be regenerated by acid hydrolysis. Where the less reactive 11-keto grouping is also present, a 20-keto group can be selectively reduced while the 11-keto remains unaffected; or, where the 11-keto is likewise reduced, it can be oxidized to a keto group, as with N-bromoacetamide or other N-halogeno-acylamide, like N-bromosuccinimide after acylation of the 20-hydroxyl with acetic, propionic, butyric, benzoic or other acid or anhydride.

Referring more particularly to specific reactions, we have found that pregnan-17α,21-diol-3,11,20-trione 21-acetate (I), reacted with methanol in the presence of selenium dioxide, yields the 3,3-dimethoxy ketal (II). Upon pyrolysis, methanol was eliminated from the ketal to yield 3-methoxy-Δ^3-pregnen-17α,21-diol-3,11-trione 21-acetate (III). The addition of bromine produced the known 4-bromopregnan-17α,21-diol-3,11,20-trione 21-acetate (IV), while dehydrobromination gave the unsaturated compound V.

Pregnan-17α-ol-3,11,20-trione (VI), pregnan-3,11,20-trione (XI) and pregnan-11β,17α-diol-3,20-dione (XVII) all gave the corresponding 3,3-dimethoxy ketals upon reaction with selenium dioxide in methanol. These in turn were converted to the known 3,11-diketo 20β-acetoxy compounds (X and XVI).

The final steps in the preparation of cortisone acetate (Δ^4-pregnen-17α,21-diol-3,11,20-trione 21-acetate) from bile acids comprise the bromination of pregnan-17α,21-diol-3,11,20-trione 21-acetate (I) in the C-4 position (V. Mattox and E. C. Kendall, J. Biol. Chem., 185, 593 (1950)), followed by the elimination of hydrogen bromide and formation of the 4,5-double bond via the dinitrophenylhydrazone or semicarbazone (V. Mattox and E. C. Kendall, ibid., 188, 287 (1951); B. Koechlin, T. Kritchevsky and T. F. Gallagher, ibid., 184, 393 (1950)), either of which ketone condensates may be converted to the 3-ketone by reaction with pyruvic acid (F. B. Hershberg, J. Org. Chem., 13, 542 (1948)).

In an attempt to find other routes which might lead to the introduction of the 4,5-double bond, we investigated the action of selenium dioxide on I. When a solution of I and selenium dioxide in methanol was warmed for a short time and then cooled, a new crystalline product deposited. Upon examination of the infra-red spectrum, the disappearance of one carbonyl group was disclosed, along with the appearance of a strong, saturated ether bond. Analytical data, plus the fact that this new compound could be easily reconverted to the starting material with aqueous acetic acid (or mineral acids), indicated that the compound was 3,3-dimethoxypregnan-17α,21-diol,11,20-trione 21-acetate (II).

This unexpected reaction of selenium dioxide in methanol is probably the normal formation of a steroid ketal in which the selenium dioxide is functioning simultaneously as the acid catalyst and as the dehydrating agent, removing the water formed and thus driving the reaction to completion.

The dimethyl ketal, II, melted at about 180–190° C. with vigorous evolution of vapor, which apparently arose from the elimination of a molecule of methanol. When a sample was pyrolyzed at 200° C. for a short length of time, a new compound was obtained, M.P. 208–210°, which was identified as 3-methoxy-Δ^3-pregnen-17α,21-diol-11,20-dione 21-acetate, III, (methyl enol ether of 4,5-dihydrocortisone acetate) by means of analysis, infra-red spectrum, bromination experiments and hydrolysis to pregnan-17α,21-diol-3,11,20-trione 21-acetate. The high degree of stability of the ketol sidechain to this pyrolytic treatment was entirely unexpected.

The enol ether (III) readily added bromine in either methylene chloride or acetic acid solution to form 4-bromo-pregnan-17α,21-diol-3,11,20-trione 21-acetate (IV); the latter solvent gave a bromide with a somewhat higher rotation, and presumably a higher purity. Either bromide preparation could be readily converted to cortisone acetate (V) via the semicarbazone procedure.

The reaction of N-bromosuccinimide with coprostanone enol acetate has been reported (B. Armbrecht and M. Rubin, Abstracts of Papers, 119th Meeting of the American Chemical Society, April 1951) to give Δ^4-cholesten-3-one directly. The first step was presumed to be allylic bromination at C-5. However, when the same reaction was attempted with the enol ether III, a bromide was obtained which had an infra-red spectrum identical with that of the bromide obtained by the addition reaction and which was also converted to cortisone acetate by the standard procedure. Therefore the bromide from III must be 4-bromopregnan-17α,21-diol-3,11,20-trione 21-acetate (IV) and not the 5-bromo compound which would be expected from allylic bromination. The 4-bromide may arise from either the addition of bromine or of N-bromosuccinimide to the double bond, although the former is a more likely possibility especially in the light of the recent investigation (E. A. Braude and E. S. Waight, J. Chem. Soc. 1116 (1952) on the addition of bromine to ethylenic double bonds by using N-bromosuccinimide.

The structure of these ketals has been established by conversion to the known 3,11-diketo-20β-hydroxy compounds, isolated as the acetates (X and XVI). 3,3-dimethoxypregnan-11,20-dione (XII) and 3,3-dimethoxypregnan-11β,17α-diol-20-one (XIII) were reduced completely to the 11β,20β-diols (XIII and XIX). After splitting the ketals with dilute acid, acetylation of the C-20 hydroxyl group and oxidation of the C-11 hydroxyl group, there were obtained the known pregnan-17α,20β-diol-3,11-dione 20-acetate (X) and pregnan-20β-ol-3,11-dione 20-acetate (XVI).

3,3-dimethoxypregnan-17α-ol-11,20-dione (VII) can be reduced partially with sodium borohydride to 3,3-dimethoxy-pregnan-17α,20β-diol-11-one (VIII). Hydrolysis of the ketal group, followed by acetylation at C-20, yields pregnan-17α,20β-diol-3,11-dione 20-acetate (X).

As already mentioned, the 3-keto group must not be conjugated to a nuclear double bond; where such double bond is present in the A-ring, the 3-ketal will not be formed. Thus cortisone acetate and Δ^4-androsten-3,17-dione failed to react. Keto groups at the 7,11,17 and 20 positions likewise failed to react, as in the case of pregnan-3α-ol-11,20-dione. It thus appears that keto groups which are conjugated to a double bond, or are joined to carbons at least one of which is tertiary, will not form ketals with alcohols in the presence of the catalysts above disclosed.

The reactions on the steroid compound following the ketalization should not be under such conditions as will cause hydrolysis of the ketal, at least not at a rate comparable to that of such reactions. Reduction at other points in the molecule is therefore preferably effected under neutral or alkaline conditions, as with alkali metal borohydrides and alkali metal aluminum hydrides (like sodium borohydride and lithium aluminum hydride), hydrogen in the presence of hydrogenation catalysts, etc.

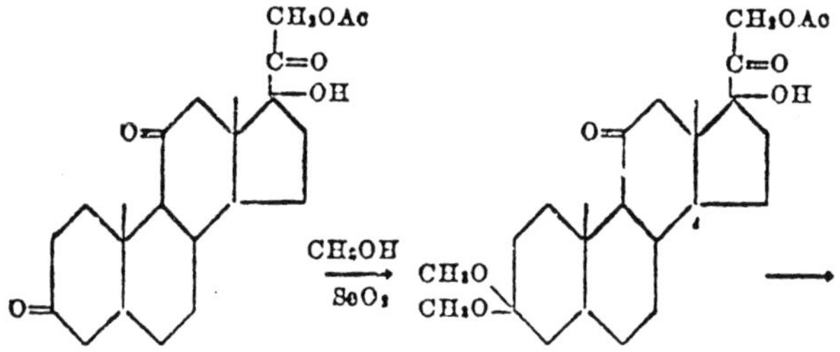

I II

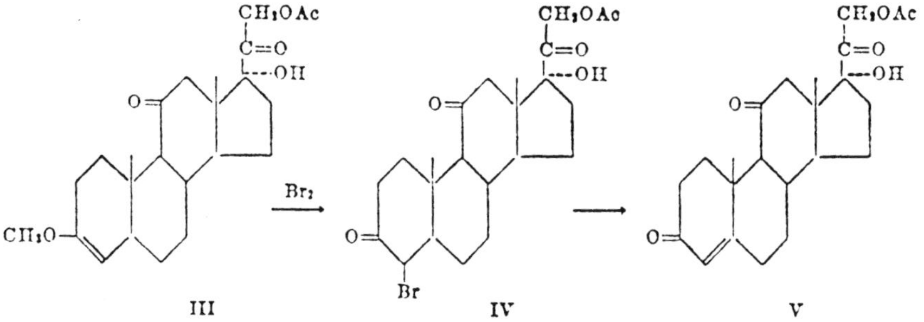

III IV V

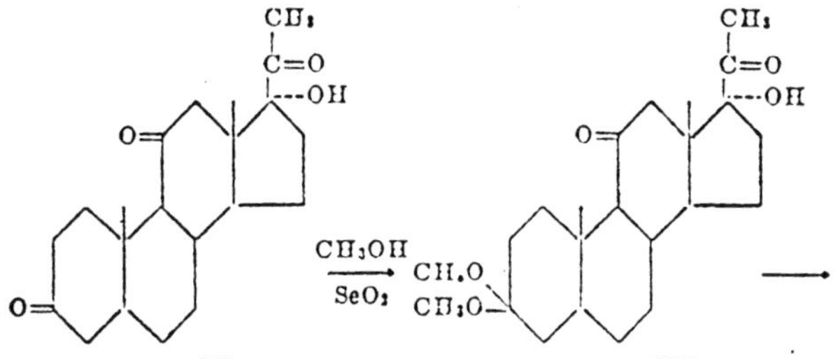

VI VII

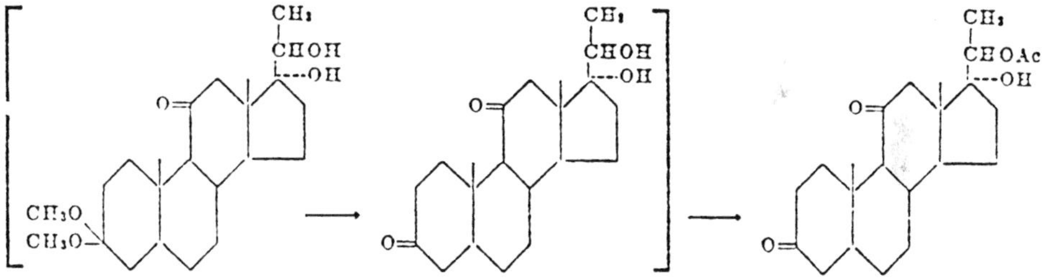

VIII IX X

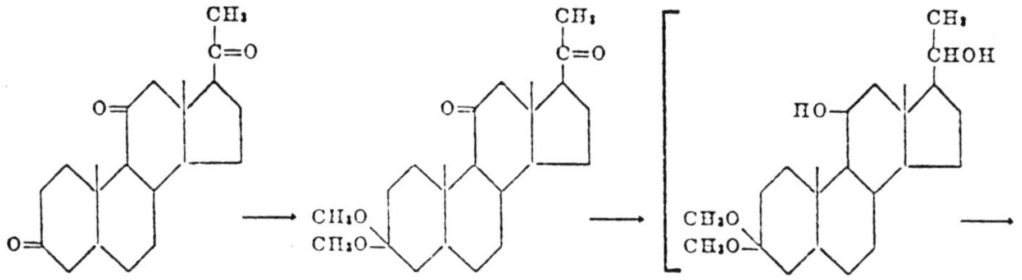

XI XII XIII

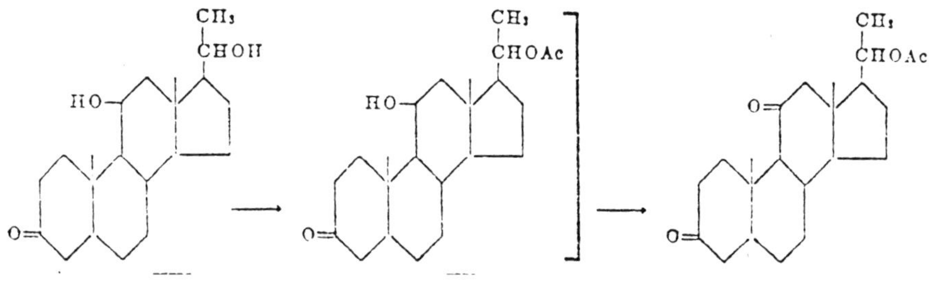

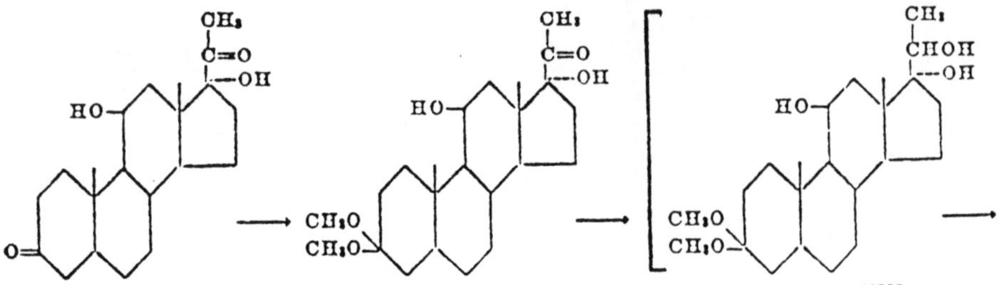

XVII XVIII XIX

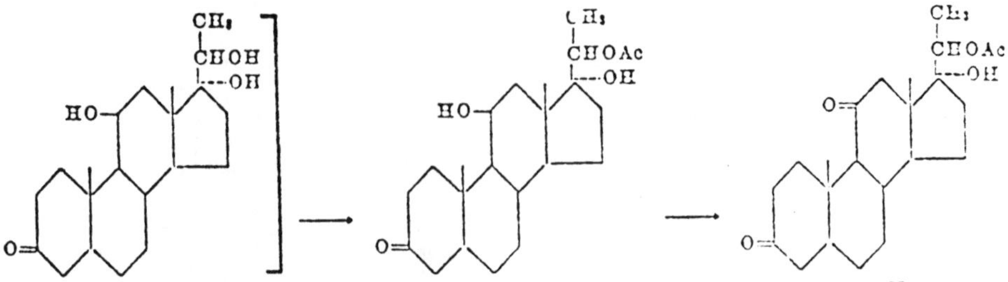

XX XXI X

In the above formulae, Ac stands for any suitable acyl group, preferably of a carboxylic acid, either aliphatic or aromatic, such as acetyl, propionyl, butyryl, isovaleryl, phenacetyl, cyclohexylacetyl, benzoyl, phthalyl, etc.

The invention is applicable to 3-keto steroids generally, including not only the different types of pregnanes illustrated by the above formulae, but also to bile acids, androstanes, etiocholanes, sapogenins, pseudosapogenins and degraded sapogenins having a 3-keto group, etc. Reactions typical of bile acids are represented by the following equations A and B, while those typical of androstanes are indicated by reactions C and D, it being noted that the equation D illustrates the synthesis of estradiol from androstane-dione:

A.

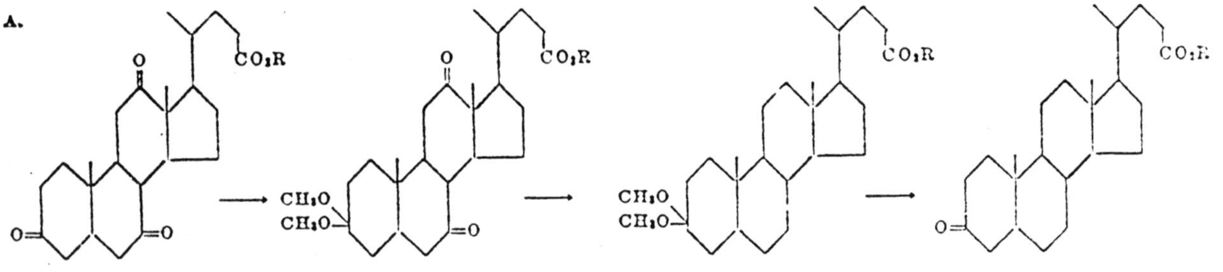

B.

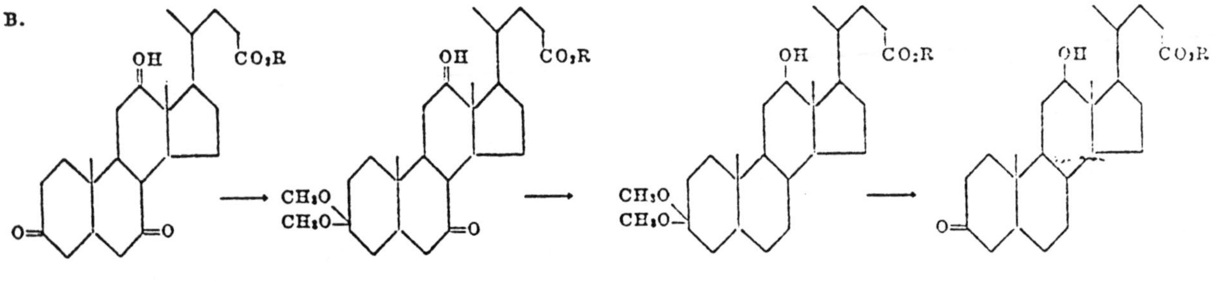

C.

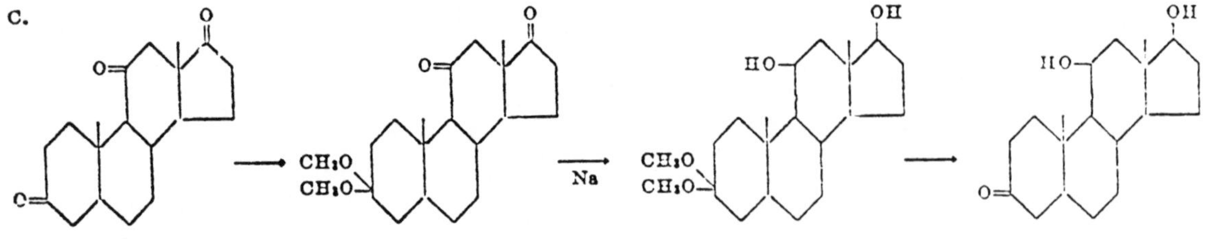

D.

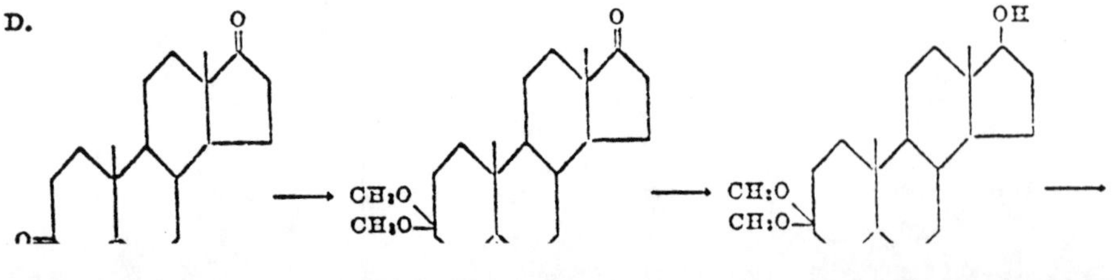

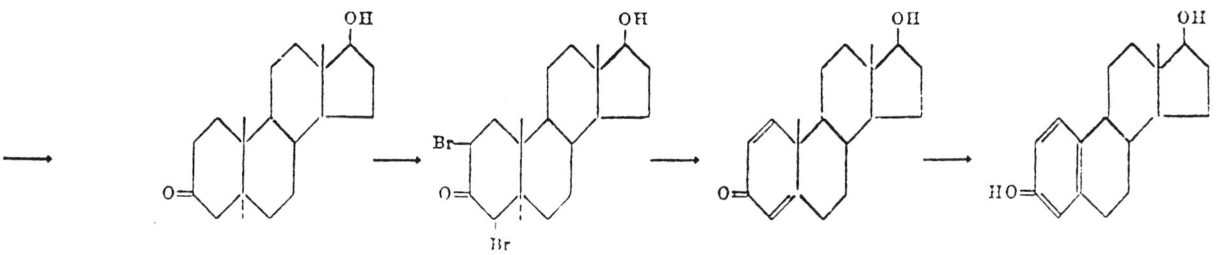

In the above formulae R stands for a hydrocarbon radical, such as lower alkyls, like methyl, ethyl and butyl, or aromatic, like benzyl, or cycloaliphatic, like cyclohexyl and cyclopentyl, the methyl or ethyl radical being usually preferred.

As indicated in equations A and B above, the 3-keto group of, for example, a 3,7-diketo steroid can be treated to remove the 7-ketonic oxygen (and/or other ketonic oxygen, when present), as by the Wolff-Kishner reduction, for example, by conversion to the semicarbazone followed by heating with sodium ethylate. As this reaction is well known, it has not been thought to be necessary to illustrate it in detail.

Our invention can be employed with compounds of both the normal and allo-series, and with compounds which are saturated or unsaturated in the B, C and D-rings.

The invention will be described in greater detail in the following examples which are presented only illustratively and not as indicating the scope of the invention.

EXAMPLE I

(a) *3,3-dimethoxypregnan-17α,21 - diol - 11,20 - dione-21-acetate (II)*.—A solution of 15.00 of pregnan-17α,21-diol-3,11,20-trione-21-acetate (dihydrocortisone acetate, I) and 15.0 g. of selenium dioxide in 350 ml. of C.P. methanol was kept at 50–55° C. for 1 hour. The precipitate obtained upon cooling the solution was collected with suction and after drying weighed 11.85 g., M.P. 179–215°. Recrystallization from methanol gave two crops; 9.72 g., M.P. 193–195° with gas evolution and 1.45 g. M.P. 184–190° with gas evolution. An analytical sample, recrystallized again from methanol melted at 181–184° with gas evolution, $[\alpha]_D^{24}+71.3°$ (acetone).

Analysis.—Calc'd for $C_{25}H_{38}O_7$: C, 66.64; H, 8.50. Found: C, 66.72; H, 8.80. Infra-red absorption studies showed the loss of a carbonyl group, and the appearance of the C—O—C group.

(b) *Hydrolysis of the 3,3-dimethyl ketal.*—A solution of 0.39 g. of II in 15 ml. of glacial acetic acid was warmed on the steam bath to about 75°, 15 ml. of water were added and the solution was allowed to stand overnight while cooling slowly to room temperature. The resulting crystals were collected, washed and dried: yield, 0.18 g., M.P. 230–234°, $[\alpha]_D^{21}+81.31°$ (acetone). Dilution of the filtrate with water yielded an additional 0.15 g., M.P. 226–229°, $[\alpha]_D^{21}+83.34°$. Total yield +94%. Neither fraction gave a melting point depression when mixed with dihydrocortisone acetate (I), and the infrared spectra were identical with that of dihydrocortisone acetate.

(c) *3-methoxy-Δ³-pregnen-17α,21 - diol - 11,20-dione-21-acetate (III)*.— A small flask containing 9.72 g. of (II) was heated gradually and with constant stirring in a Woods metal bath to a temperature of 200° over a period of about 30 minutes. Upon cooling, the solidified residue was recrystallized from acetone to yield 4.70 g. (52%) of III. M.P. 208–210°, $[\alpha]_D^{21}+120.9°$ (acetone).

Anaylsis.—Calc'd for $C_{24}H_{34}O_8$: C, 68.87; H, 8.19. Found: C, 68.91%; H, 8.51%.

Hydrolysis of 0.50 g. of III as described for the 3,3-dimethoxy compound yielded 0.36 g. (75%), M.P. 231–233°. There was no depression in M.P. on admixture with dihydrocortisone acetate, and the infra-red

(d) *4-bromopregnan-17α - diol - 3,11,20 - trione - 21-acetate (IV)*

(1) Bromination in methylene chloride: A solution of 1.00 g. of III in 40 ml. of methylene chloride was cooled in an ice bath and brominated by the dropwise addition of 0.40 g. of bromine dissolved in 10 ml. of methylene chloride. Decolorization was instantaneous and copious fumes of hydrogen bromide were evolved. The solvent was removed under reduced pressure, leaving a residue which crystallized upon the addition of acetone. Recrystallization of this material from aqueous acetone gave 0.57 g., M.P. 184–185° d., $[\alpha]_D^{21}+79.6$ (acetone).

(2) Bromination in acetic acid: A solution of 0.50 g. of III in 10 ml. of glacial acetic acid at 25° C. was brominated by the drop-wise addition of 0.20 g. of bromine in 4 ml. of acetic acid. Fumes of hydrogen bromide were again evolved. The solution was poured into water and the solid was collected on a filter and washed with water. Recrystallization from aqueous acetone gave 0.35 g. of IV, M.P. 184–186° d., $[\alpha]_D^{21}+91.4°$ (acetone).

Analysis.—Calc'd for $C_{23}H_{31}O_6Br$: Br, 16.53. Found: Br, 16.61%.

(3) Bromination with N-bromosuccinimide: A suspension of 1.00 g. of III in 100 ml. of carbon tetrachloride was heated to reflux. The addition of 0.45 g. of N-bromosuccinimide caused most of the solid to dissolve within 5 minutes and reflux was continued 25 minutes longer. The solution was cooled, chilled and the resulting solid collected with suction, washed with water and dried. Recrystallization from aqueous acetone gave 0.46 g., $[\alpha]_D^{23}+105.1°$ (acetone).

(e) *Cortisone acetate V.*—The bromides were put through the semi-carbazone formation and split as described in the literature:

V. Mattox and E. C. Kendall, Journal of Biological Chemistry, 188, 287 (1951);

B. Koechlin, T. Kritchevsky and T. F. Gallagher, ibid., 184, 393 (1950);

E. B. Hershberg, J. Org. Chem., 13, 542 (1948).

Bromide	Crude V	Recrystallized V
(a) 0.38 g. $[\alpha]_D+79.6°$	0.24 g., M.P. 200–222°.	0.13 g., M.P. 227–233° dec., ε237 14,600, $[\alpha]_D$ +201.5°.
(b) 0.38 g. $[\alpha]_D+91.4°$	0.26 g., M.P. 213–222°.	0.21 g., M.P. 228–233° dec., ε237 14,600 $[\alpha]_D$ +197.3°.
(c) 0.59 g. $[\alpha]_D+105.1°$	0.30 g., M.P. 210–223°.	0.31 g., M.P. 227–233° dec., ε237 13,200 $[\alpha]_D$ +189.1°.

All rotations were in dioxane and the u.v. determinations in 95% ethanol. The crude cortisone acetate (V) was crystallized from aqueous acetone. Infra-red spectra showed no significant differences between the three samples and a reference sample of cortisone acetate.

EXAMPLE 2

(a) *3,3 - dimethoxypregnan - 11β,17α - diol - 20 - one (XVIII)*.—A solution of 5.00 g. of pregnan-11β,17α-diol-3,20-dione and 5.0 g. of selenium dioxide in 100 ml. of C.P. methanol was kept at 50° C. for 2 hours and at room temperature (30°) for four hours. No crystals formed, whereupon a solution of 5 g. of potassium hy-

solution was poured into water. The precipitated solid was collected with suction, washed with water and dried; weight 4.56 g. Recrystallization from ether-hexane gave two crops of XVIII, 3.95 g., M.P. 164–168° with gas evolution, and 0.44 g., M.P. 156–159° with gas evolution. A sample recrystallized for analysis melted at 168–171° dec., $[\alpha]_D+23.5°$ (chloroform).

Analysis.—Calc'd for $C_{23}H_{28}O_5$: C, 70.01; H, 9.71. Found: C, 70.06; H, 9.81.

(b) *Pregnan - 11β,17α,20β - triol - 3 - one - 20-acetate (XXI).*—A solution of 3.92 g. of 3,3-dimethoxypregnan-11β,17α-diol-20-one (XVIII) in 100 ml. of C.P. methanol containing 0.4 g. of potassium hydroxide was combined with a solution of 4.00 g. of sodium borohydride in 10 ml. of water. After refluxing for 16 hours, the solution was diluted with water and extracted three times with methylene chloride. The combined extracts were washed twice with water, dried over sodium sulfate, and evaporated, leaving a colorless oil. In order to hydrolyze the dimethoxy group, this residue was taken up in 20 ml. of acetic acid, treated with 20 ml. of hot water and heated for 15 minutes on the steam bath. After cooling, the solution was diluted with water and extracted with methylene chloride. The extracts were washed with dilute sodium bicarbonate solution and water, dried over sodium sulfate, and evaporated. The residue, again an oil, was acetylated by treating with acetic anhydride in pyridine over-night at room temperature. The solution was diluted with water and extracted with methylene chloride. The extracts were washed with water, dilute hydrochloric acid, water, dilute sodium bicarbonate solution, and water. Drying over sodium sulfate and evaporation left 3.45 g. of crystalline material. Recrystallization from acetone gave two crops: 1.57 g., M.P. 248–250° and 0.43 g., M.P. 239–241°. A second crystallization of the first crop gave 1.44 g. of product, M.P. 250–252°, $[\alpha]_D^{28}+63.0°$ (chloroform).

Analysis.—Calc'd for $C_{23}H_{36}O_5$; C, 70.37; H, 9.25. Found: C, 70.76; H, 9.53.

EXAMPLE 3

(a) *3,3 - dimethoxypregnan-17α-ol-11,20-dione (VII).*—A solution of 2.00 g. of pregnan-17α-ol-3,11,20-trione (VI) and 2.00 g. of selenium dioxide dissolved in 80 ml. of C.P. methanol was allowed to stand 2 days at room temperature. The solution was made alkaline by the addition of a methanolic solution of 3 g. of potassium hydroxide and poured into water. After filtration and drying, the crude product weighed 1.87 g. The material was recrystallized from ether-hexane (in the presence of a few drops of pyridine), and gave 1.35 g. of VII, M.P. 138–141° with bubbling. Another crystallization raised the M.P. to 148–150° dec., $[\alpha]_D^{25}+35.0°$ (chloroform).

Anaylsis.—Calc'd for $C_{23}H_{36}O_5$: C, 70.37; H, 9.24. Found: C, 70.25; H, 9.41.

(b) *Pregnan - 17α,20β-diol-3,11-dione-20-acetate (X).*—(1) A solution of 1.20 g. of 3,3-dimethoxypregnan-17α-ol-11,20-dione (VII) in 40 ml. of C.P. methanol was added to a solution of 1.2 g. of sodium borohydride in 4 ml. of water, the mixture allowed to stand at room temperature (24°) for three hours, and then worked up as before. Hydrolysis of the dimethoxy group followed by acetylation, as described above, yielded 1.17 g., M.P. 183–190°. Recrystallization from ethanol gave two crops: 0.61 g., M.P. 215–222° and 0.06 g., M.P. 251–253°. A mixed M.P. of the second crop with pregnan-11β,17α,20β-triol-3-one-20-acetate (Xa) showed no depression, and the infra-red spectra were identical. A second crystallization of the first crop yielded 0.52 g. of X solvated with ethanol, M.P. 222–224°, $[\alpha]_D^{25}+59.5°$ (acetone). Reported M.P. 222–224°. (L. H. Sarett, Journal of Biological Chemistry 71,1169 (1949)).

Analysis.—Calc'd for $C_{23}H_{33}O_5$; C_2H_5OH: C, 68.77; H, 9.23. Found: C, 68.66; H, 9.61.

3-one-20-acetate (Xa) in 75 ml. of C.P. acetone and 7.5 ml. of water was cooled to 3° and treated with 0.35 g. of N-bromo-acetamide. After 18 hours at 3°, a solution of 1 g. of sodium sulfite in a minimum amount of water was added and the acetone was removed under reduced pressure. The concentrated suspension was diluted with water and the solid collected with suction weighed 0.48 g., M.P. 218–220°. Recrystallization from ethanol gave 0.42 g., M.P. 223–225°, $[\alpha]_D^{20}+59.6°$ (acetone). A mixture M.P. with the sample prepared in (1) showed no depresion.

EXAMPLE 4

(a) *3,3 - dimethoxy-pregnan-11,20-dione (XII).* — A solution of 1.00 g. of pregnan-3,11,20-trione (XI) in 40 ml. of C.P. methanol was treated with 1.00 g. of selenium dioxide and allowed to stand 2 days at room temperature. The solution was made alkaline by the addition of 1 g. of potassium hydroxide in methanol, and poured into water. Filtration yielded 0.85 g. of material melting at 136–143°. Recrystallization from hexane gave 0.75 g., M.P. 140–142°, $[\alpha]_D^{25}+130.4°$ (chloroform).

Analysis.—Calc'd for $C_{23}H_{36}O_4$: C, 73.36; H, 9.64. Found: C, 73.48; H, 9.85.

(b) *Pregnan - 20β-ol-3,11-dione-20-acetate (XVI).* — A solution of 1.70 g. of 3,3-dimethoxy-pregnan-11,20-dione in 80 ml. of C.P. methanol containing 0.2 g. of potassium hydroxide was added to a solution of 3.40 g. of sodium borohydride in 8 ml. of water. After refluxing for 16 hours, the solution was cooled and worked up as previously described. The dimethoxy group was hydrolyzed by treatment with 50% acetic acid and the residue was acetylated, again as previously described in the formation of X. This material was taken up in 100 ml. of C.P. acetone and 20 ml. of water. The solution was cooled to 3° and 1.78 g. of N-bromoacetamide was added. After 3 hours at 3°, the solution was poured into 1 liter of water containing 3 g. of sodium sulfite. Filtration yielded 1.43 g. of solid melting at 150–170°. This material was taken up in C.P. benzene and chromatographed on 17 g. of Florisil (100/200 mesh). Elution with benzene gave 0.96 g. of material, M.P. 165–198°. Two recrystallizations from methanol yielded 0.49 g., M.P. 201–203°, $[\alpha]_D^{25}+66.6°$ (acetone). Reported M.P., 201–203° (L. K. Sarett, ibid., 71, 1165 (1949)).

Analysis.—Calc'd for $C_{22}H_{34}O_4$: C, 73.76; H, 9.15. Found: C, 73.56; H, 9.45.

EXAMPLE 5

Androstan-17β-ol-3-one

A solution of 1.0 g. of 3,17-androstandione in 50 ml. of methanol and containing 1 g. of selenium dioxide, was allowed to remain in an ice-chest overnight. The formed 3,3-dimethoxy-androstan-17-one was not separated. One gram of solid potassium hydroxide and 2.5 g. of sodium borohydride in 2.5 ml. of water were added and the mixture allowed to react at room temperature for 24 hours. The solution was then poured into a large excess of water, extracted with methylene chloride. the organic layer dried and evaporated to a residue. The residue was dissolved in ether, and a small amount of selenium removed by filtration. The ether was boiled off and the organic material dissolved in 100 ml. of boiling acetone. Twenty-five ml. of dil. hydrochloric acid were added. the solution boiled for 5 minutes and then allowed to cool. Upon crystallization, 0.85 g. of androstan-17β-ol-3-one was obtained, M.P. 175–178°.

EXAMPLE 6

Etiocholan-11β,17β-diol-3-one

In a manner similar to Example 5. 1 g. of etiocholan-3,11,17-trione was treated with selenium dioxide in methanol to give the 3,3-dimethyl ketal. This was not isolated, but reduced with sodium borohydride and potas-

13

Hydrolysis of the ketal with dil. hydrochloric acid gave etiocholan-11β,17β-diol-3-one, M.P. 171–173°.

EXAMPLE 7.

A mixture of 10.0 g. of pregnan-11β,17α-diol-3,20-dione, 10.0 g. of selenium dioxide, 150 ml. of ethylene glycol and 100 ml. of alcohol-free chloroform, was stirred for 24 hours at room temperature. The reaction mixture was poured into a solution of 20 g. of potassium carbonate in 1.5 l. of water and extracted with methylene chloride. The extract was washed with water, dried with magnesium sulfate and upon evaporation left a solid residue weighing 11.06 g., M.P. 225–229°. The analytical sample of pregnan-11β,17α-diol-3,20-dione 3-ethylene ketal, crystallized from acetone-hexane, melted at 232.4–233.8°.

Analysis.—Calcd. for $C_{23}H_{36}O_6$: C, 70.307; H. 9.24. Found: C, 70.26; H, 9.67.

EXAMPLE 8

4-bromopregnan-11β,17α-diol-3,20-dione 3-ethylene ketal

(*a*) When 1.0 g. of 4-bromopregnan-11β,17α-diol-3,20-dione was treated with ethylene glycol and selenium dioxide as in Example 4(*a*), only a small amount of 4-bromopregnan-11β,17α-diol-3,20-dione 3-ethylene ketal was obtained. Even lengthening the time of reaction to six days did not substantially improve the yield.

(*b*) A mixture of 1.0 g. of 4-bromopregnan-11β,17α-diol-3,20-dione, 1.0 g. of selenium dioxide, 0.1 g. of p-toluene sulfonic acid monohydrate, 10 ml. of ethylene glycol and 25 ml. of alcohol-free chloroform was stirred at 25° for four days. Methylene chloride was added and the organic layer was washed with water, dilute sodium bicarbonate solution, water, and dried over magnesium sulfate. The solvent was removed by distillation and the residue triturated with ether. There was obtained 0.6 g. of 4-bromopregnan-11β,17α-diol-3,20-dione 3-ethylene ketal M.P. 178–179° dec.

Variations from the specific procedures hereinabove disclosed may be resorted to by those skilled in the art within the scope of the appended claims without departing from the spirit of the invention.

We claim:

1. Process for the selective protection of the 3-keto group of a polyketo steroid of the class consisting of (1) 3-keto-pregnanes having an additional keto group in at least one of the 7-, and 11-, and 20-positions, (2) 3-keto-androstanes having an additional keto group in at least one of the 11- and 17-positions, and (3) 3-keto etiocholanes having an additional keto group in at least one of the 7- and 12-positions, the 3-keto group being in each case in a non-conjugated relation to a double bond, which comprises reacting such steroid under substantially anhydrous conditions with a saturated lower aliphatic alcohol in the presence of selenium dioxide and of a strong acid, to form the 3-ketal.

14

2. Process according to claim 1, wherein the alcohol is primary.

3. Process according to claim 1, wherein the alcohol is methyl alcohol.

4. Process according to claim 1, wherein the steroid is a 3,20-diketo pregnane having a keto group also in one of the 7- and 11-positions.

5. Process according to claim 1, wherein the steroid is a 3,20-diketo-4-bromo-pregnane, and wherein the acid is p-toluenesulfonic acid.

6. Process according to claim 1, wherein the aliphatic alcohol is ethylene glycol.

7. Process according to claim 1, wherein the steroid is substituted in at least one of the 2- and 4-positions with a member of the group consisting of chlorine, bromine and iodine.

8. Process according to claim 1, wherein the steroid is a 3,20-diketo pregnane.

9. 3-ethylene ketal of pregnan-11β,17α-diol-3,20-dione.

10. Process for the manufacture of 3-ketals of a 3,20-diketo-pregnane, while leaving the 20-keto group unreacted, which comprises reacting a 3,20-diketo pregnane wherein the 3-keto group is non-conjugated to a double bond, with a lower aliphatic alcohol in the presence of selenium dioxide and of a strong acid.

11. Process for the manufacture of 3-ketals of a 3,20-diketo-pregnane, while leaving the 20-keto group unreacted, which comprises reacting a 3,20-diketo pregnane wherein the 3-keto group is non-conjugated to a double bond, with ethylene glycol in the presence of selenium dioxide and of a strong acid.

12. A 3-ethylene glycol ketal of a 3,20-diketo-pregnane having a saturated A-ring, the 20-keto group being free.

13. A 3-lower alkylene ketal of a 3,20-diketo-pregnane having a saturated A-ring, the 20-keto group being free.

14. A 3-lower aliphatic alcohol ketal of a 3,20-diketo-pregnane having a saturated A-ring, the 20-keto group of said ketal being free, and said ketal having attached to at least one of the 2- and 4-carbons a member of the group consisting of chlorine, bromine and iodine.

15. The process which comprises reacting a 3,20-diketo pregnane having a saturated A-ring and having attached to at least one of the 2- and 4-positions a member of the class consisting of chlorine, bromine, and iodine, with a lower aliphatic alcohol in the presence of selenium dioxide and of a strong acid to form the 3-ketal while leaving the 20-keto group unchanged.

16. A 3-lower aliphatic alcohol ketal of a 3,20-diketo-4-bromo-pregnane, the 20-keto group being free.

References Cited in the file of this patent

UNITED STATES PATENTS

2,294,433	Westphal _____	Sept. 1, 1942
2,647,134	Hogg _____	July 28, 1953
2,656,367	Graber _____	Oct. 20, 1953
2,666,068	Hanze _____	Jan. 12, 1954

CHAPTER FOURTEEN

1

3,030,358
PROCESS FOR REDUCTION OF Δ4 ANDROSTENE [3.2-c] PYRAZOLE COMPOUNDS
Andrew John Manson, North Greenbush, N.Y., assignor
to Sterling Drug Inc., New York, N.Y., a corporation
of Delaware
No Drawing. Filed May 11, 1961, Ser. No. 109,273
6 Claims. (Cl. 260—239.5)

This invention relates to a reduction process, and in particular is concerned with a method for preparing androstano[3.2-c]pyrazoles by reducing the corresponding 4-androsteno[3.2-c]pyrazoles.

The products of the process of the invention, androstano[3.2-c]pyrazoles, are valuable anabolic agents, and both these compounds and the starting materials for said process are disclosed in the copending application of R. O. Clinton, Serial No. 793,292, filed February 16, 1959.

It has been discovered that 17β-hydroxy-4-androsteno-[3.2-c]pyrazole and 17α-lower-alkyl derivatives thereof can be reduced to 17β-hydroxyandrostano[3.2-c]pyrazole and 17α-lower-alkyl derivatives thereof by treating the former with a liquid ammonia solution of an alkali metal (lithium, sodium, potassium, rubidium or cesium) or alkaline earth metal (calcium, strontium or barium), and with a lower-alkanol. Surprisingly, it was found that the double bond was reduced in excellent yield without affecting the pyrazole ring system or producing appreciable amounts of the 5β isomer (rings A/B cis).

The conversion brought about by the process of the invention is depicted by structural formulas as follows:

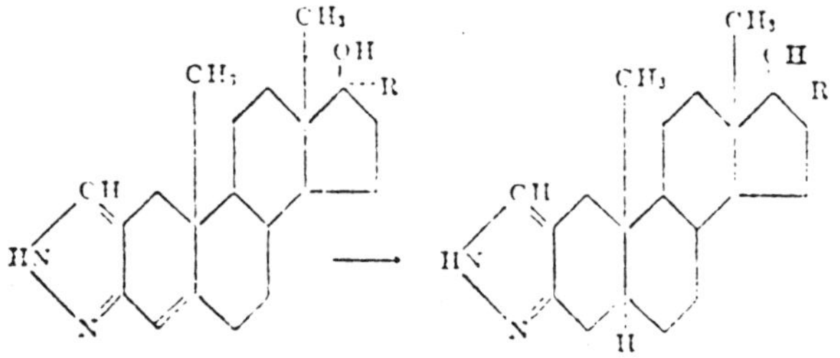

In the above formulas R stands for a hydrogen atom or a lower-alkyl radical having from one to about four carbon atoms including methyl, ethyl, propyl, isopropyl, butyl, isobutyl and the like.

The reaction medium may contain an inert solvent, such as a liquid hydrocarbon solvent or an aliphatic or cycloaliphatic ether, which serves to solubilize the steroid and as a diluent for the liquid ammonia. A preferred inert solvent is tetrahydrofuran.

To insure completion of the reaction, at least four gram atoms of alkali metal (two gram atoms of alkaline earth metal) are required per mole of steroid. It is preferred to use a large excess of the metal.

The lower-alkanol is preferably added after the steroid and metal have been dissolved in the liquid ammonia. Any lower-alkanol can be used and said lower-alkanol has from one to about six carbon atoms, thus including methanol, ethanol, 1-propanol, 2-propanol, 1-butanol, 2-butanol, tertiary-butyl alcohol, amyl alcohol, hexyl alcohol, and the like.

The quantities of liquid ammonia, inert solvent, metal and lower-alkanol relative to the amount of steroid can vary within wide limits. The following examples will illustrate the invention more fully without the latter being limited thereby.

Example 1

To a stirred solution of 1.00 g. of 17β-hydroxy-17α-methyl-4-androsteno[3.2-c]pyrazole in 200 ml. of tetra-

2

hydrofuran and 400 ml. of liquid ammonia was added 2.12 g. of lithium wire during five minutes. The dark blue mixture was stirred for forty-five minutes. A solution of 40 ml. of tertiary-butyl alcohol in 160 ml. of diethyl ether was added with stirring. After fifteen minutes 25 ml. of ethanol was added with stirring. The mixture turned colorless after several hours, and the liquid ammonia was allowed to evaporate and the mixture warm to room temperature over a period of about fifteen hours. The solvent was evaporated to yield a colorless solid residue, which was taken up in ethyl acetate-ice water. The two layers were separated and the aqueous layer was extracted with ethyl acetate. The combined organic layers were washed with water, saturated sodium chloride solution and filtered through anhydrous sodium sulfate. The solvent was evaporated to yield 1.20 g. of light tan crystals, M.P. 151–155° C., ultraviolet maximum at 224 mμ (E=4,095). Two recrystallizations from ethanol afforded: 1st crop, 0.619 g. (62%) of colorless crystals (dried at 120° C. in vacuo for 17 hours), M.P. 232.8–238.0° C., ultraviolet maximum at 224 mμ (E=4,840), [α]$_D^{25}$ (1% in CHCl₃)=+34.8°; 2nd crop, 0.142 g. (14%) of colorless crystals, M.P. 23-242° C. A mixed melting point with authentic 17β-hydroxy-17α-methylandrostano[3.2-c]pyrazole, M.P. 228-241° C., prepared as described in Clinton application Serial No. 793,292, was 230–241° C. The infrared spectrum was identical.

Example 2

To a stirred solution of 10.0 g. of 17β-hydroxy-17α-methyl-4-androsteno[3.2-c]pyrazole in 300 ml. of tetrahydrofuran and 300 ml. of liquid ammonia in a 2 l. 3-necked round-bottomed flask equipped with Dry Ice condenser with soda lime drying tube and a mechanical Hershberg stirrer, was added 20 g. of sodium during five minutes. Two layers formed: a bronze-colored upper layer and a gray opaque lower layer. The mixture was stirred for one hour, and then 100 ml. of ethanol was added with stirring through a pressure-equalized dropping funnel during fifteen minutes. The mixture was stirred at reflux for an additional six hours (the two layers were still present at this time) and then the liquid ammonia was allowed to evaporate and the mixture warm to room temperature over a period of about fifteen hours. The gray mixture containing both solid and liquid was concentrated under reduced pressure to about 200 ml. and then poured with stirring into 1500 ml. of ice-water. The mixture was filtered and the collected solid was washed with water and sucked dry to yield light yellow crystals, a portion of which was dried in vacuo at 120° C. for 64 hours to yield light yellow crystals, M.P. 157–165° C., partially resolidified, M.P. <215° C., ultraviolet maxima at 223 mμ (E=4,600), 260 mμ (E=130) (>98% reduction). Two recrystallizations from ethanol afforded 6.38 g. (63%) of colorless crystals of 17β-hydroxy-17α-methylandrostano[3.2-c]pyrazole (dried in vacuo at 120° C. for 20 hours), M.P. 232–241° C., ultraviolet maximum at 223 mμ (E=4,710), [α]$_D^{25}$ (1% in CHCl₃)=+34.9°. From the mother liquors the following additional crops were obtained after treatment with activated charcoal and several recrystallizations from ethanol: 1.18 g. of light yellow crystals (dried in vacuo at 120° C. for 17 hours), M.P. 152–155° C., resolidified, M.P. 224–245° C., ultraviolet maxima at 223 mμ (E=4,650), 260 mμ (E=96), [α]$_D^{25}$ (1% in CHCl₃)=+34.8°; 0.37 g., M.P. 153–157° C., resolidified, M.P. 222–230° C.; 0.10 g., M.P. 151–154° C., resolidified, M.P. 227–243° C.; 0.47 g., M.P. 207–242° C.

By following the foregoing procedures, 17β-hydroxy-4-androsteno[3.2-c]pyrazole, 17β-hydroxy-17α-ethyl-4-androsteno[3.2-c]pyrazole, 17β-hydroxy-17α-propyl-4-androsteno[3.2-c]pyrazole, 17β-hydroxy - 17α - isopropyl-4-androsteno[3.2-c]pyrazole, or 17β-hydroxy-17α-butyl-4-androsteno[3.2-c]pyrazole can be reduced, respectively, to 17β-hydroxyandrostano[3.2-c]pyrazole, 17β-hydroxy-17α-ethylandrostano[3.2-c]pyrazole, 17β - hydroxy - 17α-propylandrostano[3.2-c]pyrazole, 17β - hydroxy - 17α-iso-propylandrostano[3.2-c]pyrazole, or 17β-hydroxy-17α-butylandrostano[3.2-c]pyrazole.

I claim:

1. The process for preparing a compound selected from the group consisting of 17β-hydroxyandrostano[3.2-c]-pyrazole and 17β - hydroxy - 17α - lower-alkylandrostano-[3.2-c]pyrazoles which comprises treating a compound selected from the group consisting of 17β-hydroxy-4-androsteno[3.2-c]pyrazole and 17β-hydroxy-17α-lower-alkyl-4-androsteno[3.2-c]pyrazoles with a liquid ammonia solution of a metal selected from the group consisting of alkali metals and alkaline earth metals and with a lower-alkanol.

2. The process for preparing a 17β-hydroxy-17α-lower-alkylandrostano[3.2-c]pyrazole which comprises treating a 17β-hydroxy-17α-lower-alkyl-4-androsteno[3.2-c]pyra-

zole with a liquid ammonia solution of an alkali metal and with a lower-alkanol.

3. The process for preparing 17β-hydroxy-17α-methyl-androstano[3.2-c]pyrazole which comprises treating 17β-hydroxy-17α-methyl-4-androsteno[3.2-c]pyrazole with a liquid ammonia solution of an alkali metal and with a lower-alkanol.

4. The process for preparing 17β-hydroxy-17α-methyl-androstano[3.2-c]pyrazole which comprises treating 17β-hydroxy-17α-methyl-4-androsteno[3.2-c]pyrazole with a liquid ammonia solution of lithium and with a lower-alkanol.

5. The process for preparing 17β-hydroxy-17α-methyl-androstano[3.2-c]pyrazole which comprises treating 17β-hydroxy-17α-methyl-4-androsteno[3.2-c]pyrazole with a liquid ammonia solution of sodium and with a lower-alkanol.

6. The process for preparing 17β-hydroxy-17α-methyl-androstano[3.2-c]pyrazole which comprises treating 17β-hydroxy-17α-methyl-4-androsteno[3.2-c]pyrazole with a liquid ammonia solution of sodium and with ethanol.

No references cited.

CHAPTER FIFTEEN

1

2,744,120

1-DEHYDROTESTOLOLACTONE

Josef Fried and Richard W. Thoma, New Brunswick, N. J., assignors to Olin Mathieson Chemical Corporation, New York, N. Y., a corporation of Virginia

No Drawing. Application January 14, 1953, Serial No. 331,333

1 Claim. (Cl. 260—343.2)

This invention relates to microbiological oxidation, and has for its object the provision of a process for oxidizing C_{17}-substituted steroids to obtain novel and useful derivatives.

Although C_{17}-substituted steroids have been subjected to microbiological oxidation prior to this invention, the microbiological oxidation of this invention is novel in affecting the substituent in the C-17 position of the cyclopentanophenanthrene nucleus, resulting in novel and useful derivatives.

More specifically, this invention includes subjecting C_{17}-substituted steroids to the action of fungi (or enzymes thereof) of the order Moniliales (Families: Moniliaceae, Dematiaceae, Stilbaceae, Tuberculariaceae), especially of the family Tuberculariaceae (Genera: Cylindrocarpon, Fusarium, Ramularia, etc.) and preferably of the genus Cylindrocarpon (species: *radicola, album, ianthothele*). Thus, it has been found that the fungus *Cylindrocarpon radicola* ATCC 11011 has a high order of activity in the microbiological oxidation of this invention. The novel derivatives obtained by the process of this invention are valuable hormones or intermediates therefor.

In the practice of this invention, the oxidation may be effected in a growing culture by either adding the C_{17}-substituted steroid to the culture during the incubation period, or by including it in the nutrient medium prior to inoculation. In any case, assimilable sources of nitrogenous materials (for growth-promotion) and carbon-containing materials (as energy source) should be present in the culture medium. Also, an adequate, sterile air supply should be maintained during the oxidation, e. g., by the conventional techniques of (1) exposing a large surface of the medium to air, or (2) submerged culture.

As the C_{17}-substituted steroid, any cyclopentanophenanthrene (or hydrogenated cyclopentanophenanthrene) having a substituent, especially an oxy- or oxo-containing substituent, at C_{17} may be used [the term oxy-containing including, of course, both free hydroxy and etherified hydroxy (e. g., alkoxy)]. Thus, among the C_{17}-substituted steroids utilizable in the process of the invention are: progesterone; testosterone; Reichstein's Compound "S"; estriol; estradiol; testosterone fatty acid esters (e. g., acetate, propionate, enanthate); Reichstein's Compound "S" fatty acid esters (e. g., acetate, propionate, butyrate, etc.); diosgenin; diosgenin acetate; Δ^4-tigogenone; Δ^4-becogenone; $\Delta^{1,4}$-androstadiene-17-ol-3-one; Δ^5-androstenediol-1-3, 17; Δ^4-androstenedione-3,17; Δ^5-androstenediol-3,17-3 monoacetate; the 3,20-pregnanediols and allopregnanediols; pregnanedione; 11-dehydroprogesterone; desoxycorticosterone; hydroxyprogesterones, such as the 11α, 11β or 6β hydroxy compounds; ketoprogesterones, such as the 11, 12 or 6 keto compounds; and Δ^4-3-keto etiocholanic acid. Also utilizable are the known dehydro [the term "dehydro" having the accepted meaning "dehydrogenated" and not "dehydrated"] derivatives of the above-mentioned steroids,

2

e. g., those having a C=C linkage in the following positions: 6, 7; 8, 9; 9, 11; 11, 12; 8, 14; or 14, 15).

The sources of nitrogenous, growth-promoting factors are those normally employed in such processes. They may be natural organics (e. g., soybean meal, cornsteep liquor, meat extract and/or distillers solubles) or synthetics such as nitrates and ammonium compounds.

As to the energy-source material, lipids, especially (1) fat acids having at least 14 carbon atoms, (2) fats or (3) mixtures thereof, are preferred. Examples of such fats are lard oil, soybean oil, linseed oil, cottonseed oil, peanut oil, coconut oil, corn oil, castor oil, sesame oil, crude palm oil, fancy mutton tallow, sperm oil, olive oil, tristearin, tripalmitin, triolein and trilaurin; and illustrative fat acids are stearic, palmitic, oleic, linoleic and myristic acids. However, other carbon-containing materials may also be used. Examples of such materials are glycerol, glucose, fructose, sucrose, lactose, maltose, dextrins, starches and whey. These materials may be used either in purified state or as concentrates, such as whey concentrate, cornsteep liquor, or grain mashes (e. g., corn, wheat, or barley mash). Mixtures of the above may, of course, be employed. It is to be noted, however, that the C_{17}-substituted steroid is added to the fermentation medium essentially as a precursor, and not as an energy source.

The media used in the process of the invention may contain other precursors in addition to the C_{17}-substituted steroids to obtain other valuable products.

The process of the invention may result in various oxidation products. Primarily, the C_{17}-substituted steroid is oxidized in the C_{17} position to yield lactone products utilizable as hormones or intermediates therefor.

The following examples are illustrative of the invention, but are not to be construed as a limitation thereof.

EXAMPLE 1

Preparation of 1-dehydrotestololactone

(a) *Fermentation.*—A medium of the following composition is prepared: cornsteep liquor solids, 3.0 g.; $NH_4H_2PO_4$, 3.0 g.; $CaCO_3$, 2.5 g.; soybean oil, 2.2 g.; progesterone, 0.5 g.; and distilled water to make 1 liter. The medium is adjusted to pH 7.0 ± 0.1. Then, 100 ml. portions of the medium are distributed in 500 ml. Erlenmeyer flasks, and the flasks plugged with cotton and sterilized in the usual manner (i. e., by autoclaving for 30 minutes at 120° C.). When cool, each of the flasks is inoculated with 5–10% of a vegetative inoculum of *Cylindrocarpon radicola* [the vegetative inoculum being grown from stock cultures (lyophilized vial or agar slant) for 48–72 hours in a medium of the following composition: cornsteep liquor solids, 15 g.; brown sugar, 10 g.; $NaNO_3$, 6 g.; $ZnSO_4$, .001 g.; KH_2PO_4, 1.5 g.;

$MgSO_4 \cdot 7H_2O$.

0.5 g.; $CaCO_3$, 5 g.; lard oil, 2 g.; distilled water to make 1 liter]. The flasks are then placed on a reciprocating shaker (120 one and one-half inch cycles per minute) and mechanically shaken at 25° C. for 3 days. The contents of the flasks are then pooled and, after the pH of the culture is adjusted to about 4 ± 0.2 with sulfuric acid, filtered through Seitz filter pads to separate the mycelium from the fermented medium.

(b) *Extraction.*—The culture filtrate (40 liters) obtained in (a) is extracted with chloroform (40 liters) in an extractor (e. g., Podbielniak U. S. Patent 2,530,886, or improvements thereon) and the filtered chloroform extract is evaporated to dryness in vacuo. The residue (11.1 g.) is taken up in 200 ml. of 80% aqueous methanol, and the resulting solution is extracted four times with 100 ml. portions of hexane. The 80% aqueous

3

methanol solution is then concentrated in vacuo until crystals appear; and, after cooling at 0° C. for several (usually about 3–4) hours, the crystals formed are recovered by filtration. About 2.9 g. 1-dehydrotestololactone (M. P. 217–217.5° C.) are thus obtained. Concentration of the mother liquors yields additionally about 6.0 g. of the lactone. Recrystallization from acetone yields a purified 1-dehydrotestololactone having the following properties: M. P.; 218–219° C.; $[\alpha]_D^{23}$, —44° (C=1.20 in chloroform);

U.V.: $\lambda_{max}^{alc.}=242$ m$\mu(\epsilon=15750)$; I.R.: $\lambda_{max}^{nujol}=5.83\mu$ (lactone carbonyl) and 6.01 and 6.15μ ($\Delta^{1,4}$-3-ketone). Analysis: Calcd. for $C_{19}H_{24}O_3$; C, 75.97; H, 8.05; M. W. 300. Found: C, 76.29; H, 7.87; M. W. (Rast), 315. The compound has the structural formula

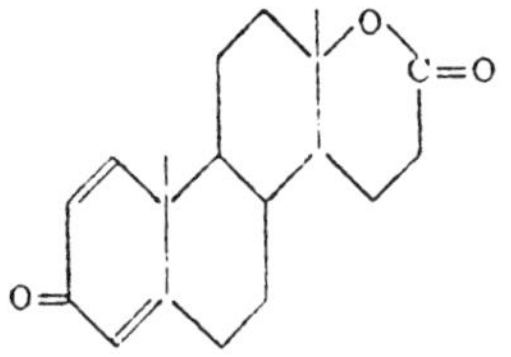

EXAMPLE 2

Preparation of estrololactone

A glass column (1 cm. diameter), filled with glass helices and maintained in a vertical position, is heated by means of an electric furnace and maintained at about 550–600° C. A hot solution of about 750 mg. 1-dehydrotestololactone in about 100 ml. mineral oil is then poured slowly through the column, and the hot effluent is collected in a round-bottom flask. The effluent is cooled, and diluted with about 200 ml. hexane; and the resulting mixture is allowed to remain at 0° C. for about 18 hours. About 496 mg. of crystalline deposit is separated by filtration, then washed with hexane. The dried crystals are then digested with warm acetone, leaving behind about 25 mg. estrololactone which is recovered by filtration.

For characterization, the estrololactone is acetylated by allowing it to remain overnight in contact with about 2 ml. of a mixture of acetic anhydride and pyridine, 1:1. The residue, after removal of the acetylating agents, is taken up in chloroform and washed successively with dilute hydrochloric acid, dilute sodium bicarbonate and water. The resulting chloroform solution is dried over sodium sulfate, and the chloroform is allowed to evaporate in vacuo to yield about 17.3 mg. crude acetate. When this crude material is dissolved in a mixture of benzene (4 ml.) and hexane (8 ml.), chromatographed on 0.5 g. sulfuric acid-washed alumina, and then eluted with benzene-hexane, 1:2, about 15 ml. oily impurities are obtained, followed by about 175 ml. solution containing the crystal-

4

line acetate. Further elution with about 50 ml. benzene-hexane (1:2) yields an additional fraction containing the crystalline acetate. The crystalline acetate is separated from the combined eluates by filtration. This crystalline acetate, on recrystallization three times from methanol, yields the pure acetate as prismatic rods mixed with heavy diamond-shaped crystals having a double melting point of 142–4° C. and 148–150° C. and U. V. absorption spectrum maxima characteristic of a phenolic acetate

$$[\lambda_{max}^{alc.}=267 \text{ m}\mu(\epsilon=1080) \text{ and } \lambda_{max}^{alc.}=275 \text{ m}\mu(\epsilon=945)]$$

The purified acetate has substantially the same melting point and I. R. spectrum as an authentic sample of estrololacetone acetate [Jacobsen, J. Biol. Chem., 171, 61 (1947)] and a mixed melting point of the two shows no depression.

EXAMPLE 3

Following the procedures of Example 1, but substituting an equivalent amount of testosterone for the progesterone of that example, the same products are obtained. 1-dehydrotestololactone thus produced was found to have the following properties: M. P. 216–218° C.; $[\alpha]_D^{22}$, —45.6° (C=1.24 in chloroform); I. R. spectrum identical with that obtained using authentic 1-dehydrotestololactone; no depression of M. P. when mixed with authentic 1-dehydrotestololactone and the melting point determined.

EXAMPLE 4

Following the procedure of Example 1, but substituting an equivalent amount of Reichstein's Compound "S" for the progesterone of that example, the same products are obtained. 1-dehydrotestololactone thus produced was found to have the following properties: M. P. 216–218° C., I. R. spectrum identical with that obtained using authentic 1-dehydrotestololactone; no depression of M. P. when mixed with authentic 1-dehydrotestololactone and the mixed melting point determined.

The invention may be variously otherwise embodied within the scope of the appended claim.

I claim:
1-dehydrotestololactone.

References Cited in the file of this patent
UNITED STATES PATENTS

2,480,246	Jacobson et al.	Aug. 30, 1949
2,499,248	Pincus et al.	Feb. 28, 1950
2,602,769	Murray et al.	July 8, 1952
2,558,023	Shull et al.	Nov. 3, 1953

OTHER REFERENCES

Jacobsen et al.: J. Biol. Chem., vol. 171, pp. 71–79 (1948).
Levy et al.: J. Biol. Chem. 171, pp. 71–79 (1947).

CHAPTER SIXTEEN

UNITED STATES PATENT OFFICE

2,236,574

BIOCHEMICAL MANUFACTURE OF KETOSTEROIDS

Heinrich Koester, Berlin-Charlottenburg, and Luigi Mamoli, Berlin-Steglitz, Germany, and Alberto Vercellone, Milan, Italy, assignors to Schering Corporation, Bloomfield, N. J., a corporation of New Jersey

No Drawing. Application May 28, 1938, Serial No. 210,778. In Germany June 3, 1937

22 Claims. (Cl. 195—12)

This invention relates to ketosteroids and compounds derivable therefrom as well as to a process of producing the same. The process of the invention consists in that steroids containing hydroxyl groups capable of dehydrogenation are subjected to the action of biochemical dehydrogenating agents and, if desired, also of biochemical hydrogenating agents.

For carrying out the biochemical dehydrogenation certain micro-organisms can be employed, for example bacteria or mold fungi or the enzymes obtainable therefrom. Among the bacteria may be mentioned for example the bacteria of the Acetobacter genus, in particular the *Acetobacter pasteurianum* and also Sorbose bacteria (*Acetobacter xylinum*: see Zentralblatt—(1896), vol. 1, pp. 1201–1202; see also Lafar "Handbuch der techn. Mykologie," vol. 5, page 565, published by Fischer, Jena, 1905–1914); among the mold fungi certain Aspergillaceae can be employed with advantage.

As particularly advantageous has proved the application of the so-called "impoverished" yeast as is obtainable for example according to Wieland, "Annalen der Chemie," vol. 492, page 183 et seq. by shaking yeast suspensions in toluene-water with oxygen.

The biochemical dehydrogenation is suitably carried out under aerobic conditions or in the presence of hydrogen acceptors such as methylene blue, quinone or the like.

To the steroid compounds coming into consideration as starting materials for the biochemical dehydrogenation belong for example the sterols and bile acids containing hydroxyl groups capable of dehydrogenation and also degradation products thereof, compounds of the type of cortin and of the animal and vegetable heart poisons containing hydroxyl groups capable of dehydrogenation. Furthermore compounds of the pregnane series containing hydroxyl groups capable of dehydrogenation can be employed as starting materials and also compounds of the oestrane and androstane series containing hydroxyl groups capable of dehydrogenation. Of the last named, compounds free from side chains may be particularly mentioned, for example, compounds such as oestratriol, octahydrooestrone and also the unsaturated compounds of the androstane series, the androstene compounds dehydroandrosterone and androstendiol.

Should other hydroxyl groups capable of dehydrogenation be contained in the starting material in addition to the hydroxyl group or groups to be dehydrogenated, the former can if necessary be protected from attack by the biochemical dehydrogenating agent by converting them intermediately, for example by esterification, etherification, halogenation or the like, into groups which can be reconverted into hydroxyl groups.

The process according to the invention for biochemical dehydrogenation is particularly advantageous in the androstene series when it is combined with the biochemical process of hydrogenation, as described for example in Berichte, vol. 70, page 470 et seq. Thus for example in this manner in one operation it is possible to proceed from dehydroandrosterone by way of androstendione to testosterone.

For this purpose the dehydroandrosterone is first subjected by means of the impoverished yeast to biochemical oxidation to androstendione and there is then added to the biochemical oxidation mixture containing androstendione a substratum which now causes the biochemical reaction to proceed in the direction of reduction. Suitable for this purpose are for example additions of carbohydrates, of degradation products of carbohydrates, such as glycerol phosphoric acid and others.

The following examples may serve to illustrate the invention without, however, limiting the same to them.

Example 1

As nutrient solution for the bacteria is employed unhopped beer wort for lager beer. The maltose content of the wort is determined and brought by dilution with water to a content of about 4%. The nutrient solution is then after the addition of calcium carbonate heated for 20 minutes at 115° C. in an autoclave and after cooling filtered clear. The nutrient solution again heated under pressure is thereupon filled into sterile large Petri dishes and inoculated with the *Acetobacter pasteurianum*. After 3 days standing at room temperature there are carefully introduced into each Petri dish which contains 300 cc. of nutrient solution, a solution of 300 mg. of androstendiol in 15 cc. of ethyl alcohol. After further standing for 2 days at room temperature again the same quantity of androstendiol is introduced and again the whole allowed to stand for 2 days at the same temperature. Thereupon the contents of the Petri dishes are combined and exhaustively treated with ether.

The ethereal solution is freed by washing from the acetic acid which has likewise been produced in the fermentation, and evaporated to dryness. The residue is precipitated with digitonin, the filtrate freed from digitonin and treated in methanol with semicarbazide acetate. The semicarbazone is isolated and split in known manner. After treatment with methanol containing acid the whole is recrystallized from ethyl acetate. The product exhibits in ethanol a rotation of

$$(\alpha)_D^{20} = +108°$$

M. P. 152° C. and is shown to be testosterone.

Example 2

With the application of the same substratum for the bacteria as described in the previous example, the alcoholic solution of the substance to be oxidized is added to the bacteria culture. 200 mg. of dehydroandrosterone are employed in the case of a quantity of substratum of 300 cc. After 3 days standing the whole is extracted with ether, the ethereal solution washed, dried and evaporated. The residue is then for removal of the unchanged dehydroandrosterone treated for 4 hours in absolute pyridine with phthalic anhydride, the reaction mixture poured into water, extracted with ether and the pyridine removed by washing with water containing acid. The acid phthalic acid ester of the dehydroandrosterone is then separated with alkali and an evaporation of the ethereal solution a crystallizate is obtained which is treated with methanol containing acid and after recrystallisation from hexane gives androstendione of rotation value

$$(\alpha)_D^{20} = +198°\,(CHCl_3)$$

and M. P. 173° C.

Example 3

As described in Examples 1 and 2 in a further process androstendiol monopropionate-17 is subjected to oxidation. 300 mg. of this product (M. P. 146 C.;

$$(\alpha)_D^{20} = -62°\,(C_2H_5OH))$$

being used for a bacteria culture with 300 cc. of substratum. After 4 days' standing at room temperature working up is carried out as described in Example 2, and also the unchanged monopropionate is removed as acid phthalic acid ester. The testosterone propionate remaining after the isomerization is then recrystallised from hexane and gives the following values: M. P. 121° C.;

$$(\alpha)_D^{20} = +87°\,(C_2H_5OH)$$

Example 4

In 1 liter of a nutrient solution containing 1% peptone, 0.2% ammonium biphosphate, 0.1% potassium biphosphate and 0.025% magnesium phosphate *Sorbose bacteria (Acetobacter xylinum)* are caused to develop. To the culture solution 10 cc. of a 2% solution of cholesterol in alcohol are added portionally. After standing for some time the reaction mixture is extracted with ether. The ethereal solution is washed with water, freed from water and evaporated to dryness. The residue is taken up with methanol and treated with semicarbazide acetate. The cholestenone semicarbazone is precipitated and filtered off. It yields after splitting in known manner the cholestenone of M. P. 80–81°;

$$(\alpha)_D^{20} = +87°$$

Example 5

3 grams of yeast (Milan flocculent ferment) are suspended in 30 cc. of water and treated with 10 cc. of N/5 Na_2HPO_4 solution and 10 cc. of N/5 KH_2PO_4 solution. The suspension is shaken for 20 hours in an oxygen atmosphere at 32° C., then 190 mg. of androstendiol, suspended in 30 cc. of water, are added and finally the mixture is shaken for a further 47 hours in an oxygen atmosphere. Thereupon the reaction mixture is extracted with ether; the ethereal solution is washed with water, caustic soda lye, N/1 hydrochloric acid and again with water. After drying over sodium sulphate the ethereal solution is evaporated to dryness.

The residue is dissolved in 30 cc. of alcohol, heated with 3 grams of glacial acetic acid and 1.5 grams of P. reagent (Girard, Helv. Chim. Acta 19, 1095 (1935)) and heated to boiling for 1 hour under reflux. After cooling, the whole is poured into 140 cc. of water, 60 grams of ice and the quantity of sodium hydroxide necessary for neutralization of 2.7 grams of glacial acetic acid. The whole is then extracted 3 times with ether in order to remove the portion free from keto groups.

To the aqueous solution are added 20 grams of 50% sulphuric acid whereby a turbidity is produced. The solution is allowed to stand for one hour and it is then extracted 3 times with ether, the ethereal solution washed with water, dried over sodium sulphate and the ether evaporated. If the residue is again treated with some ether it can be produced in crystalline form.

After recrystallization of the residue from dilute acetone a substance is obtained of M. P. 168–169° C. which is shown to be identical with androstendione.

Example 6

8 grams of yeast (Milan flocculent ferment) are suspended in 30 cc. of water, treated with 10 cc. of N/5 Na_2HPO_4 solution and 10 cc. of N/5 KH_2PO_4 solution and shaken for 20 hours in an oxygen atmosphere at 32° C. Then 200 mg. of dehydroandrosterone, suspended in 30 cc. of water are introduced and the mixture subsequently shaken for a further 48 hours in an oxygen atmosphere.

Thereupon a solution of 25 grams of invert sugar in 150 cc. of water is introduced and the reaction mixture allowed to stand in a fermentation vessel for 3 days at room temperature.

The reaction mixture is then extracted with ether and the ethereal solution washed with water, caustic soda lye, N/1 hydrochloric acid and again with water. After drying over sodium sulphate the ethereal solution is evaporated. The remaining residue is recrystallized from acetone and petrol ether. There are obtained 120 mg. of a substance of M. P. 151° C. which is shown to be identical with testosterone.

On the basis of the process according to the invention for dehydrogenation or dehydrogenation and hydrogenation it is possible in a relatively simple manner and with the production of relatively high yields to produce valuable ketosteroids which were hitherto only obtainable by relatively cumbersome methods or only in relatively small yields.

Of course, various modifications and changes in the reaction condition etc. may be made by those skilled in the art in accordance with the principles set forth herein and in the claims annexed hereto.

What we claim is:

1. Process for the manufacture of ketosteroids comprising subjecting steroids containing hydroxyl groups capable of dehydrogenation to the action of biochemical dehydrogenating agents, and isolating from the dehydrogenation mixture the keto steroids formed.

2. Process as claimed in claim 1 in which

steroid compounds free from side chains at the 17-carbon atom are employed as starting materials.

3. Process as claimed in claim 1 in which unsaturated compounds of the androstane series are employed as starting materials.

4. Process as claimed in claim 1 in which androstendiol is employed as starting material.

5. Process as claimed in claim 1 in which dehydroandrosterone is employed as starting material.

6. Process as claimed in claim 1 in which the biochemical dehydrogenation is carried out under aerobic conditions.

7. Process as claimed in claim 1 in which the biochemical dehydrogenation is carried out by means of bacteria of the genus Acetobacter.

8. Process as claimed in claim 1 in which the biochemical dehydrogenation is carried out by means of *Acetobacter pasteurianum*.

9. Process as claimed in claim 1 in which for carrying out the biochemical dehydrogenation "impoverished" yeast is employed.

10. Process for the manufacture of keto-steroids, which comprises converting at least one but less than all of the hydroxyl groups of a steroid having a plurality of hydroxyl groups capable of dehydrogenation, into a group or groups which are not attacked during the dehydrogenation defined hereinbelow, subjecting the hydroxy derivative to the action of a biochemical dehydrogenating agent, and recovering the ketonic reaction product from the reaction mixture.

11. Process for the manufacture of keto hydroxy steroids comprising subjecting steroids containing more than one hydroxyl group capable of dehydrogenation, to the action of a biochemical dehydrogenating agent, then causing a biochemical hydrogenating agent to act upon the so obtained polyketo compounds, and recovering the formed keto hydroxy compounds from the reaction mixture.

12. Process for the manufacture of keto hydroxy steroids comprising subjecting steroids containing more than one hydroxyl group capable of dehydrogenation, to the action of oxidizing bacteria of the genus Acetobacter, causing a biochemical hydrogenating agent to act upon the so obtained polyketo compounds, and isolating the formed keto hydroxy compounds from the reaction mixture.

13. Process as set forth in claim 10, in which the hydroxyl group or groups which are not to be dehydrogenated are esterified prior to the dehydrogenation.

14. Process as set forth in claim 10, in which the hydroxyl group or groups which are not to be dehydrogenated are etherified prior to the dehydrogenation.

15. Process as set forth in claim 10, in which the hydroxyl group or groups which are not to be dehydrogenated are replaced by halogen prior to the dehydrogenation.

16. Process according to claim 10, wherein the substituted hydroxyl group or groups are reconverted to the free hydroxyl group or groups after the dehydrogenation.

17. Process as set forth in claim 10, in which the hydroxyl group or groups which are not to be dehydrogenated are esterified prior to the dehydrogenation, and reconverting the substituted hydroxyl group or groups into the free hydroxyl group or groups after the hydrogenation.

18. Process as set forth in claim 10, in which the hydroxyl group or groups which are not to be dehydrogenated are etherified prior to the dehydrogenation, and reconverting the substituted hydroxyl group or groups into the free hydroxyl group or groups after the hydrogenation.

19. Process as set forth in claim 10, in which the hydroxyl group or groups which are not to be dehydrogenated are replaced by halogen prior to the dehydrogenation, and reconverting the substituted hydroxyl group or groups into the free hydroxyl group or groups after the dehydrogenation.

20. Process for the manufacture of keto hydroxy steroids which comprises subjecting steroids having more than one hydroxyl group capable of dehydrogenation, to the action of oxidizing bacteria of the genus Acetobacter, and then subjecting the obtained polyketo compounds to the action of a reducing yeast in a fermenting substratum to cause partial hydrogenation.

21. Process for the manufacture of keto hydroxy steroids which comprises subjecting steroids containing more than one hydroxyl group capable of dehydrogenation, to a biochemical dehydrogenation with the aid of an "impoverished" yeast, and thereafter adding a substratum which is capable of being fermented by the yeast to cause partial biochemical hydrogenation of the polyketone.

22. Process for the manufacture of keto hydroxy steroids which comprises subjecting steroids containing more than one hydroxyl group capable of dehydrogenation to a biochemical dehydrogenation with the aid of an "impoverished" yeast, thereafter adding a carbohydrate substratum which is capable of being fermented by the yeast to cause partial biochemical hydrogenation of the polyketone.

HEINRICH KOESTER.
LUIGI MAMOLI.
ALBERTO VERCELLONE.

CHAPTER SEVENTEEN

UNITED STATES PATENT OFFICE

2,384,335

PROCESS FOR OXIDIZING UNSATURATED POLYCYCLIC ALCOHOLS

Rupert Oppenauer. Amsterdam, Netherlands;
vested in the Alien Property Custodian

No Drawing. Application May 21, 1937, Serial No.
144,097. In the Netherlands May 26, 1936

7 Claims. (Cl. 260—397.3)

This invention relates to process for oxidizing unsaturated polycyclic alcohols; and it comprises a process in which unsaturated polycyclic alcohols, containing at least one hydroxyl group which it is theoretically possible to oxidize into a carbonyl group, said alcohols being usually of the type containing a cyclopentanopolyhydrophenanthrene nucleus, are reacted with an excess of an aldehyde or ketone in the presence of an alcoholate selected from a class consisting of aluminum alcoholate and chloro-magnesium alcoholate, the process being usually conducted at temperatures ranging from about 50° to 140° C. and in the presence of an inert solvent; all as more fully hereinafter set forth and as claimed.

The chemical investigation of hormones during recent years has shown that a great number of these physiologically and pharmacologically important substances and particularly the sex-hormones are polycyclic ketones. It has been found e. g. that progesteron which is the active substance of the corpus luteum extract is Δ-4,5 pregnendion (3,20) and that testosteron is Δ-4,5-androstenol-(17)-on-(3). These and many other hormones which are polycyclic ketones have been also prepared synthetically from cholesterol, stigmasterol etc. such as, e. g. the progesteron (Butenandt and cooperators Z. Physiol. Chem. 227, 84, 1934, Ber. 67B, 1611, 2085, 1934, and Fernholz Ber. 67, 1855, 2027, 1934), the testosteron (Ruzicka and cooperators Helv. Chim. Acta 18, 1264, 1478, 1935), the methyltestosteron (Ruzicka, Goldberg, Rosenberg Helv. Chim. Acta 18, 1487, 1945), the androstendion (Ruzicka, Wettstein, Helv. Chim. Acta 18, 986, 1935) etc.

As starting materials for the preparation of polycyclic ketones such as the above mentioned ones, containing beside a keto-group a double bond, substances were used in the already known processes which substances, leaving out of consideration possible side-chains, have a hydroxyl group in the position C3 and a double bond between C4 and C5. These substances have consequently to undergo during one stage or the other of the synthesis the same chemical changes taking place in the preparation of cholestenon from cholesterol.

For effecting this last mentioned reaction two processes have been described. Diels (Ber. 37, 3099, 1904) has melted together cholesterol and cupric oxide at 280–300° C. and obtained in this way cholestenon in a yield of 65%. On the other hand Windaus and Abderhalden (Ber. 39, 518, 1906) added to the double bond of the cholesterol the calculated quantity of bromine,

oxidized the dibromide to the dibromoketone by means of $KMnO_4$ or CrO_3 and then eliminated the bromine from this dibromoketone. They also obtained in this way a yield of cholestenon of 60 to 65%. Both processes have already been applied to the preparation of polycyclic ketones from alcohols such as e. g. the oxidation by means of CuO according to Diels in connection with the progesteron (Fernholz B. 67, 2030, 1934). In this way, however, a yield of only 4% was obtained which can be readily understood, bearing in mind the drastic treatment.

The second process (via the bromine derivatives) is the method generally in use up till now for the synthesis of polycyclic unsaturated ketones. In this way crystallized progesteron e. g. was obtained from Δ-5, 6-pregnenol-(3)-on-(20) in a yield of 35–40% (Butenandt B. 69, 443, 1936). This method was also applied to the preparation of testosteron and methyl testosteron, however with relatively low yields never exceeding 50% (Ruzicka, loc. cit.). These great losses are due, on the one hand, to the complicated reaction (2 intermediary products) and on the other hand all optimal conditions must be taken into consideration as exactly as possible when executing these reactions, which conditions are, however, different from one case to the other (vide Butenandt Ber. 67, 2087, 1934), Fernholz (Ber. 67, 2029, 1934).

Other processes for economically effecting the oxidation are unknown up till now. It is true that Schönheimer (J. Biol. Chem. 110, 461, 1935) has described a modification of the last mentioned process in which he obtains cholestenon in a good yield starting from the cholesterol dibromide (the intermediate product of bromination). In this way, however, the losses during the whole reaction are only partly avoided and, moreover, this method is not applicable with the same successful result to substances which may be prepared by my process.

The object of my invention is to effect this oxidation in a completely new and extraordinarily simple way whereby a substantially quantitative yield is obtained. I have found that unsaturated polycyclic alcohols are capable of being oxidized to the corresponding ketones by yielding 2 atoms of hydrogen per molecule and per hydroxyl group to other substances involved in this reaction and containing keto or aldehyde groups in the presence of certain alcoholates. At least one hydroxyl group of the unsaturated alcohol is converted into a carbonyl group. In this way e. g. the compounds of the cholesterol type are oxidized to those of the cholestenon type and as a matter of fact in such a delicate way that the yield is practically theoretical. My method is particularly adapted to the production of the corresponding ketones from unsaturated polycyclic alcohols containing a cyclopentano-polyhydrophenanthrene nucleus.

My new process is in every respect superior to the methods known till now. My process consists herein that the sterol alcohol to be oxidized is treated in the presence of tertiary metal alcoholates, preferably tertiary alcoholates of aluminium or of magnesium chloride with an excess of hydrogen acceptor. Preferably the reaction is carried out at an increased temperature (50–140° C.) in order to increase the reaction speed, and, moreover, in order to increase the solubility of the intermediary reaction products in an inert solvent, such as benzene, which may be added.

As hydrogen acceptors I may use ketones and aldehydes of the aliphatic, alicyclic and aromatic series.

Without limiting my process to a specific theory I have assumed that the reaction takes place in such a way that, from the polycyclic alcohol (I) e. g. with acetone, under the action of the aluminium or magnesium alcoholate, an addition compound (II) is formed which splits into the α,β-unsaturated ketone (III) and propyl alcohol.

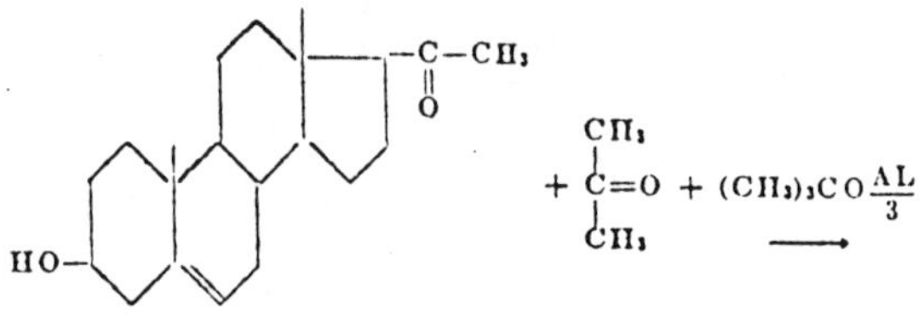

I
Pregnenolon

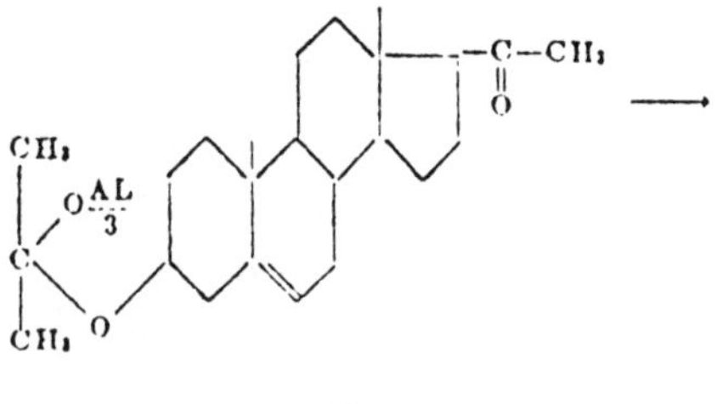

II

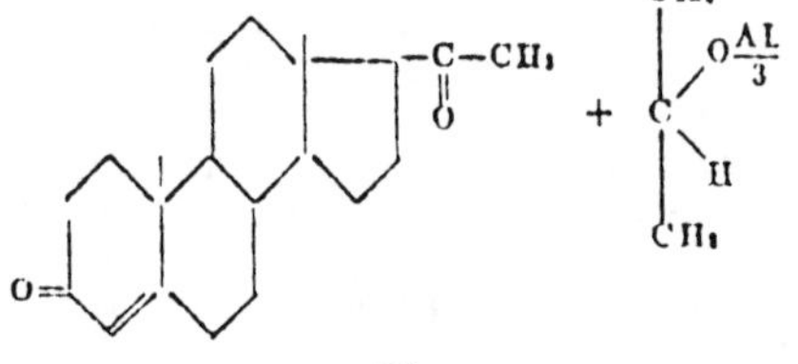

III
Progesteron

My method may be applied to unsaturated polycyclic hydroxy ketones in which it is theoretically possible for at least one of the hydroxyl groups contained therein to be oxidized to a carbonyl group (e. g. dehydroandrosteron, pregnenolon, etc. which can be oxidized in this way to diketones), as well as to unsaturated polycyclic hydroxy-esters (e. g. the acetate-(17) of the androstendiol) as well as to sterol alcohols (e. g. cholesterol). It is particularly surprising that the ester group of the hydroxy-esters is not saponified during this operation since it is known

that esters as a rule react with alcoholates under saponification (vide Windaus and cooperators Ann. 520, 100, 1925). Also the presence of a tertiary OH-group in the molecule is not objectionable in my process so that it is possible to prepare by my method e. g. methyl testosteron from 17-methyl androstendiol-(3,17) in a substantially theoretic yield (compare Ruzicka Helv. Chim. Acta 18, 1487, 1935). By means of my new method special substances can be prepared by synthesis which could not be made up till now, due to the fact that during the drastic oxidation of substances having several double bonds, secondary reactions take place in the known methods. E. g. the ergostatrienon could not yet be prepared till now and its synthesis with a large yield according to my new process is described in Example 5. For carrying the aluminium or magnesium chloride to the hydroxyl groups to be oxidized, tertiary alcohols come mainly into consideration, such as e. g. trimethyl carbinol, amylene hydrate, triphenyl carbinol.

The advantages of my new process are that:

1. The yields are approximately twice as high as in the known processes.

2. The reaction can be effected very simply and requires only a very short reaction time in comparison to the known methods.

3. The method can be applied to crude concentrates with the same success. E. g. a progesteron concentrate can be prepared from the mother liquors of the ketones obtained during the manufacture of the dehydro androsteron from cholesterol or sitosterol and this was technically absolutely impossible till now.

The unsaturated polycyclic ketones prepared in this way may be applied in therapeutics.

My invention is elucidated by but not at all restricted to the following examples:

1. Preparation of cholestenon from cholesterol

10 grams of cholesterol are dissolved in 100–150 cm.³ of acetone under heating and a solution of 20 grams of tertiary aluminium butylate in 300 cm.³ of anhydrous benzene is added hereto. This mixture is heated under reflux cooling during 7 hours; the aluminium is removed by shaking out with diluted sulphuric acid, the benzene layer is washed with water, dried with sodium sulphate and then evaporated to dryness. Substantially pure cholestenon remains behind which is obtained in crystallized form by recrystallization, e. g. from methanol in a yield of 90–95% of the theory.

2. Preparation of androstendion from dehydroandrosteron

2 grams of dehydroandrosteron are heated under reflux cooling with 2 grams of aluminate of amylene hydrate and 80 grams of acetophenone in 150 cm.³ of benzene during 14 hours. The reaction products are then hydrolized with diluted sulphuric acid and the washed and dried benzene solution is evaporated to dryness. The residue is fractionally distilled in high vacuum (cathode-vacuum) and the fraction distilling over at 120–140° C. is recrystallized from ether. Androstendion (melting point 170–172° C.) is obtained in a yield of 80–86% of the theory.

3. Preparation of methyl testosteron from methyl androstendiol

0.6 gram of 17-methyl Δ-5.6 androstendiol (3, 17) is heated under reflux cooling during 20 hours in 50 cm.³ of benzene and 12 cm.³ of acetone with 3 grams of tertiary chloro magnesium butylate, which may be prepared by conversion of acetone with methyl magnesium chloride. The further treatment takes place as in Example 1 and methyl testosteron (melting point 160–162° C.) is obtained in a yield of more than 75% of the theory.

4. Preparation of testosteron acetate from androstendiol acetate

0.7 gram of 17-mono acetate of the androstendiol (3, 17) is heated under reflux cooling in 30 cm.³ of toluene and 8 cm.³ of acetone with 1 gram of tertiary aluminium butylate during 5 hours. The further treatment takes place as in Examples 1 and 2 and testosteron acetate (melting point 135–139° C.) is obtained in a yield of 80–90% of the theory.

5. Preparation of ergostatrienon from ergosterol

1.5 grams of ergosterol are dissolved under heating in 120 cm.³ of gasoline (boiling point 100–125° C.) and heated under reflux cooling after addition of 20 grams of acetone and 1 gram of tertiary aluminium butylate during 8 hours. The further treatment is effected as in Example 1, and 1.12 grams of crystallized ergostatrienon (M. P. 131–132.5° C.) are obtained as needles.

What I claim is:

1. Process for the manufacture of unsaturated ketones of the cyclopentano polyhydrophenanthrene series from the corresponding unsaturated secondary alcohols, which comprises subjecting such alcohol to the action of an excess of a compound from the group consisting of aldehydes and ketones in the presence of tertiary aluminum butylate.

2. The process of manufacturing polycyclic ketones which comprises subjecting an unsaturated alcohol of the cyclopentano-polyhydrophenanthrene series in which it is theoretically possible for at least one hydroxyl group to be replaced by a keto group to the action of an excess of an organic compound selected from the group consisting of aldehydes and ketones in the presence of an alcoholate selected from a class consisting of the tertiary aluminum and chloromagnesium alcoholates.

3. The process of manufacturing polycyclic ketones which comprises subjecting an unsaturated polycyclic alcohol selected from a class consisting of the sterols, the hydroxy-ketones and hydroxy-esters of the cyclopentano-polyhydrophenanthrene series in which it is theoretically possible for at least one hydroxyl group to be replaced by a keto group to the action of an excess of an organic compound selected from the group consisting of aldehydes and ketones in the presence of an alcoholate selected from a class consisting of the tertiary aluminum and chloromagnesium alcoholates.

4. The process of manufacturing polycyclic ketones which comprises subjecting an unsaturated organic compound selected from a class consisting of dehydroandrosteron, pregnenolon, the 17-acetate of androstendiol and cholesterol to the action of an excess of an organic compound selected from the group consisting of aldehydes and ketones in the presence of an alcoholate selected from a class consisting of the tertiary aluminum and chloro-magnesium alcoholates.

5. The process of manufacturing polycyclic ketones which comprises subjecting an unsaturated secondary alcohol of the cyclopentano-polyhydrophenanthrene series to the action of an excess of an organic compound selected from the group consisting of aldehydes and ketones in the presence of tertiary aluminum butylate.

6. The process of manufacturing polycyclic ketones which comprises subjecting an unsaturated secondary alcohol of the cyclopentano-polyhydrophenanthrene series to the action of an excess of an organic compound selected from the group consisting of aldehydes and ketones in the presence of an alcoholate selected from a class consisting of the teritary aluminum and chloro-magnesium alcoholates.

7. The process of manufacturing polycyclic ketones which comprises subjecting an unsaturated secondary polycyclic alcohol of the cyclopentano-polyhydrophenanthrene series to the action of an organic compound selected from a class consisting of aldehydes and ketones in the presence of a tertiary alcoholate selected from a class consisting of the aluminum and chloro-magnesium alcoholates, the reaction taking place in an inert solvent and at a temperature ranging from 50° to 140° C.

RUPERT OPPENAUER.

UNITED STATES PATENT OFFICE

2,374,369

SATURATED AND UNSATURATED 17-HYDROXYANDROSTANES, THEIR DERIVATIVES AND SUBSTITUTION PRODUCTS AND PROCESS OF MAKING SAME

Karl Miescher, Rieben and Albert Wettstein, Basel, Switzerland, assignors to Ciba Pharmaceutical Products, Incorporated, Summit, N. J., a corporation of New Jersey

No Drawing. Original application December 26, 1940, Serial No. 371,832. Divided and this application October 22, 1942, Serial No. 462,989. In Switzerland December 23, 1939

11 Claims. (Cl. 260—397.4)

It has been found that saturated and unsaturated 17-hydroxy-androstanones or their derivatives (for example, esters, ethers) or substitution products with saturated or unsaturated hydrocarbon residues may be obtained by treating androstane-17-ones, containing only double bonds in the rings A and B, with agents capable of transforming the group —CO— into the group —CR(OH)—, R representing hydrogen or a saturated or unsaturated hydrocarbon radical, treating the 17-carbinols obtained if desired with esterfying or etherifying agents, hereupon reacting the products with oxidising agents, capable of introducing into the α-position of a double bond a member of the group of oxygen and oxygen containing groups, and, finally, if desired, allowing hydrolysing and/or oxidising or dehydrogenating agents, respectively, to act upon the products thus obtained.

The parent materials named may be obtained, for example, by the degradation of the side chain in dimethyl - cyclopentano - polyhydrophenanthrene compounds containing side chains and corresponding nuclear double bonds as described in patent application Serial No. 371,058, filed December 20, 1940 (now Patent No. 2,319,012, granted May 11, 1943). The double bonds may be located in particular in the 2, 3, 4, or 5 position.

Agents which are capable of transforming the group —CO— into the group —CR(OH)—, R having the meaning given above, are reducing agents in the widest sense of the term, as well as, for example, metallo-hydrocarbon compounds, such as Grignard's reagents, alkali-hydrocarbon compounds and the like, which, in addition to reducing the 17-keto group, are capable of introducing in the same position an additional saturated or unsaturated hydrocarbon radical, for example, a methyl, ethyl, allyl, or acetylene group. The 17-carbinols thus obtained, particularly those having secondary alcohol groups, are converted, if desired, into their corresponding esters or ethers in known manner by the action of esterifying or etherifying agents. In this instance, particular use is made of esterifying agents which are capable of introducing aliphatic acid radicals, such as those of formic, acetic, propionic, n- or isobutyric, n- or iso-valeric, caproic, capric, palmitic, or stearic acids, furthermore aromatic, fatty aromatic or inorganic acid radicals, examples being benzoic acid, cinnamic acid or substituted carbonic acid radicals. For the etherification, aliphatic or aliphatic-aromatic alcohols or phenols, for example, methyl, ethyl, benzyl alcohols, triarylmethyl-carbinols and the like, are introduced.

Upon the reaction products thus obtained oxidising agents are now caused to react which are capable of introducing in a manner of itself known in the α-position to a double bond, oxygen or groups containing oxygen, such as oxo, hydroxy or substituted hydroxyl groups. For this purpose, as is known, for example chromic acid, selenium dioxide, lead tetracylates, etc. may be used. In order, for example, to convert substituted hydroxyl groups into free hydroxyl groups, further treatment is given if desired with hydrolysing agents, in which case it is also possible, by cautious working, to hydrolyse partially only the newly introduced substituents in rings A or B, but not the possibly substituted hydroxyl group in the 17 position; therefore, in these instances, it is advantageous if the 17-carbinol group has already been substituted by a difficultly hydrolysable radical.

In this manner, compounds of the dimethyl-cyclopentanopolyhydrophenanthrene series have been obtained which contain a free, esterified or etherified hydroxyl group and furthermore, if desired, also a hydrocarbon radical in the 17 position, and which contain in rings A or B, keto groups or free or esterified hydroxyl groups the α-position to double bonds. From the compounds which carry hydroxyl groups, the desired ketones, saturated or unsaturated 17-hydroxyandrostanones, their derivatives or substitution products, may then be obtained in a manner of itself known by the action of oxidising or dehydrogenating agents.

The following formulae explain some of the above reactions without in any way limiting their scope;

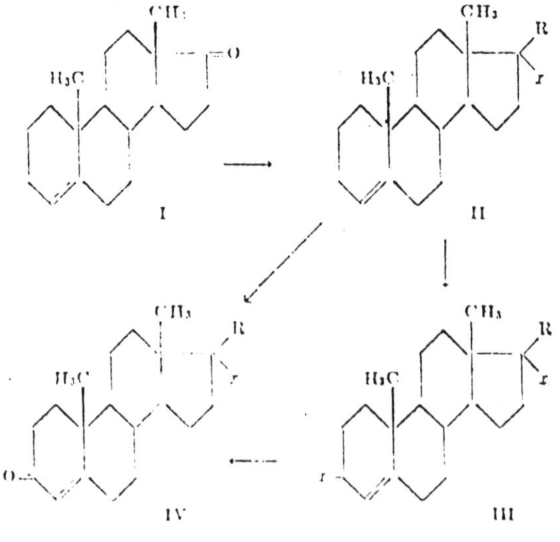

x = free or substituted hydroxyl group.
R = hydrogen, saturated or unsaturated hydrocarbon radical.

Example 1

1 part of Δ⁴-androstene-17-one of Formula I (prepared, for example, according to the instructions given in U. S. Patent No. 2.319.012. by splitting the side chain in Δ⁴-cholestene) is dissolved in 25 parts of pure alcohol and is hydrogenated by means of a nickel catalyst, prepared, for example according to the methods of Rupe or Raney. After 1 molecule of hydrogen has been absorbed, the hydrogenation is stopped, the catalyst is removed by filtration, the filtrate is evaporated in vacuo, and the residue is dissolved in 6 parts of absolute pyridine. 2 parts of propionic acid anhydride are now added. The solution is maintained for 16 hours at room temperature, after which it is poured into 50 parts of water. The ester which crystallises out after the decomposition of the anhydride is filtered off at the pump, washed with water and dried in a vacuum exsiccator. By recrystallisation from hexane, pure Δ⁴-androstene-17-ol-propionate is obtained in colourless crystalline form. It corresponds with the Formula II. in which x stands for —OCO—C₂H₅ and R for H.

Instead of by a catalytic method other reduction methods known to be suitable for the conversion of a keto group into a carbinol group may be used, for example nascent hydrogen, like an alkali metal and an alcohol, further an organo-metal compound prone to the formation of unsaturated hydrocarbons, like iso-propyl magnesium iodide, or even biochemical or electrochemical means. In place of propionic acid anhydride, other propionylating agents may naturally be used, for example, a propionic acid halide, or other desired esters or even ethers may be formed.

In place of the radical of propionic acid, other ester or ether radicals may be introduced, for example those named before, or the new carbinol group may rest unprotected if suitable oxidising agents, for example selenium dioxide, are chosen for the following oxidation.

If, instead of using Δ⁴-androstene-17-one as parent substance, a parent substance which is unsaturated in another position be used, for example, Δ²-, Δ³- or Δ⁵-androstene-17-one, the corresponding unsaturated product is analogously obtained.

Thus quite generally as intermediates androstane derivatives are obtained, containing in the rings A and B only a double bond in which the carbon atom 5 may participate, and in 17-position a free, esterified or etherified hydroxyl group: for example the Δ⁴-androstene-17-ol-acylates.

1 part of this Δ⁴-androstene-17-ol-propionate is dissolved in 50 parts of glacial acetic acid: a solution of 1.2 parts of chromium trioxide in a little water is added, and the mixture is stirred for 12 hours at room temperature, after which 400 parts of water are added. The reaction mixture is extracted exhaustively with ether, the ethereal solution is washed with a solution of bicarbonate and then with water and is then dried and evaporated in vacuo. From the residue, testosterone propionate (Δ⁴-androstene-3-one-17-ole-propionate of Formula IV, in which x stands for —OCO—C₂H₅ and R for H), together with the corresponding 3-oxo- and 3:6-dioxo-compounds, is obtained by fractional crystallisation, adsorption or sublimation.

In place of chromic acid, selenium dioxide or a lead tetraacylate, for example, may be used for the oxidation. In this case, a Δ⁴-3-hydroxy- or -acyloxy-androstene-17-ole-propionate of the Formula III is primarily obtained, which may subsequently be converted into testosterone propionate, if necessary after partial hydrolysis of only the 3-ester group, by the action of oxidising or dehydrogenating agents in a manner of itself known.

Example 2

1 part of Δ⁴-androstene-17-one of Formula I is dissolved in ether and this solution is allowed to drop into a boiling solution of excess of methyl magnesium iodide in ether. After the reaction is complete, water and acid are added cautiously, the ethereal solution is removed, washed and evaporated. From the residue Δ⁴-17-methyl-androstene-17-ole of Formula II (x stands for OH and R for CH₃) is obtained.

In a completely analogous manner compounds containing instead of a methyl other saturated or unsaturated hydrocarbon radicals may be obtained, for example the 17-ethyl, 17-ethinyl- or 17-allyl-androstene-17-oles with a double bond in 2, 3, 4, 5-position etc., by reaction with for example ethyl, ethinyl or allyl magnesium halides on the androstene-17-ones.

17-ethinyl-androstenoles like the Δ⁴-17-ethinyl-androstene-17-ole, the Δ⁵-17-ethinyl-androstene-17-ole etc., may also be prepared advantageously by the action of sodium acetylide, for example in liquid ammonia or amylene hydrate.

By energetic action of esterifying or etherifying agents the new tertiary carbinol groups in 17-position may be converted into ester or ether groups in known manner.

Thus quite generally as intermediates androstane derivatives may be obtained, containing in the rings A and B only a double bond in which the carbon atom 5 may participate, and in 17-position a free, esterified or etherified hydroxyl groups and hydrocarbon radical.

The Δ⁴-17-methyl-androstene-17-ole described above is converted in a manner fully analogous to that described in Example 1 for Δ⁴-androstene-17-ole-propionate, for example, by means of chromic acid, directly into 17-methyl-testosterone of Formula IV (x stands for OH: R for CH₃), or also, for example, by the action of selenium dioxide or of a lead tetraacylate into Δ⁴-17-methyl-androstene-3:17-diole or its 3-mono esters. These, then, if necessary after hydrolysis, may also be converted into 17-methyl-testosterone in a manner of itself known, by means of oxidising or dehydrogenating agents. If, instead of Δ⁴-17-methyl-androstene-17-ole, corresponding compounds containing for example, an ethyl, ethinyl, ethenyl, or allyl group in the 17-position be used as parent materials, 17-ethyl-, 17-ethinyl-, 17-ethenyl-, or 17-allyl-testosterone is obtained in an analogous manner.

This application is a division of our application Serial No. 371,832 filed December 26, 1940.

What we claim is:

1. A process of the character described, which comprises the steps of reacting an androstene-17-one of the formula

with a metallo-hydrocarbon compound and with a hydrolyzing agent, whereby the group

$$-C=O$$

in the 17-position is converted into the group

$$-CR(OH)$$

R standing for a hydrocarbon radical.

2. A process of the character described, which comprises the steps of reacting an androstene-17-one of the formula

with a metallo-hydrocarbon compound and with a hydrolyzing agent, whereby the group

$$-C=O$$

in the 17-position is converted into the group

$$-CR(OH)$$

R standing for a hydrocarbon radical, and then reacting the resultant compound with chromic acid, whereby a product of the formula

R representing the aforesaid hydrocarbon radical, results.

3. A process of the character described, which comprises the steps of reacting an androstene-17-one of the formula

with an organo-metallic compound of the Grignard type and with a hydrolyzing agent, whereby the group

$$-C=O$$

in the 17-position is converted into the group

$$-CR(OH)$$

R standing for a hydrocarbon radical.

4. A process of the character described, which comprises the steps of reacting an androstene-17-one of the formula

with a hydrocarbon-substituted metal halide and with a hydrolyzing agent, whereby the group

$$-C=O$$

in the 17-position is converted into the group

$$-CR(OH)$$

R standing for a hydrocarbon radical.

5. A process of the character described, which comprises the steps of reacting Δ⁴-androstene-17-one with an alkyl magnesium halide and with a hydrolyzing agent, and then reacting the resultant Δ⁴-17-alkyl-androstene-17-ole with chromic acid to produce 17-alkyl testosterone.

6. A process of the character described, which comprises the steps of reacting Δ⁴-androstene-17-one with an alkyl magnesium halide and with a hydrolyzing agent, and then reacting the resultant Δ⁴-17-alkyl-androstene-17-ole with selenium dioxide to produce Δ⁴-17-alkyl-androstene-3:17-diole.

7. A process of the character described, which comprises the steps of reacting Δ⁴-androstene-17-one with methyl magnesium halide and with a hydrolyzing agent, and then reacting the resultant Δ⁴-17-methyl-androstene-17-ol with chromic acid to produce 17-methyl testosterone.

8. A process of the character described, which comprises treating an androstene-17-one of the formula

with a metallo-organic compound capable of transforming the group —CO— into the group —CCH₃(OH)—, and causing the product thus obtained to react with chromic acid.

9. A compound of the formula

wherein R stands for a hydrocarbon radical and R' stands for a member of the group consisting of hydroxyl and a group which upon hydrolysis is converted into hydroxyl.

10. Δ⁴-17-methyl-androstene-17-ol of the formula

11. Δ⁴-17-ethinyl-androstene-17-ol of the formula

KARL MIESCHER.
ALBERT WETTSTEIN.

UNITED STATES PATENT OFFICE

2,374,370

SATURATED AND UNSATURATED 17-HY-
DROXYANDROSTANES, THEIR DERIVA-
TIVES AND SUBSTITUTION PRODUCTS
AND PROCESS OF MAKING SAME

Karl Miescher, Riehen, and Albert Wettstein,
Basel, Switzerland, assignors to Ciba Pharmaceutical Products, Incorporated, Summit, N. J.,
a corporation of New Jersey

No Drawing. Original application December 26,
1940, Serial No. 371,833, now Patent No.
2,311,067, dated February 16, 1943. Divided and
this application October 22, 1942, Serial No.
462,990. In Switzerland December 23, 1939

11 Claims. (Cl. 260—397.5)

It has been found that saturated or unsaturated 17-hydroxy-androstanones, their derivatives (for example, esters or ethers) or their substitution products with saturated or unsaturated hydrocarbon radicals may be obtained by treating an androstane-17-one, containing in the rings A and B merely free or substituted tertiary hydroxyl groups, with agents capable of transforming the group —CO— into the group —CR(OH)—, R representing hydrogen or a saturated or unsaturated hydrocarbon radical, causing the products thus obtained to react with water, acid or alcohol eliminating agents in order to eliminate the free of substituted tertiary hydroxyl groups in rings A or B, hereupon treating with oxidising agents, and finally, if desired, further treating with hydrolysing and/or oxidising, dehydrogenating, water and acid eliminating agents. During this process, the 17-carbinols may be converted if desired either during, before or after the elimination of the tertiary hydroxyl groups in rings A and B, into their esters or ethers by the action of esterifying or etherifying agents.

The parent substances mentioned may be obtained, for example, by the degradation of the side chain in corresponding dimethyl-cyclopentanopolyhydrophenanthrene compounds containing side chains according to the description in patent application Serial No. 371,058, filed Dec. 20, 1940 (now Patent No. 2,319,012, granted May 11, 1943). They contain, particularly in the 5-position, or, for example, in the 8-position, a tertiary hydroxyl group which may also be esterified by inorganic or organic acids or may be etherified by phenols or alcohols.

Agents which are capable of transforming the —CO— group into the —CR(OH)— group, R having the meaning given above, are reducing agents in the widest sense of the term, as well as, for example, metallo-hydrocarbon compounds, such as Grignard compounds, alkali-hydrocarbons and the like, which, in addition to the reduction of the 17-keto group, are capable of introducing in the same position an additional saturated or unsaturated hydrocarbon radical, for example, a methyl, ethyl allyl, or acetylene group. The 17-carbinols thus obtained, particularly those containing secondary alcohol groups, are, if desired, in this stage or only after the elimination of the tertiary hydroxyl groups, converted into their corresponding esters or ethers in known manner by the action of esterifying or etherifying agents. In this instance particular use is made of esterifying agents which are capable

of introducing aliphatic acid radicals, such as those of formic, acetic, propionic, n- or iso-butyric, n- or iso-valeric, capric, caproic, palmitic, or stearic acids, as well as aromatic, fatty aromatic or inorganic acid radicals, for example, benzoic acid, cinnamic acid or substituted carbonic acid radicals. For the purpose of etherification, aliphatic or aliphatic-aromatic alcohols or phenols are introduced, for example, methyl, ethyl, benzyl alcohols, triaryl-methyl carbinols and the like. The products are now treated in known manner with water, alcohol or acid eliminating agents, whereby, for example 4:5-or 5:6-unsaturated compounds are formed.

Upon the unsaturated reaction products obtained oxidising agents are now caused to react, in particular those capabe of introducing oxygen or groups containing oxygen in known manner in the α-position to the double bond. For this purpose, as known for example, chromic acid, selenium dioxide, or lead tetraacylates may be used, which lead to compounds containing oxo, hydroxy or substituted hydroxyl groups in the α-position to the double bond. In place of these, however, oxidising agents may also be caused to react upon the unsaturated products which are capable of adding oxygen or groups containing oxygen directly or indirectly to the double bond itself. For this purpose are suitable, for instance, peroxides, such as hydrogen peroxide, if desired, in the presence of alkalis or metal oxides, furthermore per-acids, halogens, metal oxides, such as osmium tetroxide, if desired, in the presence of chlorates, also permanganates, lead tetracylates or halogen-silver benzoate complexes. In order to convert, for example, newly introduced epoxy groupings or substituted hydroxyl groups into free hydroxyl groups, the reaction products are further treated with hydrolysing agents, it being also possible, by cautious working, only partially to hydrolyse the substituents in rings A or B but not the possibly substituted hydroxyl group in the 17-position. Therefore, in these cases, it is advantageous if the 17-carbinol group has already been substituted by a difficultly hydrolysable radical.

In this way, compounds of the dimethyl-cyclopentanopolyhydrophenanthrene series have been obtained which contain a free, esterified or etherified hydroxyl group and furthermore, if desired, also a hydrocarbon radical in the 17-position, and which contain in rings A or B keto groups or free or esterified hydroxyl groups in the α-position to double bonds, or else two adjacent free or esterified hydroxyl groups in rings A or

B. From the compounds which contain hydroxyl groups, the desired ketones, saturated or unsaturated 17-hydroxy-androstanones, their derivatives or substitution products, may subsequently be obtained in a manner of itself known by the action of agents which eliminate water or acid or by the action of oxidising or dehydrogenating agents.

The following scheme illustrates by means of formulae one of the above reactions without in any way restricting it:

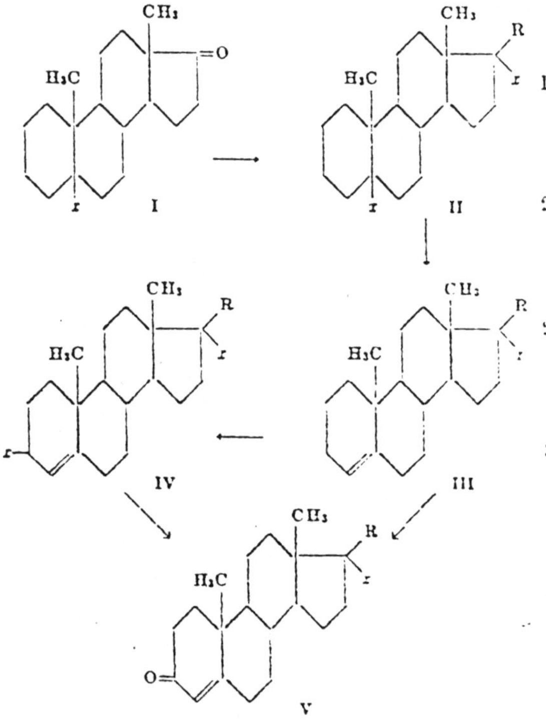

x=free or substituted hydroxyl groups.
R=hydrogen, saturated or unsaturated hydrocarbon radical.

Example 1

1 part of 5-hydroxy-androstane-17-one of Formula I (x=OH; prepared, for example, according to U. S. Patent No. 2,319,012 by splitting the side chain in 5-hydroxy-cholestane) is hydrogenated in 25 parts of pure alcohol by means of a nickel catalyst, prepared, for example, according to the method of Rupe or Raney. After 1 molecule of hydrogen has been absorbed, the hydrogenation is stopped, and the catalyst is removed by filtration. The filtrate is then evaporated in vacuo and the residue is dissolved in di-isopropyl ether and allowed to crystallise. In this manner, androstane-5:17-diole is obtained of Formula II (x=OH; R=H). This compound is now heated for 2 hours with 10 parts of boiling propionic acid anhydride, the secondary hydroxyl group thus being acylated but the tertiary being split off as water. The reaction mixture is then poured into water and, after the anhydride has decomposed, the ester which crystallises is filtered off at the pump, washed with water and dried in the vacuum exsiccator. By recrystallisation from hexane, Δ⁴-androstene-17-ole-propionate is obtained in colourless crystals (Formula III: x=—OCO.C₂H₅; R=H), in addition to some Δ⁵-androstene-17-ole-propionate.

In place of a catalytic method, other reduction methods known to be suitable for the conversion of a keto group into a carbinol group may be used, for example, nascent hydrogen like an alkali metal and an alcohol, an organo-metal compound prone to the formation of unsaturated hydrocarbons, like iso-propyl magnesium iodide, or even biochemical or electrochemical methods. Instead of propionic acid anhydride, other propionylating agents may naturally be used, for instance, a propionic acid halide, or other esters or even ethers may be prepared.

In place of the radical of propionic acid, other ester or ether radicals may be introduced, for example those named before, or the new carbinol group may rest unprotected if suitable oxidising agents, for example, selenium dioxide, are chosen for the following oxidation.

Instead of eliminating the tertiary hydroxyl group during the acylation of the secondary hydroxyl, the elimination may be carried out before the acylation, for example, by means of an alcoholic solution of hydrogen halide, or after the acylation has been carried out gently, for example, by means of propionic acid anhydride in pyridine at room temperature.

Instead of using 5-hydroxy-androstane-17-one as parent material, use may be made of a compound having a substituted hydroxyl group, for example, an esterified or etherified hydroxyl, in the 5-position, for instance, a 5-halogen-androstane-17-one. In this case agents which eliminate acid or alcohol, for example, alkalies or carbonic acid salts, are allowed to react with the reaction product, thus obtaining the same end products.

If, in place of the 5-hydroxy-androstane-17-one, a parent material be used which is hydroxylated in another position, for instance, 3-hydroxy-androstane-17-one, its esters or ethers, the corresponding unsaturated product is obtained.

Thus quite generally as intermediates androstane derivatives may be obtained containing in the rings A and B, for example in 5-position, merely free or substituted tertiary hydroxyl groups, which are eliminated later, and in 17-position a free, esterified or etherified hydroxyl group, for example, an acylated hydroxyl group.

1 part of this Δ⁴-androstene-17-ole-propionate described is dissolved in 50 parts of glacial acetic acid, a solution of 1.2 parts of chromium trioxide in a little water is added and the whole is stirred at room temperature for 12 hours. 400 parts of water are now added and the reaction mixture is extracted exhaustively with ether; the ethereal solution is washed with bicarbonate solution and with water, is dried and then evaporated in vacuo. By fractional crystallisation, absorption or sublimation, testosterone propionate (Δ⁴-androstene-3-one-17-ole-propionate, of Formula V; x=—OCO—C₂H₅; R=H), together with the corresponding 6-oxo- and 3:6-dioxo-compounds, is obtained from the residue.

In place of chromic acid, selenium dioxide or a lead tetraacylate, for example, may be used for the oxidation. In this case, a Δ⁴-3-hydroxy- or acyloxy-androstene-17-ole-propionate of Formula IV is primarily obtained, which subsequently, if necessary, after partial hydrolysis of only the 3-ester group, may also be converted into testosterone propionate in a manner of itself known by the action of oxidising or dehydrogenating agents.

Example 2

A solution of excess of methyl-magnesium iodide in ether is dropped into a solution of 1 part of 5-chloro-androstane-17-one of Formula I (prepared, for example, according to U. S. Patent No. 2,319,012 by splitting the side chain in 5-chloro-cholestane). After the reaction has taken place, water and acid are cautiously added, the ethereal solution is removed, washed and evaporated. The residue is heated to the boil for 1 hour with 20 parts of methanolic caustic potash solution of 5 per cent strength in order to obtain complete elimination of hydrochloric acid from the 5-chloro-17-methyl-androstane-17-ole of Formula II (x=OH;Cl; R=CH₃) which is formed as an intermediate product. The solution is poured into water, extracted with ether, the ethereal solution is washed with water, dried and evaporated. Δ⁴-17-methyl-androstene-17-ole of Formula III (x=OH; R=CH₃) is obtained from the residue.

In a completely analogous manner, compounds containing instead of a methyl other saturated or unsaturated hydrocarbon radical may be obtained, for example, the 17-ethyl-, 17-ethinyl- or 17-allyl-androstane-17-oles with free or substituted tertiary hydroxyl groups, for example in 5, 8 or 9-position by reaction with, for example, ethyl, ethinyl or allyl magnesium halides on the correspondingly substituted androstane-17-ones.

By energetic action of esterifying or etherifying agents, for example, the new tertiary carbinol groups in 17-position may be converted into ester or ether groups in known manner.

So quite generally as intermediates androstane derivatives may be obtained containing in the rings A and B, for example in 5-position, merely free or substituted tertiary hydroxyl groups, which are eliminated later, and in 17-position a free, esterified (like acylated) or etherified hydroxyl group and a hydrocarbon residue, like a methyl or an ethinyl group.

The Δ⁴-17-methyl-androstene-17-ole, described above, is converted directly into 17-methyl-testosterone of Formula V (x=OH; R=CH₃) in a manner fully analogous to that described in Example 1 for the Δ⁴-androstene-17-ole-propionate, for example, by means of chromic acid, or it may be converted into Δ⁴-17-methyl-androstene-3:17-diole or its 3-monoesters (Formula IV), for example, by the action of selenium dioxide or a lead tetraacylate. These may then, if necessary, after hydrolysis, be converted also into 17-methyl-testosterone in a manner of itself known, by means of oxidising or dehydrogenating agents. If, in place of the Δ⁴-17-methyl-androstene-17-ole, corresponding compounds, containing, for example, an ethyl, ethenyl, ethinyl, or allyl group in the 17-position be used as parent materials, then, for example, the 17-ethyl-, 17-ethenyl-, 17-ethinyl-, or 17-allyl-testosterone is obtained in an analogous manner.

Instead of the introduction of a keto or free or substituted hydroxyl group in the α-position to the double bond, two hydroxyl groups may also be added at the latter. To this end, the Δ⁴-17-methyl-androstene-17-ole is treated, for example, in ethereal solution with an ethereal solution of 1.1 equivalents of osmium tetroxide, allowing the reaction mixture to stand 5 days at room temperature, after which the solution is evaporated completely at a bath temperature of 30° C. The residue is heated for 2 hours with an aqueous-alcoholic solution of sodium sulphite. For the reductive hydrolysis of the osmic acid ester other reducing agents, for example, acid agents such as ascorbic acid, or formic acid, may also be used. The reduction mixture is poured into water and

extracted exhaustively with chloroform; the chloroform solution is purified from the last traces of colloidal osmium by means of an acid absorption agent and is then evaporated to dryness. The crude 17-methyl-androstane-4:5:17-triole is obtained from the residue.

Instead of the direct addition of two hydroxyl groups at the double bond, an oxide ring may first of all be added or one or both of the hydroxyl groups in substituted form, for example, in the acylated state, the reagents already described, for example, being used in a manner of itself known for this purpose. The oxide rings or substituted hydroxyl group may subsequently be hydrolysed if desired, the latter either completely or partially.

For the last stage of the process, an agent capable of eliminating water is allowed to react upon the 17-methyl-androstane-4:5:17-triole. If the hydroxyl group or groups be present in the esterified form in the 4 and/or 5-position, which, for example, is the case if peracetic acid, a lead tetraacylate or a halogen-silver benzoate complex has been used for the hydroxylation, then, instead of an agent eliminating water, an agent eliminating acid is used, for example, alkali, or zinc dust in toluene. In this manner 17-methyl-androstane-4-one-17-ole is obtained.

This application is a division of our application Serial No. 371,833 filed December 26, 1940.

What we claim is:

1. A process of the character described, which comprises the step of reacting an androstane-17-one of the formula

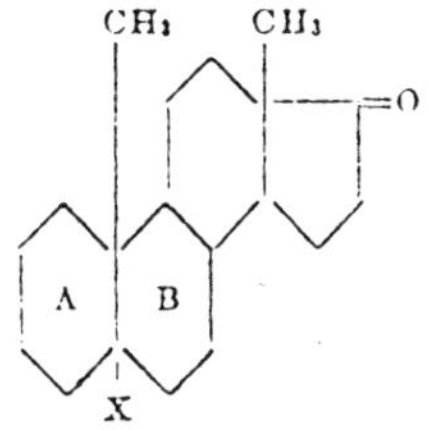

wherein X represents a substituent which is selected from the class consisting of tertiary hydroxyl and a group which upon hydrolysis is converted into tertiary hydroxyl, rings A and B containing no further substituent, with a Grignard reagent and with aqueous acid, whereby the group

$$-C=O$$

in the 17-position is converted into the group

$$-CR(OH)$$

R standing for a hydrocarbon radical.

2. A process of the character described, which comprises the steps of reacting an androstane-17-one of the formula

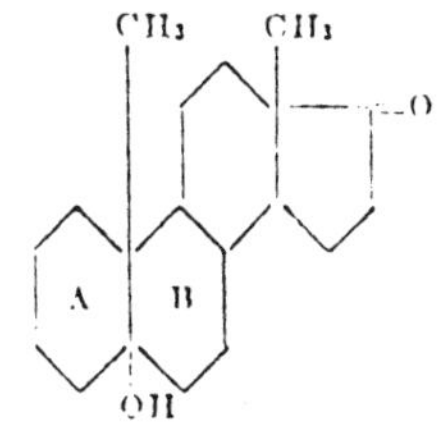

wherein rings A and B contain no further substituent, with a Grignard reagent and with aqueous acid, whereby the group

$$-C=O$$

in the 17-position is converted into the group

$$-CR(OH)$$

R standing for a hydrocarbon radical, and then dehydrating the resultant product, whereby the HO— group indicated in the above formula is eliminated and a double bond is introduced in lieu thereof.

3. A process of the character described, which comprises the steps of reacting an androstane-17-one of the formula

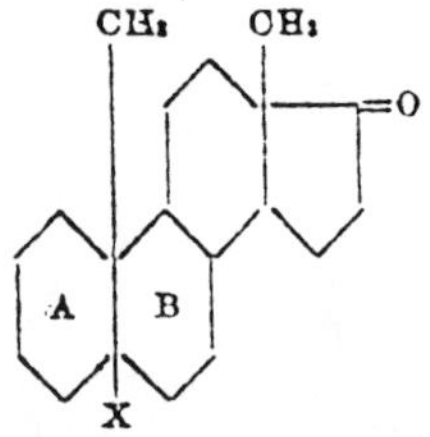

wherein X represents an esterified tertiary hydroxyl group, rings A and B containing no further substituent, with a Grignard reagent and with aqueous acid, whereby the group

$$-C=O$$

in the 17-position is converted into the group

$$-CR(OH)$$

R standing for a hydrocarbon radical, and then reacting the resultant product with an alkali, whereby the esterified tertiary hydroxyl group is eliminated and a double bond is introduced in lieu thereof.

4. A process of the character described, which comprises the steps of reacting an androstane-17-one of the formula

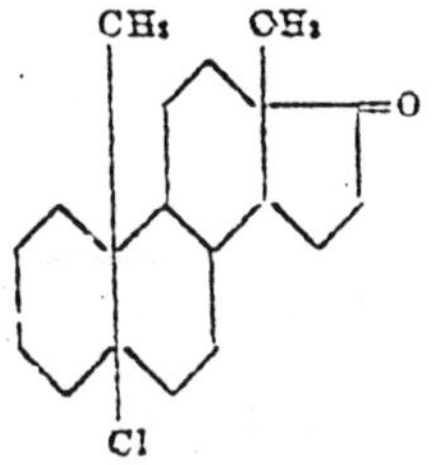

with a hydrocarbon-substituted metal halide and with aqueous acid whereby the

$$-C=O$$

group is converted into the

$$-CR(OH)$$

group, R standing for a hydrocarbon radical, then reacting the resultant product with an alkali, whereby the Cl is eliminated and a double bond is introduced in lieu thereof.

5. A process of the character described, which comprises the steps of reacting an androstane-17-one of the formula

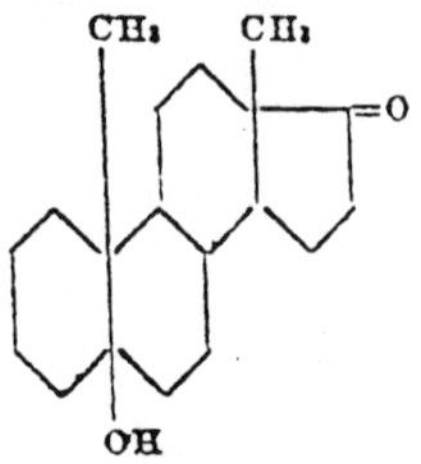

with a hydrocarbon-substituted metal halide and with aqueous acid whereby the

$$-C=O$$

group is converted into the

$$-CR(OH)$$

group, R standing for a hydrocarbon radical, then dehydrating the resultant product, whereby the OH in 5-position is eliminated and a double bond introduced in lieu thereof.

6. A process of the character described, which comprises the steps of reacting 5-chloro-androstane-17-one with a compound of the formula R.MgI and with aqueous acid, treating the resultant 5-chloro-17-R-androstane-17-ole with methanolic KOH, and then reacting the resultant Δ^4-17-R-androstene-17-ole with chromic acid, whereby 17-R-testosterone is produced, R standing for a hydrocarbon group.

7. A process of the character described, which comprises the steps of reacting 5-chloro-androstane-17-one with a compound of the formula R.MgI and with aqueous acid, treating the resultant 5-chloro-17-R-androstane-17-ole with methanolic KOH, and then reacting the resultant Δ^4-17-R-androstene-17-ole with selenium dioxide, whereby 17-R-androstene-3,17-diol is produced, R standing for a hydrocarbon group.

8. A process of the character described, which comprises the steps of reacting 5-chloro-androstane-17-one with methyl magnesium iodide and with aqueous acid, treating the resultant 5-chloro-17-methyl-androstane-17-ole with methanolic KOH, and then reacting the resultant Δ^4-17-methyl-androstene-17-ole with chromic acid, whereby 17-methyl-testosterone is produced.

9. A compound of the formula

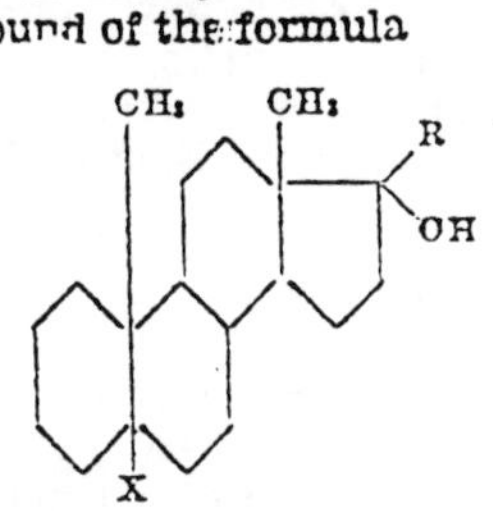

wherein X represents a member of the group consisting of tertiary hydroxyl and a group which upon hydrolysis is converted into tertiary hydroxyl, and R stands for a hydrocarbon radical.

10. A compound of the formula

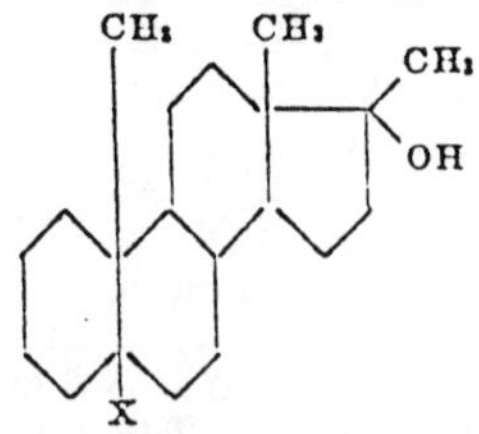

wherein X represents a member of the group consisting of tertiary hydroxyl and a group which upon hydrolysis is converted into tertiary hydroxyl.

11. The 5-chloro-17-methyl-androstane-17-ole.

KARL MIESCHER.
ALBERT WETTSTEIN.

UNITED STATES PATENT OFFICE

2,386,331

3-DERIVATIVES OF THE SATURATED AND UNSATURATED ANDROSTANE-3-ONE-17-OLS SUBSTITUTED IN 17-POSITION AND PROCESS OF MAKING SAME AS WELL AS THE CORRESPONDING FREE KETONES

Karl Miescher, Riehen, Switzerland, assignor to Ciba Pharmaceutical Products Incorporated, Summit, N. J., a corporation

No Drawing. Application November 10, 1943, Serial No. 509,776. In Switzerland December 10, 1938

8 Claims. (Cl. 260—239.5)

This application is a continuation in part of my copending application Serial No. 306,184, filed November 25, 1939.

It is known that saturated and unsaturated androstanolones containing a substituent, for example a saturated or unsaturated hydrocarbon radical, in the 17-position and a keto group in the 3-position, may be obtained by treating corresponding 3-oxy-compounds with oxidizing agents. Such a final oxidation, however, has shown itself in many cases to be undesirable. It has now been found that it may be avoided if metallo-organic compounds are allowed to react on 3-enolates or 3-acetals of saturated or unsaturated androstandiones, and, if required, the derivatives thus obtained are hydrolyzed.

As parent substances, for example the 3-enol ethers, like 3-methyl- or 3-ethyl-enol ethers as well as the 3-enol esters and the 3-acetals, for example the 3-glycolates or 3-propandiolates, of androstendiones or androstandiones or their derivatives may be used. These can be prepared according to the data of the publication of A. Serini and A. Klöster in "Berichte der deutschen chemischen Gesellschaft," vol. 71, page 1766 (1938).

Suitable metallo-organic compounds are, for example, the magnesium organo compounds, such as alkyl- (like methyl-, ethyl-), alkylene- (like allyl-), aralkyl- (like benzyl-) or aryl- (like phenyl-) magnesium halides, further zinc-alkyl compounds and the like.

As products of the present invention there may be named for example the 3-derivatives like 3-enolates (3-enol-ethers or -esters) or 3-acetals of the saturated and unsaturated androstane-3-one-17-ols containing in 17-position saturated hydrocarbon radicals like alkyl groups (methyl, ethyl groups) or hydrocarbon radicals containing double bonds like allyl- or benzyl-groups. Furthermore their hydrolysation products containing free 3-keto-groups are also obtained.

Example 1

A solution of 63 gms. of androstendione-3-mono-enol-ethylether in toluene is allowed to drop into an ethereal solution of 72 gms. of methyl-magnesium bromide. The mixed solutions are then boiled for some time. After the reaction is complete, the solution is decomposed with excess of ammonium chloride solution and the layers are separated. The 3-enol ether of the 17-methyl-testosterone is obtained after concentration of the organic solution and may easily be converted by an acid agent into the known 17-methyl-testosterone. In an analogous manner

also the 17-ethyl-, -allyl-, or -benzyl-testosterones are obtained. The corresponding Grignard-reagents may be replaced for example by zinc derivatives.

Instead of the androstendione-3-mono-enol-ethylether one may start also from other androstendione-3-mono-enol-ethers, for example the methyl-, propyl-, benzyl- or trityl-ethers or even from corresponding 3-mono-enolesters or -acetals.

The 17-methyl-dihydro-testosterone, for example, may be obtained in a similar manner for example from the 3-glycol-acetal, other 3-mono-acetals, 3-mono-enolethers or -esters of androstandione.

The alcohols epimeric in 17-position may also be separated from the mother liquors of the reaction product.

Example 2

35 gms. of androstendione-3-mono-ethyleneglycol-acetal (M. Pt. 200°, obtainable by condensation of androstendione with ethyleneglycol in presence of acid as catalyst), 25 gms. of magnesium, some activated magnesium-copper-alloy and 500 cc. of ether are stirred in a flask. Into this, 70 cc. of allyl-bromide are dropped, when gentle reaction takes place. After the reaction has started, boiling is continued for 2 hours if necessary by externally warming the flask with warm water. The reaction mixture is then cooled with ice and treated with 200 cc. of water. Diluted sulfuric acid is added till acid to congo and the whole shaken at 35° C. to split the 17-allyl-testosterone-3-ethyleneglycol-acetal contained in the ether. The ether layer is then separated, dried and evaporated. From the residue there is obtained by chromatography the known 17-allyl-testosterone. In a similar manner other 3-acetals of saturated or unsaturated androstane-3-one-17-ols containing in 17-position a saturated or unsaturated hydrocarbon radical, e. g. 17-methyl-testosterone-3-acetals or 17-methyl-dihydrotestosterone-3-acetals, and their hydrolysation products are obtained.

What I claim is:

1. Process for the manufacture of a member of the group consisting of the saturated and unsaturated androstanolones substituted in 17-position and derivatives thereof, comprising allowing an allyl-magnesium halide to react on a member of the group consisting of the 3-acetals of saturated and unsaturated androstandiones, and then hydrolyzing the derivatives obtained.

2. The 3-acetals of the saturated and unsaturated androstane-3-one-17-ols containing in 17-

position a member of the group consisting of saturated hydrocarbon radicals and hydrocarbon radicals containing double bonds.

3. The 3-acetals of the saturated and unsaturated androstane-3-one-17-ols containing in 17-position an alkyl group.

4. The 3-acetals of the saturated and unsaturated androstane-3-one-17-ols containing in 17-position a methyl group.

5. The 3-acetals of the saturated and unsaturated androstane-3-one-17-ols containing in 17-position an allyl group.

6. The 17-methyl-testosterone-3-acetals.

7. The 17-methyl-dihydrotestosterone-3-acetals.

8. 17-allyl-testosterone-3-ethyleneglycol - acetal.

KARL MIESCHER.